PHYSICAL THERAPY CASE FILES®
Orthopaedics

Jason Brumitt, PT, PhD, SCS, ATC, CSCS
Assistant Professor
School of Physical Therapy
College of Health Professions
Pacific University
Hillsboro, Oregon

Series Editor: Erin E. Jobst, PT, PhD
Associate Professor
School of Physical Therapy
College of Health Professions
Pacific University
Hillsboro, Oregon

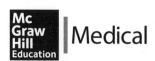 Medical

New York   Chicago   San Francisco   Lisbon   London   Madrid   Mexico City
Milan   New Delhi   San Juan   Seoul   Singapore   Sydney   Toronto

Physical Therapy Case Files®: Orthopaedics

Note: The work of Kristi A. Greene, Michael D. Rosenthal, Michael D. Ross, and Shane A. Vath was performed outside the scope of their employment as U.S. government employees. The work represents their personal and professional views and not necessarily those of the U.S. government.

1 2 3 4 5 6 7 8 9 0   DOC/DOC   18 17 16 15 14 13

ISBN 978-0-07-176377-6
MHID 0-07-176377-5

Notice

Medicine is an ever-changing science. As new research and clinical experience broaden our knowledge, changes in treatment and drug therapy are required. The authors and the publisher of this work have checked with sources believed to be reliable in their efforts to provide information that is complete and generally in accord with the standard accepted at the time of publication. However, in view of the possibility of human error or changes in medical sciences, neither the editors nor the publisher nor any other party who has been involved in the preparation or publication of this work warrants that the information contained herein is in every respect accurate or complete, and they disclaim all responsibility for any errors or omissions or for the results obtained from use of the information contained in this work. Readers are encouraged to confirm the information contained herein with other sources. For example and in particular, readers are advised to check the product information sheet included in the package of each drug they plan to administer to be certain that the information contained in this work is accurate and that changes have not been made in the recommended dose or in the contraindications for administration. This recommendation is of particular importance in connection with new or infrequently used drugs.

This book was set in Goudy by Cenveo® Publisher Services.
The editors were Catherine A. Johnson and Christina M. Thomas.
The production supervisor was Catherine H. Saggese.
Project management was provided by Yashmita Hota, Cenveo® Publisher Services.
The designer was Janice Bielawa.
RR Donnelley was the printer and binder.

Library of Congress Cataloging-in-Publication Data

Brumitt, Jason.
    Physical therapy case files. Orthopaedics / Jason Brumitt.
       p. ; cm.
    Orthopaedics
    Includes bibliographical references and index.
    ISBN 978-0-07-176377-6 (pbk.) — ISBN 0-07-176377-5 (pbk.)
    I. Title. II. Title: Orthopaedics.
    [DNLM: 1. Physical Therapy Modalities—Case Reports.   2. Needs Assessment—Case Reports.
  3. Orthopaedic Procedures—methods—Case Reports.   WB 460]
    616.7'06—dc23
                                      2012039901

CONTENTS

Lane Bailey, PT, DPT, CSCS
Physical Therapist and Clinical Research Assistant
Proaxis Therapy
Greenville, South Carolina

David S. Bailie, MD
The Orthopaedic Clinic, (TOCA)
Scottsdale, Arizona

Jolene Bennett, PT, OCS, Cert MDT, ATC
Spectrum Health Rehabilitation Services
Grand Rapids, Michigan

Jake Bleacher, PT, MSPT, OCS, Cert SMT, MTC, CSCS
The Ohio State University Sports Medicine Center and Rehabilitation
    Services at Care Point in Gahana
Ohio State's Wexner Medical Center
Staff Physical Therapist
Gahanna, Ohio

Kyle Botten, PT, DPT, CSCS
Wise Physical Therapy and Sports Medicine
Grove City, Pennsylvania

Jason Brumitt, PT, PhD, SCS, ATC, CSCS
Assistant Professor
School of Physical Therapy
College of Health Professions
Pacific University
Hillsboro, Oregon

Shelly Coffman, PT, DPT, OCS, FAAOMPT, CSCS
Clinical Director
360° Sports Medicine and Spine Therapy
Portland, Oregon

R. Barry Dale, PhD, PT, DPT, ATC, SCS, OCS, CSCS
UC Foundation Associate Professor
University of Tennessee at Chattanooga
Chattanooga, Tennessee

Carl DeRosa, PT, PhD, FAPTA
Fellow, American Physical Therapy Association
Professor, Physical Therapy
Nothern Arizona University
Flagstaff, Arizona

Todd S. Ellenbecker, DPT, MS, SCS, OCS, CSCS
Clinic Director
Physiotherapy Associates, Scottsdale Sports Clinic
National Director of Clinic Research
Physiotherapy Associates
Director of Sports Medicine ATP World Tour
Scottsdale, Arizona

Johanna Gabbard, PT, DPT, OCS, FAAOMPT
Adjunct Professor
US Army-Baylor University
Doctoral Program in Physical Therapy
Army Medical Department Center and School
Fort Sam Houston, Texas

Caryn Gehrke, PT, DPT
Wise Physical Therapy and Sports Medicine
Grove City, Pennsylvania

Kristi A. Greene, MPT, OCS
Senior Physical Therapist
Kaiser Permanente Medical Center
Vallejo, California

Laurie Griffin, PT, DPT, OCS
Howard Head Sports Medicine
Vail, Colorado

Barbara J. Hoogenboom, EdD, PT, SCS, ATC
Associate Professor
Clinical Doctorate of Physical Therapy Program
Grand Valley State University
Grnad Rapids, Michigan

Douglas Lauchlan, MSc, BSc, MCSP, FHEA
Senior Lecturer in Physiotherapy
Department of Psychology and Allied Health Sciences
School of Health & Life Sciences
Glasgow Caledonian University
Scotland, United Kingdom

Janice K. Loudon, PT, PhD, SCS, ATC
Associate Professor
Division of Physical Therapy
Duke University Medical Center
Durham, North Carolina

Robert C. Manske, DPT, SCS, MEd, ATC, CSC
Associate Professor
Department of Physical Therapy
Wichita State University
Physiotherapy Associates Wichita
Wichita, Kansas

Danny J. McMillian, PT, DSc, OCS, CSCS
Clinical Associate Professor
School of Physical Therapy
University of Puget Sound
Tacoma, Washington

Erik P. Meira, PT, SCS, CSCS
Clinic Director
Black Diamond Physical Therapy
Portland, Oregon

Jandra Mueller, PT, DPT
Physical Therapist
Fysiotherapie Hawaii, Inc.
Honolulu, Hawaii

Melissa Murray, PT, DPT
Physical Therapist
Pediatric Therapy Services
Gresham, Oregon
Consonus Health Services
Newberg, Oregon

Matt Mymern, PT, DPT, SCS, CSC
Howard Head Sports Medicine
Vail, Colorado

Luke T. O'Brien, PT, Grad. Cert. Sports Physiotherapy, SCS, PES
Howard Head Sports Medicine
Vail, Colorado

Thomas J. Olson, PT, DPT, SCS
Howard Head Sports Medicine
Vail, Colorado

Mark V. Paterno, PT, PhD, MBA, SCS, ATC
Coordinator of Orthopaedic and Sports Physical Therapy
Associate Professor
Sports Medicine Biodynamics Center
Division of Occupational Therapy and Physical Therapy
Cincinnati Children's Hospital Medical Center
Cincinnati, Ohio

Paul Reuteman, DPT, OCS, ATC
Clinical Associate Professor
Program of Physical Therapy
University of Wisconsin–La Crosse
La Crosse, Wisconsin
Staff Physical Therapist
Faculty, Sports Physical Therapy Residency Program
Gundersen Lutheran Sports Medicine
Onalaska, Wisconsin

Michael D. Rosenthal, PT, DSc, SCS, ECS, ATC, CSCS
Director of Physical and Occupational Therapy
Naval Medical Center
San Diego, California

Michael D. Ross, PT, DHSc, OCS
Assistant Professor
Department of Physical Therapy
University of Scranton
Scranton, Pennsylvania

Christy Schuckman, PT, ATC
Cincinnati Reds Physical Therapist
Staff Physical Therapist Beacon Orthopedics
Cincinnati, Ohio

Ellen Shanley, PhD, PT, OCS, CSCS
Adjunct Assistant Professor
Clemson Bioengineering Department
Clemson University
Clemson, South Carolina
Adjunct Assistant Professor
Department of Physical Therapy
Arnold School of Public Health
University of South Carolina
Columbia, South Carolina

Laura Stanley, PT, DPT
Physical Therapist
Proaxis Therapy
Greenville, South Carolina

Casey A. Unverzagt, PT, DPT, OCS, SCS
Wise Physical Therapy and Sports Medicine
Slippery Rock, Pennsylvania

Shane A. Vath, PT, DSc, SCS
Physical Therapy Department
Naval Hospital Camp Lejeune
Camp Lejeune, North Carolina

Ted Weber, PT, DPT, OCS
Axis Sports Medicine
Eagle, Colorado

Paul E. Westgard, PT, DPT, OCS, SCS, CSCS
Howard Head Sports Medicine
Vail, Colorado

ACKNOWLEDGMENTS

First, I would like to thank Erin Jobst for providing me the opportunity to be the editor of the *Physical Therapy Case Files: Orthopaedics*. Her vision and leadership has helped create a special book that I believe will be an invaluable text for students in an entry-level physical therapy program as well as a relevant clinical reference for experienced physical therapists. I am extremely lucky to work with her and to continue to learn from her!

Next, I would like to thank each contributor, for without you, this text would not be possible. You have shared your knowledge, expertise, and time to define evidence-based practice patterns that will benefit our patients and better our profession.

Finally, I would like to thank my wife Renee for supporting my professional goals and pursuits. For my children, Rex, Halsey, and Stone—you are too young to appreciate this now, but as you get older I hope that you realize that you can do anything. Dream big!

Jason Brumitt, PT, PhD, SCS, ATC, CSCS

As the physical therapy profession continues to evolve and advance as a doctoring profession, so does the rigor of entry-level physical therapist education. Students must master fundamental foundation courses while integrating an understanding of new research in all areas of physical therapy. Evidence-based practice is the use of current best evidence in conjunction with the expertise of the clinician and the specific values and circumstances of the patient in making decisions regarding assessment and treatment. Evidence-based practice is a major emphasis in physical therapy education and clinical practice. However, the most challenging task for students is making the transition from didactic classroom-based knowledge to its application in developing a physical therapy diagnosis and implementing appropriate evidence-based interventions. Ideally, instructors who are experienced and knowledgeable in every diagnosis and treatment approach could guide students at the "bedside" and students would supplement this training by self-directed independent reading. While there is certainly no substitute for clinical education, it is rare for clinical rotations to cover the scope of each physical therapy setting. In addition, it is not always possible for clinical instructors to be able to take the time necessary to guide students through the application of evidence-based tests and measures and interventions. Perhaps an effective alternative approach is teaching by using clinical case studies designed with a structured clinical approach to diagnosis and treatment. At the time of writing the *Physical Therapy Case Files* series, there were no physical therapy textbooks that contain case studies that utilize and reference current literature to support an illustrated examination or treatment. In my own teaching, I have designed case scenarios based on personal patient care experiences, those experiences shared with me by my colleagues, and searches through dozens of textbooks and websites to find a case study illustrating a particular concept. There are two problems with this approach. First, neither my own nor my colleagues' experiences cover the vast diversity of patient diagnoses, examinations, and interventions. Second, designing a case scenario that is not based on personal patient care experience or expertise takes an overwhelming amount of time. In my experience, detailed case studies that incorporate application of the best evidence are difficult to design "on the fly" in the classroom. The twofold goal of the *Physical Therapy Case Files* series is to provide resources that contain multiple real-life case studies within an individual physical therapy practice area that will minimize the need for physical therapy educators to create their own scenarios and maximize the students' ability to implement evidence into the care of individual patients.

The cases within each book in the *Physical Therapy Case Files* series are organized for the reader to either read the book from "front to back" or to randomly select scenarios based on current interest. A list of cases by case number and by alphabetical listing by health condition is included in Section III to enable the reader to review his or her knowledge in a specific area. Sometimes a case scenario may include a more abbreviated explanation of a specific health condition or clinical test than was provided in another case. In this situation, the reader will be referred to the case with the more thorough explanation.

Every case follows an organized and well thought-out format using familiar language from both the World Health Organization's International Classification of Functioning, Disability, and Health (ICF) framework[1] and the American Physical Therapy Association's *Guide to Physical Therapist Practice*.[2] To limit redundancy and length of each case, we intentionally did not present the ICF framework or the *Guide's* Preferred Practice Patterns within each case. However, the section titles and the language used throughout each case were chosen to guide the reader through the evaluation, goal-setting, and intervention process and how clinical reasoning can be used to enhance an individual's activities and participation.

The front page of each case begins with a patient encounter followed by a series of open-ended questions. The discussion following the case is organized into *seven* sections:

1. **Key Definitions** provide terminology pertinent to the reader's understanding of the case. **Objectives** list the instructional and/or terminal behavioral objectives that summarize the knowledge, skills, or attitudes the reader should be able to demonstrate after reading the case. **PT considerations** provides a summary of the physical therapy plan of care, goals, interventions, precautions, and potential complications for the physical therapy management of the individual presented in the case.

2. **Understanding the Health Condition** presents an abbreviated explanation of the medical diagnosis. The intent of this section is *not* to be comprehensive. The etiology, pathogenesis, risk factors, epidemiology, and medical management of the condition are presented in enough detail to provide background and context for the reader.

3. **Physical Therapy Patient/Client Management** provides a summary of the role of the physical therapist in the patient's care. This section may elaborate on how the physical therapist's role augments and/or overlaps with those of other healthcare practitioners involved in the patient's care, as well as any referrals to additional healthcare practitioners that the physical therapist should provide.

4. **Examination, Evaluation, and Diagnosis** guides the reader how to organize and interpret information gathered from the chart review (in inpatient cases), appreciate adverse drug reactions that may affect patient presentation, and structure the subjective evaluation and physical examination. Not every assessment tool and special test that could possibly be done with the patient is included. For each outcome measure or special test presented, available reliability, validity, sensitivity, and specificity are discussed. When available, a minimal clinically important difference (MCID) for an outcome measure is presented because it helps the clinician to determine the "the minimal level of change required in response to an intervention before the outcome would be considered worthwhile in terms of a patient/client's function or quality of life."[3]

5. **Plan of Care and Interventions** elaborates on a few physical therapy interventions for the patient's condition. The advantage of this section and the previous section is that each case does *not* exhaustively present every outcome measure, special test, or therapeutic intervention that *could be* performed. Rather, only selected outcome measures or examination techniques and interventions are chosen. This is done

to simulate a real-life patient interaction in which the physical therapist uses his or her clinical reasoning to determine the *most appropriate* tests and interventions to utilize with that patient during that episode of care. For each intervention that is chosen, the evidence to support its use with individuals with the same diagnosis (or similar diagnosis, if no evidence exists to support its use in that particular patient population) is presented. To reduce redundancy, standard guidelines for aerobic and resistance exercise have not been included. Instead, the reader is referred to guidelines published by the American College of Sports Medicine,[4] Goodman and Fuller,[5] and Paz and West.[6] For particular case scenarios in which standard guidelines are deviated from, specific guidelines are included.

6. **Evidence-Based Clinical Recommendations** includes a minimum of three clinical recommendations for diagnostic tools and/or treatment interventions for the patient's condition. To improve the quality of each recommendation beyond the personal clinical experience of the contributing author, each recommendation is graded using the Strength of Recommendation Taxonomy (SORT).[7] There are over one hundred evidence-grading systems used to rate the quality of individual studies and the strength of recommendations based on a body of evidence.[8] The SORT system has been used by several medical journals including *American Family Physician, Journal of the American Board of Family Practice, Journal of Family Practice,* and *Sports Health.* The SORT system has been chosen for two reasons: it is simple and its rankings are based on patient-oriented outcomes. The SORT system has only three levels of evidence: A, B, and C. Grade A recommendations are based on consistent, good-quality patient-oriented evidence (*e.g.*, systematic reviews, meta-analysis of high-quality studies, high-quality randomized controlled trials, high-quality diagnostic cohort studies). Grade B recommendations are based on inconsistent or limited-quality patient-oriented evidence (*e.g.*, systematic review or meta-analysis of lower-quality studies or studies with inconsistent findings). Grade C recommendations are based on consensus, disease-oriented evidence, usual practice, expert opinion, or case series (*e.g.*, consensus guidelines, disease-oriented evidence using only intermediate or physiologic outcomes). The contributing author of each case provided a grade based on the SORT guidelines for each recommendation or conclusion. The grade for each statement was reviewed and sometimes altered by the editors. Key phrases from each clinical recommendation are bolded within the case to enable the reader to easily locate where the cited evidence was presented.

7. **Comprehension Questions and Answers** include two to four multiple-choice questions that reinforce the content or elaborate and introduce new, but related concepts to the patient's case. When appropriate, detailed explanations about why alternative choices would not be the best choice are also provided.

My hope is that these real-life case studies will be a new resource to facilitate the incorporation of evidence into everyday physical therapy practice in various settings and patient populations. With the persistent push for evidence-based healthcare to promote quality and effectiveness[9] and the advent of evidence-based reimbursement guidelines, case scenarios with evidence-based recommendations will be an added benefit as physical therapists continually face the threat of decreased reimbursement rates for their services and will need to demonstrate evidence supporting their services. I hope physical therapy educators, entry-level physical therapy students, practicing physical therapists, and professionals preparing for Board Certification in clinical specialty areas will find these books helpful to translate classroom-based knowledge to evidence-based assessments and interventions.

Erin E. Jobst, PT, PhD

1. World Health Organization. International Classification of Functioning, Disability and Health (ICF). Available at: http://www.who.int/classifications/icf/en/. Accessed August 7, 2012.

2. American Physical Therapy Association. *Guide to Physical Therapist Practice (Guide)*. Alexandria, VA: APTA; 1999.

3. Jewell DV. *Guide to Evidence-Based Physical Therapy Practice*. Sudbury, MA: Jones and Barlett; 2008.

4. ACSM's *Guidelines for Exercise Testing and Prescription*. 8th ed. Wolters Kluwer/Lippincott Williams & Wilkins; 2010.

5. Goodman CC, Fuller KS. *Pathology: Implications for the Physical Therapist*. 3rd ed. Philadelphia, PA: W.B. Saunders Company; 2009.

6. Paz JC, West MP. *Acute Care Handbook for Physical Therapists*. 3rd ed. St. Louis, MO: Saunders Elsevier; 2009.

7. Ebell MH, Siwek J, Weiss BD, et al. Strength of Recommendation Taxonomy (SORT): a patient-centered approach to grading evidence in the medical literature. *Am Fam Physician*. 2004;69: 548-556.

8. Systems to rate the strength of scientific evidence. Summary, evidence report/technology assessment: number 47. AHRQ publication no. 02-E015, March 2002. Available at: http://www.ahrq.gov/clinic/epcsums/strengthsum.htm. Accessed August 7, 2012.

9. Agency for Healthcare Research and Quality. Available at: www.ahrq.gov/clinic/epc/. Accessed August 7, 2012.

Introduction

Physical therapists have numerous active and passive treatment options available to administer, perform, or prescribe to a patient with an orthopaedic musculoskeletal injury. However, in the age of evidence-based practice, physical therapists must be able to justify the use of an intervention based on the best available research evidence, their clinical experience (selecting an intervention based on sound clinical reasoning), and the individual patient's values. The purpose of this text is to illustrate how evidence-based practice principles should guide the examination, evaluation, and treatment of the patient with orthopaedic dysfunction.

This text contains 34 orthopaedic cases from an international selection of some of the top physical therapy researchers, educators, and master clinicians. Cases include a spectrum of diagnoses including pediatric conditions, sports injuries, chronic conditions, and back pain. Each case presents the best practice patterns supported by the strongest available research for the management of common orthopaedic musculoskeletal conditions. Some cases may challenge the experienced therapists' notions regarding the appropriateness of their current practice strategies. For example, this text addresses concepts such as whether joint mobilization to the glenohumeral joint is indicated or necessary for individuals with adhesive capsulitis and whether custom orthotics are effective for persons with plantar fasciitis.

While the physical therapy profession has made (and continues to make) advances in the clinical management of orthopaedic conditions, there are still conditions, such as low back pain, that challenge and frustrate both therapists and patients. In some cases, emerging evidence is helping to guide treatment, often with excellent results. For example, Carl DeRosa, PT, PhD presents how the use of a clinical prediction rule can guide treatment selection for adults with acute low back pain (Case 14). In other musculoskeletal conditions of the spine, numerous patient/client management strategies have been advocated with inconclusive or inconsistent results. To illustrate this point, Cases 15 to 18 present a case scenario of a single patient with a herniated nucleus pulposus in the lumbar spine. While each of the four cases illustrates a unique approach to diagnosis and treatment (mechanical traction, McKenzie or Mechanical Diagnosis Therapy, muscle energy technique, and the Ola Grimsby approach), each has varying levels of support in the literature. These four cases side by side illustrate to students and clinicians how the same patient may be approached quite differently with therapists attempting to implement the principles of evidence-based practice. While the popularity and reported success of these approaches provide clinicians with a starting point, clinicians must critically analyze established and emerging peer-reviewed published literature to determine the best approach or combination of approaches for the physical therapy management of each condition.

We hope that the cases presented here help improve the ability of students, new therapists, and even experienced therapists to examine, evaluate, and treat patients. Our hope is that these cases inspire reflections on clinical practice, incite new questions to be asked, and push physical therapists to continually pursue new knowledge.

Thirty-Four Case Scenarios

Subacromial Impingement

Christy Schuckman

An 18-year-old right-hand dominant male presents to an outpatient physical therapy clinic with a physical therapy prescription from an orthopaedic physician to evaluate and treat right shoulder subacromial impingement. The patient states he started to experience shoulder pain approximately four weeks ago. He attributes the cause to playing tennis three times during the past week after not playing at all over the winter. His right shoulder pain increases with reaching forward, reaching behind his back, lifting any type of weight with his right arm and playing tennis. He also reports not being able to reach behind his back to loop his belt or tuck his shirt in, activities he could previously do without difficulty. The only position that relieves his shoulder pain is keeping his arm at his side. His physician started him on a course of nonsteroidal anti-inflammatory drugs, which has helped decrease the pain intensity. X-rays (performed in the physician's office) of the acromioclavicular and glenohumeral joints were negative for any bony abnormalities or structural deficits. The patient's medical history is otherwise unremarkable.

▶ Based on the patient's diagnosis, what do you anticipate may be the contributing factors to his condition?
▶ What examination signs may be associated with this diagnosis?
▶ What are the most appropriate physical therapy interventions?
▶ What possible complications may limit the effectiveness of physical therapy?

KEY DEFINITIONS

SCAPULAR DYSKINESIS: Visible alterations in scapular position and movement patterns

SUBACROMIAL IMPINGEMENT SYNDROME: Compression, entrapment, or mechanical irritation of the rotator cuff tendons beneath the coracoacromial arch

Objectives

1. Describe subacromial impingement syndrome.

2. Identify possible causes of subacromial impingement.

3. Discuss signs and symptoms of subacromial impingement based on examination findings.

4. Prescribe appropriate joint range of motion and/or muscular flexibility exercises for an individual with subacromial impingement syndrome.

5. Prescribe appropriate resistance exercises for a person with subacromial impingement syndrome.

Physical Therapy Considerations

PT considerations during management of the individual with a diagnosis of subacromial impingement syndrome:

▶ **General physical therapy plan of care/goals:** Decrease pain; increase glenohumeral joint range of motion; increase muscle flexibility; increase rotator cuff and scapular muscle strength; improve function with activities of daily living

▶ **Physical therapy interventions:** Patient education regarding shoulder anatomy and pathomechanics of the diagnosis; modalities as needed to decrease pain; manual therapy to decrease pain and improve joint and muscular flexibility; range of motion and flexibility exercises; resistance exercises to increase muscular strength and endurance; proprioceptive exercises to promote joint and muscular control

▶ **Precautions during physical therapy:** Monitor vital signs; address precautions or contraindications for exercise based on patient's pre-existing condition(s)

▶ **Complications interfering with physical therapy:** Patient noncompliance with exercise program

Understanding the Health Condition

Shoulder pain affects 16% to 21% of the adult population in the United States, second only to low back pain in total prevalence of musculoskeletal conditions.[1-4] Subacromial impingement syndrome (SAIS) accounts for 44% to 60% of all conditions causing shoulder pain.[3,5,6] An impingement syndrome involves degeneration and/or mechanical compression of soft tissue structures.[3] In the case of SAIS, the rotator cuff, the long head of the biceps, and the subacromial bursa are compressed between the acromion, the coracoacromial ligament, and the humeral head.[3,7,8]

The **etiology of SAIS is multifactorial**—caused by extrinsic and/or intrinsic mechanisms. Extrinsic mechanisms of compression include anatomical factors, biomechanical factors, or a combination of both.[9] Anatomical variations that can narrow the subacromial space include variations in the shape of the acromion,[9-13] orientation of the slope or angle of the acromion,[9,14-17] and osseous changes to the acromioclavicular (AC) joint or coracoacromial ligament.[9,13,18,19] Subacromial and AC joint spurs are other anatomical factors that can contribute to rotator cuff impingement.[9] Biomechanical factors leading to subacromial impingement include abnormal scapular and humeral kinematics, postural abnormalities, rotator cuff and scapular muscle weakness, and decreased flexibility of the pectoralis minor or posterior shoulder tissues.[9] Intrinsic mechanisms of rotator cuff tendinopathy that may lead to SAIS result from tendon degradation due to the natural aging process,[9,20-23] poor vascularity,[9,24-28] altered biology,[9,20,29-31] and inferior mechanical properties resulting in damage with tensile or shear loads.[9,32-35] Patients with rotator cuff tendinopathy have been found to have decreased total collagen content, increased proportion of type III collagen fibers, and greater cell death within the tendons compared to normal tendons.[9,31,36,37] These factors can contribute to thinning and weakening of the rotator cuff tendons, leading to impingement.[9,38,39]

Nonsurgical treatment options for SAIS include physical therapy, oral medications, and injections. While further research is needed, there have been studies demonstrating decreased pain and increased function with nonsurgical rehabilitation programs for individuals with SAIS.[40] If nonsurgical interventions fail to resolve the patient's symptoms, a surgical decompression of the subacromial space is indicated.[3]

Physical Therapy Patient/Client Management

There are multiple physical therapy interventions for SAIS based on the patient's presentation. These interventions may include modalities, manual therapy, therapeutic exercise (which includes stretching and resistance training), postural education, and patient education on how to prevent recurring problems in the future.[3,9,40] In some cases, a patient may not benefit from physical therapy interventions and will need to be referred to an orthopaedic physician for a surgical consult. A standard of practice is to provide physical therapy for 3 to 6 weeks (~6-12 visits) before considering a surgical consultation.[3]

Examination, Evaluation, and Diagnosis

When evaluating an individual with SAIS, it is important to start with a thorough subjective evaluation. The patient's history often contains a description of repetitive overhead work or athletic activity involving overhead movements that aggravate the patient's shoulder pain.[3] A patient may complain of pain in the anterior aspect of the shoulder with movements that decrease the size of the subacromial space, causing impingement of the subacromial bursa, long head of the biceps, or rotator cuff tendons. The patient's functional limitations should be discussed, since these are usually the primary reasons for which the patient has sought treatment. In addition to changes in objective measurements, improvements in functional tasks (*e.g.*, being able to loop a belt or tuck in his shirt behind his back) can be used to document progress in physical therapy. Questions should also be asked about previous medical history, current medications, and any diagnostic imaging that has been performed.

A comprehensive objective evaluation begins with screening the cervical spine to rule out referred symptoms from the neck as the etiology of his shoulder pain. Unrestricted cervical active range of motion and a clear neurologic screen of the upper quadrant (testing of dermatomes, myotomes, and deep tendon reflexes from C5-C8) help rule out cervical spine involvement.[3,41] A summary of the objective examination for the patient with suspected SAIS is presented in Table 1-1.

Table 1-1 SUMMARY OF OBJECTIVE EXAMINATION FOR PATIENT WITH SUSPECTED SAIS

Test	Patient Position and Movement	Positive Findings
Posture observation	Standing posterior view	Posterior view: atrophy of infraspinatus and supraspinatus; winging of scapula
	Standing lateral view	Lateral view: thoracic kyphosis, shoulder protraction
Active range of motion	1. Standing shoulder flexion 2. Standing shoulder abduction 3. Standing external rotation (ER) with elbow at 90° 4. Standing internal rotation (IR): ask patient to place hand behind back; measure level of thumb to highest spinous process	Painful arc of motion (60°-120°) with shoulder flexion Pain at end range of shoulder flexion and/or shoulder abduction Decreased IR on affected side, as demonstrated by inability to reach spinous process equal to that of unaffected shoulder
Passive range of motion	1. Supine shoulder flexion 2. Supine shoulder abduction 3. Supine shoulder ER at 90° abduction 4. Supine shoulder IR at 90° abduction	Decreased IR on affected side
Manual muscle testing: 1. Teres minor and infraspinatus 2. Subscapularis 3. Supraspinatus 4. Serratus anterior 5. Middle trapezius 6. Lower trapezius	Therapist applies force in direction opposite of muscle action. 1. Standing ER with arm at side and elbow at 90° 2. Standing IR with arm at side and elbow at 90° 3. Standing shoulder horizontal abduction at 40° anterior to the frontal plane 4. Seated with shoulder at 120° of flexion 5. Prone with shoulder at 90° horizontal abduction with ER 6. Prone with arm parallel to body and shoulder at 145° horizontal abduction	All muscles tested have the potential to be graded as weak, but the most common weaknesses are found in the supraspinatus (mostly due to pain) and scapular muscles (serratus anterior, middle trapezius and lower trapezius)

The physical therapist should carefully observe the patient's standing posture from posterior and lateral views. From the posterior view, note any atrophy of the rotator cuff muscles in the infraspinatus and supraspinatus fossas. Compare the heights of the shoulders and look for the presence of scapular winging with the patient's arms by his side. Due to increased upper trapezius activity and decreased serratus anterior strength, the patient's involved shoulder may be elevated and scapular winging present.[42] From the lateral view, evaluate for the presence of excessive thoracic kyphosis and shoulder protraction.[43] Patients with SAIS often have increased thoracic kyphosis and decreased thoracic mobility that contribute to altered movement patterns.[42,44] The shoulder affected by SAIS is often in a protracted position due to the increased thoracic kyphosis and a tight pectoralis minor muscle.[45] Both of these postural abnormalities contribute to a decreased subacromial space and impingement of the underlying tissues.[9,45]

During an active range of motion movement screen of the shoulder, patients with SAIS may demonstrate **scapular dyskinesis**. Scapular dyskinesis refers to visible alterations in scapular position and movement patterns.[46] Dyskinesis of the shoulder may be caused by adaptive shortening of the pectoralis minor muscle,[42,43,47,48] posterior shoulder tightness,[9,49] decreased scapular and rotator cuff strength,[9,45] and increased thoracic kyphosis.[9,42,44,50] Generally, the affected shoulder demonstrates decreased scapular posterior tilting, decreased upward rotation, and increased internal rotation of the scapula.[9,42] This results in failure of the anterior aspect of the acromion to move away from the humeral head during shoulder flexion, contributing to a reduction in subacromial space and rotator cuff impingement.[9,42] A method for identifying scapular dyskinesis is the scapula dyskinesis test (SDT, Fig. 1-1).[46]

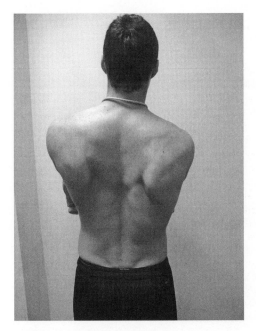

Figure 1-1. Scapula dyskinesis test. The patient performs 5 repetitions of shoulder flexion with weights in his hand, while the therapist observes the patient's scapular motion. Note the obvious scapular winging on the right.

The patient performs 5 repetitions of bilateral, active, weighted shoulder flexion followed by bilateral, active, weighted shoulder abduction while the physical therapist observes from the posterior and superior views.[46] The shoulder of a patient with a positive scapula dyskinesis test demonstrates scapular winging, dysrhythmia, or both.[3,46,51]

Evaluating muscle strength during the objective portion of the examination helps to further determine the contributing factors to SAIS. Weakness of the serratus anterior, lower trapezius, and middle trapezius muscles can lead to altered scapular kinematics in patients with SAIS.[3,9,42,52] The serratus and trapezius muscles stabilize the scapula and produce scapular upward rotation, external rotation, and/or posterior tilting of the scapula to allow the humeral head to clear the acromion with elevation.[9,53] Patients with SAIS often complain of increased pain and decreased strength with shoulder flexion. This is due to scapular weakness and altered kinematics on the affected side, which leads to rotator cuff impingement in the subacromial space. In a study performed by Tate et al.,[54] manually repositioning the scapula (using the Scapula Reposition Test) resulted in less pain during impingement testing and increased strength in athletes with a positive impingement test. The Scapula Reposition Test involves manually posterior tilting, externally rotating, and retracting the scapula to allow normal scapular mechanics that occur with shoulder elevation to prevent impingement of the rotator cuff (Fig. 1-2). In addition

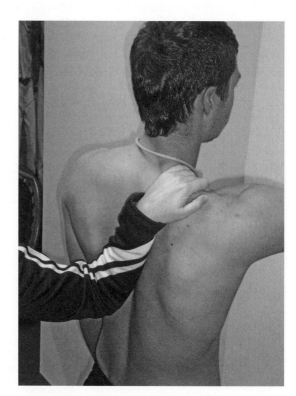

Figure 1-2. Physical therapist performing the Scapula Reposition Test.

to strength testing of the scapular stabilizers, manual muscle tests of the supraspinatus, teres minor, infraspinatus, and subscapularis muscles should also be performed. These muscles frequently demonstrate weakness and strength testing may cause increased pain in patients with SAIS.[3]

Special tests for the shoulder (Table 1-2) should be performed at the end of the musculoskeletal examination. Impingement tests that may help confirm the diagnosis of SAIS are the Neer test, Hawkins test, and empty can test. Tate et al.[3] reported that patients with SAIS demonstrate the following: (1) a positive Neer, Hawkins, or empty can test, (2) a painful shoulder arc of motion, and (3) pain or weakness with resisted shoulder external rotation with the arm at the side. Kelly et al.[55] found the Hawkins test to be the most accurate for diagnosing any degree of SAIS. In a study done by Calis et al.,[56] the Hawkins test was also found to be the most sensitive for diagnosing shoulder impingement, followed by Neer impingement test. Additional special tests should be performed to rule out labral tears, shoulder instability, and rotator cuff tears.

Table 1-2   SPECIAL TESTS ASSOCIATED WITH IMPINGEMENT SYNDROME[57]

Special Test	Patient Position	Findings
Neer impingement test	With the patient seated or standing, the physical therapist passively forward flexes the shoulder while stabilizing the scapula with the other hand	Positive test: pain with full forced flexion is a positive sign of supraspinatus impingement
Hawkins impingement test	With the patient seated or standing, the physical therapist passively flexes the shoulder to 90° and internally rotates the shoulder with elbow flexed to 90°	Positive test: pain is a positive sign of supraspinatus tendonitis/ impingement
Empty can test	With patient seated or standing, the patient flexes the shoulder to 90° in the scapular plane with full internal rotation (thumb down) and resists downward pressure placed at the wrist by the physical therapist	Positive test: pain and/ or muscle weakness is a positive sign of supraspinatus tendonitis/ impingement
Scapula dyskinesis test	Standing, the patient performs 5 repetitions of shoulder flexion with weight in hand (2.3 kg for patients weighing >68.0 kg and 1.4 kg for patients weighing <68.0 kg)[3]	Patients are rated as having normal scapular motion, subtle abnormalities, or obvious abnormalities. Abnormalities are defined as winging or dysrhythmia[3]
Scapula reposition test	With the patient standing, the physical therapist applies a moderate force to the patient's scapula to encourage posterior tilting and external rotation of the scapula	Manually repositioning the scapula reduces pain and increases shoulder elevation strength in patients with impingement

Plan of Care and Interventions

Physical therapy interventions for patients with SAIS should address deficits and limitations found in the objective examination. **Therapeutic exercise** has been found to have a positive effect in retraining muscle imbalances and restoring normal movement patterns.[3,40,58] Manual therapy techniques assist in decreasing pain, improving range of motion, and increasing function in these patients.[3]

Several studies have evaluated the effectiveness of therapeutic exercise programs for SAIS. Tate et al.[3] evaluated a 6- to 8-week three-phase intervention for patients with SAIS that included: progressive strengthening, manual stretching, thrust and non-thrust manipulations to the shoulder and spine, patient education, activity modification, and a daily home exercise program of stretching and strengthening as shown in Table 1-3. Eight of the ten subjects reported successful outcomes based on symptomatic and functional improvement after completion of the treatment program. The outcome measures used to define success included: the three pain subscale questions of the Penn Shoulder Scale, the Disabilities of the Arm, Shoulder and Hand (DASH) questionnaire, and the Global Rating of Change (GRC) question that allowed subjects to rate the perceived change in their shoulder condition since starting the strengthening program.[3]

Bernhardsson et al.[58] demonstrated that a 12-week eccentric strengthening program decreased pain and improved function in patients with SAIS. The exercise regimen targeted the supraspinatus and infraspinatus muscles, emphasizing the eccentric phase of strengthening for these two muscles, along with scapular stabilizing exercises to promote correct movement patterns.[58]

The studies by Tate et al.[3] and Bernhardsson et al.[58] focused on specific exercise programs and types of exercises for the treatment of SAIS. A recent systematic review in 2010 evaluated eight studies that used various strengthening

Table 1-3 EXAMPLE SAIS TREATMENT PROGRAM	
Treatment Technique	Treatment Specifics
Motor control/ strengthening	Phase 1: rotator cuff strengthening with humerus in neutral position Phase 2: add shoulder flexion exercises, focus on more aggressive strengthening of serratus anterior (Fig. 1-3) and trapezius Phase 3: higher-level strengthening and endurance training at multiple levels of shoulder flexion; incorporate trunk strengthening
Manual therapy	Manual stretching techniques focusing on improving flexibility of the posterior shoulder and inferior glenohumeral capsule Thrust and non-thrust manipulation techniques directed at the thoracic spine to improve thoracic extension
Self-stretches	Stretches performed independently by the patient to increase mobility of the glenohumeral capsule and flexibility of the pectoral and thoracic spinal muscles
Home exercise program	Selective combination of strengthening exercises and self-stretches to be performed once daily at home, using same repetitions and resistance as was performed in the clinic

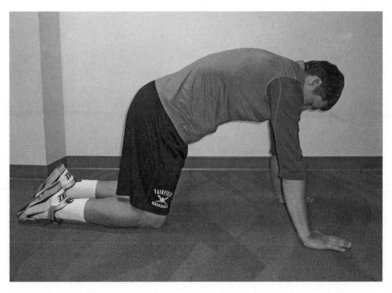

Figure 1-3. Serratus anterior strengthening exercise in quadruped: push-up plus. Patient moves from quadruped position to pictured push-up plus position.

and stretching exercises, manual therapies, and modalities in the treatment of SAIS.[40] The review concluded that there is limited evidence to support the use of exercise in the treatment of SAIS to relieve pain and improve function.[40] As with any diagnosis, exercises and treatment strategy should focus on improving the patient's objective and functional deficits. For the patient with SAIS in this case study, after 2 weeks of treatment, the physical therapist should reassess his pain intensity with reaching in various directions and lifting objects, and his progress toward being able to loop his belt and tuck a shirt in behind his back. If his symptoms remain unchanged, the treatment strategy and focus of exercises may need to be altered.

Evidence-Based Clinical Recommendations

SORT: Strength of Recommendation Taxonomy

A: Consistent, good-quality patient-oriented evidence
B: Inconsistent or limited-quality patient-oriented evidence
C: Consensus, disease-oriented evidence, usual practice, expert opinion, or case series

1. Intrinsic and extrinsic factors contribute to the development of subacromial impingement syndrome (SAIS). **Grade A**

2. Patients with SAIS may demonstrate scapular dyskinesis. **Grade B**

3. Therapeutic exercise helps retrain muscle imbalances, restore normal movement patterns, and decrease pain in patients with SAIS. **Grade B**

COMPREHENSION QUESTIONS

1.1 An outpatient physical therapist evaluates a patient suffering from right shoulder subacromial impingement syndrome (SAIS). While observing the patient's active range of motion, the therapist notes altered right scapular movement. Weakness in which muscles is *most* likely to be responsible for this scapular dyskinesis?

    A. Supraspinatus, infraspinatus, teres minor

    B. Supraspinatus, serratus anterior, lower trapezius

    C. Serratus anterior, lower trapezius, middle trapezius

    D. Middle trapezius, pectoralis minor, biceps brachii

1.2 SAIS involves degradation and/or mechanical compression of *which* of the following soft tissue structures?

    A. Rotator cuff

    B. Long head of the biceps

    C. Subacromial bursa

    D. All of the above

ANSWERS

1.1 **C.** Weakness of the serratus anterior, lower trapezius, and middle trapezius muscles can lead to altered scapular kinematics in patients with SAIS.[25,26,27,42,46] The serratus anterior and trapezius muscles stabilize the scapula and cause scapular upward rotation, external rotation, and/or posterior tilting of the scapula to allow the humeral head to clear the acromion with shoulder elevation.[31,42]

1.2 **D.** Impingement syndrome involves degeneration and/or mechanical compression of soft tissue structures.[46] In the case of SAIS, the rotator cuff, long head of the biceps, and the subacromial bursa are compressed between the acromion, the coracoacromial ligament, and the humeral head.[28,33,46]

REFERENCES

1. Picavet HS, Schouten JS. Musculoskeletal pain in the Netherlands: prevalences, consequences and risk groups, the DMC(3)-study. *Pain.* 2003;102:167-178.

2. Pope DP, Croft PR, Pritchard CM, Silman AJ. Prevalence of shoulder pain in the community: the influence of case definition. *Ann Rheum Dis.* 1997;56:308-312.

3. Tate AR, McClure PW, Kareha S, Irwin D. Effect of the scapula reposition test on shoulder impingement symptoms and elevation strength in overhead athletes. *J Orthop Sports Phys Ther.* 2008;38:4-11.

4. Urwin M, Symmons D, Allison T, et al. Estimating the burden of musculoskeletal disorders in the community: the comparative prevalence of symptoms at different anatomical sites, and the relation to social deprivation. *Ann Rheum Dis.* 1998;57:649-655.

5. van der Widnt DA, Koes BW, de Jong BA, Bouter LM. Shoulder disorders in general practice: incidence, patient characteristics, and management. *Ann Rheum Dis.* 1995;54:959-964.

6. Vecchio PC, Kavanagh RT, Hazleman BL, King RH. Community survey of shoulder disorders in the elderly to assess the natural history and effects of treatment. *Ann Rheum Dis*.1995;54:152-154.

7. Ludewig PM, Reynolds JF. The association of scapular kinematics and glenohumeral joint pathologies. *J Orthop Sports Phys Ther*. 2009;39:90-104.

8. Neer CS II. Impingement lesions. *Clin Orthop Relat Res*.1983;173:70-77.

9. Seitz AL, McClure PW, Finucane S, Boardman ND III, Michener LA. Mechanisms of rotator cuff tendinopathy: intrinsic, extrinsic, or both? *Clin Biomech*. 2011;26:1-12.

10. Bigliani LU, Ticker JB, Flatow EL, Soslowsky LJ, Mow VC. The relationship of acromial architecture to rotator cuff disease. *Clin Sports Med*. 1991;10:823-838.

11. Epstein RE, Schweitzer ME, Frieman BG, Fenlin JM Jr, Mitchell DG. Hooked acromion: prevalence on MR images of painful shoulder. *Radiology*. 1993;187:479-481.

12. Gill TJ, McIrvin E, Kocher MS, Homa K, Mair SD, Hawkins RJ. The relative importance of acromial morphology and age with respect to rotator cuff pathology. *J Shoulder Elbow Surg*. 2002;11: 327-330.

13. Ogawa K, Yoshida A, Inokuchi W, Naniwa T. Acromial spur: relationship to aging and morphologic changes in the rotator cuff. *J Shoulder Elbow Surg*. 2005;14:591-598.

14. Aoki M, Ishii S, Usui M. The slope of the acromion and rotator cuff impingement. *Orthop Trans*. 1986;10:228.

15. Edelson JG. The 'hooked' acromion revisited. *J Bone Joint Surg Br*. 1995;77:284-287.

16. Toivonen D, Tuite MJ, Orwin JF. Acromial structure and tears of the rotator cuff. *J Shoulder Elbow Surg*. 1995;4:376-383.

17. Vaz S, Soyer J, Pries P, Clarac JP. Subacromial impingement: influence of coracoacromial arch geometry on shoulder function. *Joint Bone Spine*. 2000;67:305-309.

18. Farley TE, Neumann CH, Steinbach LS, Petersen SA. The coracoacromial arch: MR evaluation and correlation with rotator cuff pathology. *Skeletal Radiol*. 1994;23:641-645.

19. Nicholson GP, Goodman DA, Flatow EL, Bigliani LU. The acromion: morphologic condition and age-related changes. A study of 420 scapulas. *J Shoulder Elbow Surg*.1996;5:1-11.

20. Iannotti JP, Zlatkin MB, Esterhai JL, Kressel HY, Dalinka MK, Spindler KP. Magnetic resonance imaging of the shoulder. Sensitivity, specificity, and predictive value. *J Bone Joint Surg Am*. 1991;73: 17-29.

21. Milgrom C, Schaffler M, Gilbert S, van Holsbeeck M. Rotator-cuff changes in asymptomatic adults. The effect of age, hand dominance and gender. *J Bone Joint Surg Br*. 1995;77:296-298.

22. Sher JS, Uribe JW, Posada A, Murphy BJ, Zlatkin MB. Abnormal findings on magnetic resonance images of asymptomatic shoulders. *J Bone Joint Surg Am*. 1995;77:10-15.

23. Tempelhof S, Rupp S, Seil R. Age-related prevalence of rotator cuff tears in asymptomatic shoulders. *J Shoulder Elbow Surg*. 1999;8:296-299.

24. Biberthaler P, Wiedemann E, Nerlich A, et al. Microcirculation associated with degenerative rotator cuff lesions. In vivo assessment with orthogonal polarization spectral imaging during arthroscopy of the shoulder. *J Bone Joint Surg Am*. 2003;85-A:475-480.

25. Brooks CH, Revell WJ, Heatley FW. A quantitative histological study of the vascularity of the rotator cuff tendon. *J Bone Joint Surg Br*. 1992;74:151-153.

26. Fukuda H, Hamada K, Yamanaka K. Pathology and pathogenesis of bursal-side rotator cuff tears viewed from en bloc histologic sections. *Clin Orthop Relat Res*. 1990;254:75-80.

27. Goodmurphy CW, Osborn J, Akesson EJ, Johnson S, Stanescu V, Regan WD. An immunocytochemical analysis of torn rotator cuff tendon taken at the time of repair. *J Shoulder Elbow Surg*. 2003;12:368-374.

28. Rudzki JR, Adler RS, Warren RF, et al. Contrast-enhanced ultrasound characterization of the vascularity of the rotator cuff tendon: age-and activity-related changes in the intact asymptomatic rotator cuff. *J Shoulder Elbow Surg*. 2008;17:96S-100S.

29. Kumagai J, Sarkar K, Uhthoff HK. The collagen types in the attachment zone of rotator cuff tendons in the elderly: an immunohistochemical study. *J Rheumatol.* 1994;21:2096-2100.

30. Riley GP, Harrall RL, Constant CR, Chard MD, Cawston TE, Hazleman BL. Glycosaminoglycans of human rotator cuff tendons: changes with age and in chronic rotator cuff tendinitis. *Ann Rheum Dis.* 1994;53:367-376.

31. Riley GP, Harrall RL, Constant CR, Chard MD, Cawston TE, Hazleman BL. Tendon degeneration and chronic shoulder pain: changes in the collagen composition of the human rotator cuff tendons in rotator cuff tendinitis. *Ann Rheum Dis.* 1994;53:359-366.

32. Bey MJ, Song HK, Wehrli FW, Soslowsky LJ. Intratendinous strain fields of the intact supraspinatus tendon: the effect of glenohumeral joint position and tendon region. *J Orthop Res.* 2002;20:869-874.

33. Herbert LJ, Moffet H, McFadyen BJ, Dionne CE. Scapular behavior in shoulder impingement syndrome. *Arch Phys Med Rehabil.* 2002;83:60-69.

34. Hung CJ, Jan MH, Lin YF, Wang TQ, Lin JJ. Scapular kinematics and impairment features for classifying patients with subacromial impingement syndrome. *Man Ther.* 2010;15:547-551.

35. Reilly P, Amis AA, Wallace AL, Emery RJ. Mechanical failures in the initiation and propagation of tears of the rotator cuff. Quantification of strains of the supraspinatus tendon in vivo. *J Bone Joint Surg Br.* 2003;84:594-599.

36. Tuoheti Y, Itoi E, Pradhan RL, et al. Apoptosis in the supraspinatus tendon with stage II subacromial impingement. *J Shouler Elbow Surg.* 2005;14:535-541.

37. Yuan J, Murrell GA, Wei AQ, Wang MX. Apoptosis in rotator cuff tendinopathy. *J Orthop Res.* 2002;20:1372-1379.

38. Lake SP, Miller KS, Elliott DM, Soslowsky JL. Effect of fiber distribution and realignment on the nonlinear and inhomogeneous mechanical properties of human supraspinatus tendon under longitudinal tensile loading. *J Orthop Res.* 2009;27:1596-1602.

39. Cholewinski JJ, Kusz DJ, Wojciechowski P, Cielinski LS, Zoladz MP. Ultrasound measurement of rotator cuff thickness and acromio-humeral distance in the diagnosis of subacromial impingement syndrome of the shoulder. *Knee Surg Sports Traumatol Arthrosc.* 2007;16:408-414.

40. Kelly SM, Wrightson PA, Meads CA. Clinical outcomes of exercise in the management of subacromial impingement syndrome: a systemic review. *Clin Rehabil.* 2010;24:99-109.

41. Wainner RS, Fritz JM, Irrgang JJ, Boninger ML, Delitto A, Allison S. Reliability and diagnostic accuracy of the clinical examination and patient self-report measures for cervical radiculopathy. *Spine.* 2003;28:52-62.

42. Ludewig PM, Cook TM. Alterations in shoulder kinematics and associated muscle activity in people with symptoms of shoulder impingement. *Phys Ther.* 2000;80:276-291.

43. Kendall FP, Provance PG, McCreary EK. *Muscles, Testing and Function: With Posture and Pain.* 4th ed. Baltimore: Lippincott, Williams and Wilkins; 1993.

44. Kebaetse M, McClure P, Pratt NA. Thoracic position effect on shoulder range of motion, strength, and three-dimensional scapular kinematics. *Arch Phys Med Rehabil.* 1999;80:945-950.

45. Borstad JD, Ludewig PM. The effect of long versus short pectoralis minor resting length on scapular kinematics in healthy individuals. *J Orthop Sports Phys Ther.* 2005;35:227-238.

46. McClure P, Tate AR, Kareha S, Irwin D, Zlupko E. A clinical method for identifying scapular dyskinesis, part 1: reliability. *J Athl Train.* 2009;44:160-164.

47. Borstad JD. Resting position variables at the shoulder: evidence to support a posture-impairment association. *Phys Ther.* 2006;86:549-557.

48. Huang CY, Wang VM, Pawluk RJ, et al. Inhomogeneous mechanical behavior of the human supraspinatus tendon under uniaxial loading. *J Orthop Res.* 2005;23:924-930.

49. Borich MR, Bright JM, Lorello DJ, Cieminski CJ, Buisman T, Ludewig PM. Scapular angular positioning at end range internal rotation in cases of glenohumeral internal rotation deficit. *J Orthop Sports Phys Ther.* 2006;36:926-934.

50. Wang CH, McClure P, Pratt NE, Nobilini R. Stretching and strengthening exercises: their effect on three-dimensional scapular kinematics. *Arch Phys Med Rehabil.* 1999;80:923-929.

51. Tate AR, McClure P, Kareha S, Irwin D, Barbe MF. A clinical method for identifying scapular dyskinesis, part 2: validity. *J Athl Train.* 2009;44:165-173.

52. Lewis JS, Wright C, Green A. Subacromial impingement syndrome: the effect of changing posture on shoulder range of movement. *J Orthop Sports Phys Ther.* 2005;35:72-87.

53. McQuade KJ, Dawson J, Smidt GL. Scapulothoracic muscle fatigue associated with alterations in scapulohumeral rhythm kinematics during maximum resistive shoulder elevation. *J Ortho Sports Phys Ther.* 1998;28:74-80.

54. Tate AR, McClure PW, Kareha S, Irwin D. Effect of the Scapula Reposition Test on shoulder impingement symptoms and elevation strength in overhead athletes. *J Orthop Sports Phys Ther.* 2008;38:4-11.

55. Kelly SM, Brittle N, Allen GM. The value of physical tests for subacromial impingement syndrome: a study of diagnostic accuracy. *Clin Rehabil.* 2010;24:149-158.

56. Calis M, Akgun K, Birtane M, Karacan I, Calis H, Tuzun F. Diagnostic values of clinical diagnostic tests in subacromial impingement syndrome. *Ann Rheum Dis.* 2000;59:44-47.

57. Magee DJ. *Orthopedic Physical Assessment.* 3rd ed. Philadelphia: WB Saunders Co; 1997.

58. Bernhardsson S, Klintberg IH, Wendt GK. Evaluation of an exercise concept focusing on eccentric strength training of the rotator cuff for patients with subacromial impingement syndrome. *Clin Rehabil.* 2011;25:69-78.

Shoulder Labral Tear

Lane Bailey
Ellen Shanley

A 16-year-old elite-level volleyball player was participating in a regional tournament when she sustained an injury to her dominant left upper extremity while attempting to spike a ball. The patient continued to play despite left shoulder pain, a feeling of the shoulder "slipping in and out," and a decrease in striking power. Immediately following the tournament, she sought the care of her family physician that performed x-rays, which were negative for shoulder dislocation and bony pathology. The athlete's medical history was positive for vague left shoulder pain over the past season and an eating disorder, for which she is currently under the care of a sports psychiatrist. She now presents to physical therapy 3 days after her injury with a referring diagnosis of a "SLAP tear." You are asked to evaluate and treat the patient for a safe return to volleyball activities.

▶ What are the examination priorities?
▶ What are the key examination tests that should be performed to identify the specific pathology and impairments?
▶ What are the most appropriate physical therapy interventions?
▶ What precautions should be taken *during* physical therapy?
▶ What are possible complications interfering with the patient's progress in physical therapy?

KEY DEFINITIONS

BICEPS-LABRAL COMPLEX: Integration of the long head of the biceps tendon into the superior glenoid labrum

CONCAVITY-COMPRESSION: Stabilizing mechanism in which compression provided by the rotator cuff muscles is applied through the convex humeral head into the concave glenoid fossa, thereby resisting translational forces

SHOULDER INSTABILITY: Clinical condition in which excessive translation of the humeral head occurs on the glenoid fossa, potentially resulting in subluxation or dislocation

Objectives

1. Understand the functional anatomy of the glenohumeral joint and biceps-labral complex.

2. Ask relevant patient history questions to elucidate the prognosis and treatment plan of care.

3. Identify critical examination findings that should be evaluated prior to patient treatment.

4. Identify reliable and valid physical examination tools to aid in patient diagnosis and prognosis.

5. Provide appropriate interventions that will allow the patient to safely return to sport.

6. Determine when the athlete is prepared to return to volleyball competition with functional return-to-sport tests.

Physical Therapy Considerations

PT considerations during management of the athlete with a labral tear:

▶ **General physical therapy plan of care/goals:** Protect patient from incurring subsequent injury; identify anatomical source(s) of pathology; improve muscular balance and flexibility to restore shoulder stability

▶ **Physical therapy interventions:** Patient education regarding local anatomy, pathomechanics, and activity modifications; modalities to manage pain; manual therapy and selective stretching to improve identified areas of hypomobility; increase joint stability through rotator cuff and periscapular muscle strengthening

▶ **Precautions during physical therapy:** Avoid aggressive overhead activity that places excessive stress on the labrum in early phases of therapy; careful progression from a neutral position to full overhead shoulder elevation as strength and symptoms allow

▶ **Complications interfering with physical therapy:** Components of patient's current and past medical history (*i.e.*, eating disorder, poor nutrition/diet) that will impact the treatment plan and overall prognosis; difficulty in establishing collaborative lines of communication with the patient and other healthcare professionals involved in her care

Understanding the Health Condition

The glenohumeral joint is highly mobile, allowing for wide ranges of motion to occur about the shoulder. As a result, the natural stability of the joint is decreased due to a lack of bony congruency. Glenohumeral stability is dependent upon a crucial balance of both passive and active restraints. Passive restraints include the osseous congruency between the glenoid fossa and humeral head and contributions from the capsuloligamentous structures. The rotator cuff muscles improve joint stability through muscular contraction by tightening the capsule, which forces the humeral head to compress into the glenoid. This action provides increased dynamic stability at the joint. Scapular position is an extrinsic factor that influences shoulder stability by positioning the glenoid fossa for maximal osseous congruency during dynamic movements. Scapular position impairments have been associated with individuals who have postural deficits and shoulder pathology.

The glenoid fossa covers approximately 20% to 30% of the humeral head[1] and serves as the socket to the glenohumeral joint. The fibrocartilaginous glenoid labrum enhances joint congruency by increasing the depth of the socket by up to 50%.[2,3] The labrum attaches along the peripheral edges of the pear-shaped glenoid fossa and acts to improve joint stability by providing a lateral "bumper" to keep the humeral head centered on the glenoid fossa. The labrum also improves shoulder stability by increasing concavity compression by up to 10%[4] and by maintaining negative intra-articular pressure. The thin film of synovial fluid that is contained between the articular surfaces produces a negative pressure within the enclosed joint capsule. This negative pressure acts as a vacuum to resist distraction forces of the humerus, thereby maintaining normal arthrokinematics. Labral defects can allow fluid exchange between the joint and adjacent tissues, resulting in a loss of negative intra-articular pressure and joint stability.

Perhaps just as important, the labrum serves as an attachment site for the glenohumeral joint capsule and the ligaments that stabilize the glenohumeral joint, particularly in extreme ranges of motion. The glenohumeral ligaments are fibrous bands intrinsic to the joint capsule that resist translational forces that oppose their anatomical positions. Rotator cuff tendons blend with the glenohumeral joint capsule prior to their attachment to the humerus. This blending of muscular tissues with the inert capsule helps increase stability by tensioning the joint capsule during contraction, causing the humeral head to approximate within the glenoid fossa. The muscles of the rotator cuff maintain a delicate balance of both the anterior-posterior and superior-inferior force couples that are responsible for proper joint alignment. Deficits to any of these relationships may potentially jeopardize the integrity of glenohumeral joint stability.

Injuries to the superior labrum that extend anterior to posterior at the proximal biceps insertion were first described by Andrews et al.[5] in 1985 and later by Snyder et al.,[6] who coined the term superior labrum anterior to posterior (SLAP) to describe these lesions. Research suggests that the incidence[7] and prevalence[8] of SLAP lesions are higher among active individuals, particularly those who engage in overhead activities.[9,10] The mechanical impact of SLAP lesions has been studied using cadaver models that showed significant increases in humeral head translation when compared to those with intact labrums.[3,11] Several mechanisms that may contribute to the high rate of superior labral injury have been proposed: traction overload of the biceps during the deceleration phase of throwing[5]; shear forces exerted on the biceps-labral complex during the maximal cocking phase of throwing[12]; posterior shoulder tightness[13]; and, compression shearing caused by a fall on outstretched hand.[14] SLAP lesions can result in pain and loss of function with potential for significant disability and decreased performance.

There are four basic types of SLAP lesions based on differences in anatomical variance.[6] Additional classifications have been proposed.[15,16] However, the type I-IV SLAP lesions established by Snyder et al.[6] are most commonly used within the literature. A type I SLAP lesion refers to fraying of the inner rim of the superior glenoid labrum. These lesions are considered to be degenerative in nature due to a decreasing blood supply associated with increased age.[17] Type II tears are the most common and clinically significant, accounting for the majority of SLAP lesions found in overhead athletes.[18-21] Type II tears occur when the superior labrum is detached from the biceps insertion at the superior glenoid tubercle. These tears may be further divided into anterior, posterior, or a combination of anterior and posterior relative to the long head of biceps tendon.[22] As a result of the traction force being applied by the biceps (e.g., deceleration during throwing activities), these injuries commonly result in elevation of the labrum away from the glenoid fossa. Concomitant injuries of shoulder instability and rotator cuff pathology may also be present with SLAP lesions, warranting thorough physical screening. Bucket-handle tears of the superior labrum are categorized as type III SLAP lesions that extend from anterior to posterior on the face of the glenoid fossa.[17] These lesions alone do not cause superior elevation of the labrum away from the glenoid fossa; however, entrapment and joint "locking" may ensue if the lesion is severe. Type IV SLAP tears are also classified as bucket-handle lesions. These defects extend into the biceps tendon, resulting in a split proximal attachment. Type III and IV lesions are often the result of episodes of traumatic instability.[23,24] Additional categories have been expanded to include lesions associated with the presence of shoulder instability,[15] loose bodies, and articular damage.[25] For additional detail regarding the other varieties of SLAP lesions, the reader is encouraged to seek more thorough resources.[15,16]

It has been estimated that a high-level volleyball athlete performs up to 40,000 spikes in a single season.[26] Considering this large volume of repetitive stress, it is not surprising that 62% of these athletes report shoulder pain within the hitting zone (the arc of motion the athlete uses for impacting the ball).[27] In addition, volleyball-related overuse shoulder injuries result in an average of 6.5 weeks of lost training and/or competition time.[28] These factors suggest the need for addressing functional deficits and restoring proper mechanics for safe return to sport. Functionally, the ideal initiation of the overhand spike originates from the torso, which is responsible for the majority of the forces imparted to the ball. These forces are then potentiated up the kinetic chain to the hand. Thus, the upper extremity relies on sufficient core muscle strength to generate the forces necessary to produce the desired performance outcome. The scapula serves as a "funnel" for the efficient transfer of this kinetic energy from the trunk to the upper extremity, and is furthermore responsible for providing a stable base of support so that the hand can be properly positioned in space at the moment of impact.[29]

There are sufficient biomechanical similarities between various overhead sports such as volleyball and baseball. However, the contact point in the volleyball spiking motion is much higher than the release point of a baseball pitcher, resulting in greater maximal glenohumeral abduction for the volleyball spiker.[30] During the acceleration phase of the spike, the trunk uncoils, elevating and externally rotating the shoulder joint, which generates high tension in the inferior joint capsule.[30] The inferior glenohumeral ligament is maximally stressed in this elevated position, which increases the potential of capsular avulsion injuries as a result of repetitive microtrauma.[30]

Functionally, volleyball athletes have demonstrated decreased external rotation strength of the dominant hitting arm when compared to the opposite arm.[27] Thirty percent of these athletes also exhibit infraspinatus muscle atrophy on physical examination.[27] Suprascapular nerve pathology (*e.g.*, paralabral cysts, neuropraxia) has been provided as a rationale for these asymmetries due to repetitive neural tension and/or compression at the spinoglenoid notch.[31] However, additional study is required to validate these claims. Sufficient external rotation strength is vital to the deceleration phase of overhead throwing and spiking. Decreased strength of the external rotators is thought to contribute to the high prevalence of shoulder injury within this population. Therapeutic interventions should focus on addressing these deficits prior to returning to play.

Physical Therapy Patient/Client Management

The conservative management of shoulder pain should be tailored to the individual's symptoms, clinical presentation, and functional goals. Therapeutic interventions that have proven beneficial for nonoperative care of individuals with SLAP lesions include scapular stabilization exercises, rotator cuff strengthening, and posterior-inferior capsule stretching.[8] Depending on the extent of soft tissue and joint inflammation, the patient may also benefit from physician-prescribed nonsteroidal anti-inflammatory drugs (NSAIDs) and/or intra-articular glucocorticoid injection. Predicting which patients will respond positively to conservative care is often difficult and poorly understood. Indications for surgical intervention include failure of physical therapy interventions to improve patient symptoms, strength, joint stability, and shoulder function. The choice for operative care is usually a collective agreement made by the entire orthopaedic team; however, the final decision is often made by the patient and treating physician.

Examination, Evaluation, and Diagnosis

A thorough patient history is the foundation of the clinical examination and provides valuable information regarding the mechanism of injury, likely impairments, and rehabilitation prognosis. Patients with SLAP lesions commonly complain of diffuse shoulder pain, instability, and "clicking" or "popping" that is exacerbated with overhead activity.[23] Understanding the prevalence of this type of injury is particularly helpful when evaluating a patient with a suspected SLAP lesion because active individuals[24] and overhead athletes[32] have exhibited high injury rates. Based on the mechanism of injury, the physical therapist may also be able to gain valuable insight into the specific pathological tissue involvement. For example, falls on outstretched hands (FOOSH injuries) are likely to be traction injuries of the biceps-labral complex resulting from an inferior humeral subluxation or dislocation episode.[33] In contrast, the eccentric load placed on the biceps during pitching is often a shear or traction type of injury that causes the superior labrum to "peel-back" from the glenoid (type II lesion).[13] Reports of a traumatic unstable event, severe weakness, and/or intense pain may indicate the presence of concomitant pathologies. The prevalence of additional injuries associated with SLAP lesions has been well documented.[23,24,32] These pathologies include partial- and full-thickness rotator cuff tears, as well as Bankart and Hill-Sachs lesions. If additional injury is suspected, the physical therapist should examine the integrity of these specific tissues. Patient reports are useful in guiding the clinical examination by revealing potential injury and diminishing the necessity to investigate unlikely pathologies.

For both competitive and recreational athletes, the only functional sign(s) of a SLAP lesion may be a sudden decrease in physical performance. Functional deficits can include a loss in striking power, throwing velocity, target accuracy, and level of consistency. Other relevant questions to ask are those specifically related to diet and the presence of systemic disease. These factors can significantly influence tissue healing rates and patient prognosis, thereby demanding modification of the rehabilitation timeline. Based on the severity of comorbidities, the patient may require referral to other healthcare disciplines (*e.g.*, physician, psychiatrist, registered dietician) to receive treatments that are outside the scope of physical therapy practice. In this case, the patient's eating disorder may prolong the rate of tissue healing. Her condition could significantly impact the overall prognosis by lengthening the time required to safely return to sport. Interviews should be adapted to glean this type of relevant information, which helps direct the physical examination and tailor the plan of care.

The physical examination begins with careful observation of the patient's posture, scapular position, and assessment of muscle volume. Procedures include superficial palpation to provide feedback and reinforcement to support (or contradict) the therapist's clinical observations. Although a rare complication of labral pathology, spinoglenoid cysts can cause significant infraspinatus muscle atrophy due to the neural compression exerted at the spinoglenoid notch. Magnetic resonance imaging may be ordered to confirm the presence of a cyst. Careful neurovascular and cervical examination helps clarify involvement of the neck and upper thorax.

The physical examination includes careful consideration to each of the following: active and passive range of motion and flexibility, passive physiologic joint mobility, strength, and tissue irritability and apprehension. The therapist should carefully observe active range of motion (AROM) of the shoulders for symmetrical quantity and quality. Motion is also observed for normal kinematics and contributions from the thoracic spine, scapulothoracic articulation, and glenohumeral joint. Cardinal plane AROM is typically preserved in isolated SLAP lesions.[33] However, pain is often noted in positions of rotator cuff impingement and end-range humeral rotation. Previous investigators have found that thoracic posture influences scapular position, resulting in altered movement patterns of the upper extremity during shoulder elevation.[34] Altered scapular position such as medial border winging and inferior angle prominence are physical examination findings of scapular dyskinesis, which has been associated with labral pathology.[35] It remains unclear whether scapular dyskinesis is the predisposing impairment or the consequence of labral pathology. The presence of these impairments is suggestive of scapular instability and/or excessive muscle tightness.[36] Although it is standard practice to suggest that the patient's scapular dyskinesis might benefit from therapeutic interventions to improve scapular position and decrease risk for injury, no empirical evidence is available to confirm this assumption. Qualitative observational evaluations of scapular dyskinesis have been reported to reliably associate with kinematic analyses.[37-39]

Deficits in passive range of motion of the shoulder may also cause altered movement patterns and create compensatory strategies. Restrictions common in overhead athletes include glenohumeral internal rotation deficit (GIRD), decreased cross-body adduction, and scapular dyskinesis.[13] Overhead athletes, including volleyball players,[40] have shown a higher frequency of GIRD in the dominant arm. Presence of GIRD and decreased cross-body adduction are clinical measures of posterior shoulder tightness that have been associated with a higher incidence[41] and prevalence of injury.[42] These impairments can influence range of motion and function by placing excessive stress on the labrum. Factors thought to influence these motions include posture, posterior-inferior capsular tightness, and humeral torsion.[13,33,43,44] If these limitations are not identified and addressed, the patient may be unable to reach her optimal level of performance, and possibly be at risk for subsequent injury.[41]

Next, the physical therapist should use manual joint glides to clinically assess the resting glenohumeral relationship as well as the degree of capsular extensibility. Individuals with posterior shoulder tightness have demonstrated excessive anterior humeral resting positions on the glenoid fossa.[45,46] Contributions to altered positions are thought to result from increased stiffness of the inferior glenohumeral ligament (IGHL) and posterior capsule.

Due to the loss of negative intra-articular pressure and excessive translation of the humeral head that can occur with a SLAP tear, the passive stability of the glenohumeral joint may be impaired. Table 2-1 lists common physical examination tests to aid in the diagnosis of a SLAP lesion or glenohumeral joint instability.[47] Principles of diagnostic test sensitivity and specificity should be employed to accurately identify the patient's specific impairments and pathology. For example, tests that are more sensitive should be performed first to help focus the physical examination and avoid unnecessary procedures.

Table 2-1   PHYSICAL EXAMINATION TESTS FOR SHOULDER INSTABILITY AND SLAP LESIONS

Test (Purpose)	Patient Positioning	Performance of Test	Sensitivity	Specificity
Sulcus sign (joint stability)	Seated or standing	Therapist grasps the elbow and produces an inferior traction force	17%	93%
Biceps load I (SLAP tear)	Supine with 90° of shoulder abduction and 90° of elbow flexion	Therapist resists elbow flexion at maximal shoulder external rotation	91%	97%
Biceps load II (SLAP tear)	Supine with shoulder in 120° of abduction and 90° of elbow flexion	Therapist resists elbow flexion at maximal shoulder external rotation	90%	97%
Speed test (labral tear)	Standing with the elbow fully extended and forearm fully supinated	Therapist resists shoulder flexion from 0° to 60°	9%-18%	74%-87%
Load and shift (joint stability)	Supine with examiner stabilizing the clavicle and superior border of the scapula	Therapist provides humeral compression into the glenoid fossa and independently applies posteriorly and anteriorly directed forces at glenohumeral joint	Not available	Not available
Apprehension test (joint stability)	Supine with shoulder abducted to 90° and elbow flexed to 90°. Therapist maximally externally rotates shoulder.	Therapist provides anteriorly directed force through the posterior shoulder	30%-40%	63%-87%
Surprise test (joint stability)	Supine with therapist providing a posteriorly directed force through the humeral head	Therapist moves the patient to 90° of shoulder abduction and the posterior force is released	64%-92%	89%-99%
Crank test (labral tear)	Supine or seated with shoulder in 160° of elevation in the scapular plane	Therapist applies compression and then rotates between internal and external rotation	58%-91%	72%-93%
Clunk test (labral tear)	Supine with shoulder maximally abducted	Therapist applies a posterior to anterior force to the shoulder with humeral external rotation	44%	68%

Based on criteria established by Richards et al.,[48] the load and shift test and the sulcus sign are often graded on a 0-III scale. For anterior/posterior translations, a grade of "I" equals 0 to 1 cm translation up the glenoid face; grade II equals 1 to 2 cm translation, or to the glenoid rim; and, grade III equals greater than 2 cm translation over the rim.[49] For an inferior sulcus sign, grade 0 equals no translation; grade I equals 0 to 1 cm translation; grade II equals 1 to 2 cm translation; and, grade III equals greater than 2 cm translation.[49]

Careful muscular strength and endurance testing is critical because individuals with labral pathology, shoulder pain, and joint instability often display weakness, particularly in the scapular stabilizers (e.g., rhomboids, serratus anterior) and rotator cuff muscles.[33] Neuromuscular control and endurance testing are additional components of muscle integrity that should be incorporated. Deficits that are not apparent during maximal isometric contraction may become more evident following fatiguing tasks. Hand-held dynamometry is an objective measurement tool that carries significant face validity when conveying strength deficits to the patient. Anecdotally, the presence of night pain in addition to weakness is *not* consistent with an isolated SLAP tear and may be indicative of a concomitant rotator cuff pathology.[23] Further diagnostic testing is required if this clinical presentation is present.

Other considerations during the physical examination should include levels of tissue irritability and patient apprehension. These factors may negatively influence the outcomes of other tests, based upon the patient's response. As a general rule, selective tissue testing should begin with procedures that are less aggravating, reserving those that are more provocative to the end of the examination. For example, patients with SLAP lesions and concomitant shoulder instability may become highly fearful and reactive when placed in an "apprehension test" position (Table 2-1). Eliciting these symptoms earlier in the exam may result in excessive guarding and the inability to fully investigate the patient's entire pathological involvement. These guidelines should also aid in gaining patient trust and participation compliance.

Plan of Care and Interventions

The rehabilitation program of a patient presenting with a SLAP lesion should be focused on restoring and enhancing the dynamic stability of the glenohumeral joint. Emphasis should also be placed on improving scapular mechanics and addressing any deficits within the kinetic chain (e.g., core stability, balance, and lower extremity strength). A clear understanding of the pathology and mechanism of injury should be considered prior to developing the plan of care. For example, the treatment of compressive injuries (e.g., FOOSH) should be modified to avoid excessive joint loading, while the treatment of traction injuries should discourage biceps activation due to potential migration of the superior labrum.

Several investigators have reported successful postoperative outcomes of SLAP repair.[19,50-53] However, little evidence exists regarding the effectiveness of **conservative physical therapy management** for these lesions. A 2010 study by Edwards et al.[8]

documented that 49% of individuals with SLAP lesions treated nonoperatively with physical therapy had successful outcomes as determined by subjective measures and functional return to sport participation. Approximately 67% of the overhead athletes who were treated with nonoperative care were able to return to the same or higher level of competition. These findings are difficult to reconcile with the results reported in surgical intervention studies. The therapeutic interventions in this study included **selective tissue stretching of the posterior-inferior capsule.** Sleeper and cross-body adduction stretches have been recommended for overhead athletes to improve the clinical impairments of posterior shoulder tightness commonly seen within this population.[54] Research investigating the effects of these stretches suggests a resolution of shoulder pain in overhead athletes following a course of therapy (~7 weeks).[55] Table 2-2 describes several flexibility exercises commonly prescribed for individuals with SLAP lesions.

In addition to stretching, soft-tissue mobilizations and joint mobilization techniques may be helpful in restoring passive mobility to the posterior shoulder. Glides directed toward the posterior and inferior joint capsule provide valuable feedback regarding the mobility of the posterior capsule and IGHL. Individuals with excessive or asymmetrical stiffness may benefit from manual joint mobilizations and selective tissue stretching of the posterior shoulder. Tightness of the dynamic posterior restraints of glenohumeral stability (teres minor, latissimus dorsi, and infraspinatus) is thought to contribute to motion restrictions.[13,56] Foam

Table 2-2 SOFT TISSUE FLEXIBILITY INTERVENTIONS FOR POSTERIOR SHOULDER TIGHTNESS		
Intervention	Patient Position	Exercise Performance
Cross-body stretch	Sidelying on the affected side with the shoulder elevated to 90°. The table (with a wedge, if necessary) should be used to block the scapula. (Fig. 2-1A)	The patient applies passive overpressure into horizontal adduction until a gentle stretch is felt. This position is held for 30 s and 3 sets are performed.
Sleeper stretch	Sidelying on the affected side with the shoulder elevated to 90°. The table (with a wedge, if necessary) should be used to block the scapula. (Fig. 2-1B)	The patient applies passive overpressure into humeral internal rotation until a gentle stretch is felt. This position is held for 30 s and 3 sets are performed.
Prayer latissimus dorsi stretch	Quadruped with hands positioned above head (Fig. 2-1C)	The patient sits back onto heels until a gentle stretch is felt. This position is held for 30 s and 3 sets are performed.
Latissimus dorsi and subscapularis mobilizations with foam roller	Sidelying on the affected side with the foam roller positioned under the axillary fold. The top leg is crossed in front to provide mobility. (Figs. 2-1D and E)	The patient uses the top leg to move up and down the foam roll to provide passive mobilization. Humeral internal and external rotation should be performed when over the subscapularis.

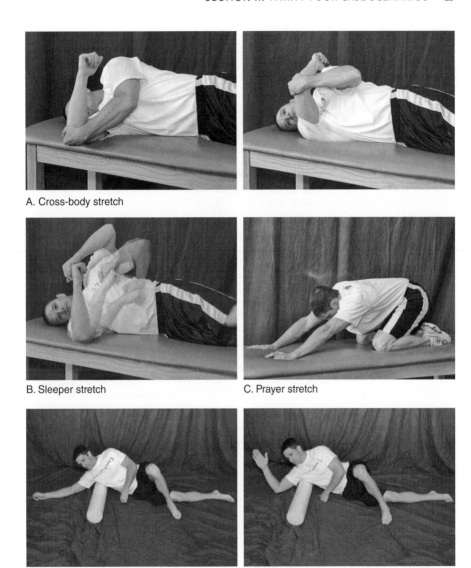

A. Cross-body stretch

B. Sleeper stretch

C. Prayer stretch

D. Foam roll - latissimus

E. Foam roll - subscapularis

Figure 2-1. Soft-tissue flexibility interventions for posterior shoulder tightness.

roller mobilizations are useful to selectively mobilize and potentially lengthen these active restraints.

Overhead motions place large distraction forces on the humerus. Because so much stress is repetitively exerted on the upper extremity, the athlete must have adequate flexibility, strength and stability in order to safely return to sport after injury. **Scapular stabilization exercises, rotator cuff strengthening, and kinetic chain activities** have been effectively used to conservatively manage overhead athletes with SLAP lesions.[8] Table 2-3 presents strengthening exercises for individuals with

Table 2-3   STRENGTHENING INTERVENTIONS FOR INDIVIDUALS WITH SLAP LESIONS

Intervention	Patient Position	Exercise Performance
Internal and external humeral rotation	Standing holding the band with towel roll under a 90° flexed elbow • Internal rotation starts with humerus in neutral rotation (Fig. 2-2A) • External rotation begins with the affected arm tucked in at the abdomen (Fig. 2-2B)	The shoulder is actively internally rotated to the abdomen for internal rotation and externally rotated just past neutral for external rotation. Progression of these activities should be performed at 90° of shoulder flexion.
Scapular stabilizations: I's, T's, and Y's	Prone on floor, table or stability ball with upper extremities within the coronal plane. • I's—arms are held out to the side at approximately 30° humeral abduction. (See Case 8, Fig. 8-13) • T's—arms are held out to the side at 90° of horizontal abduction. (See Case 8, Fig. 8-14) • Y's—arms are held out to approximately 150°-160° flexion. (See Case 8, Fig. 8-15)	• I's—shoulders are extended (~10°-20°) while simultaneously performing full scapular retraction and depression. • T's—shoulders are horizontally abducted (~10°-20°) while simultaneously performing full scapular retraction and depression. • Y's—shoulders are flexed and abducted (~10°-20°) while simultaneously performing full scapular retraction and depression.
Closed kinetic chain upper extremity stability exercise	Plank (push-up) position with the hands 15 in apart for smaller individuals and 36 in apart for larger individuals. (Fig. 2-2C)	While maintaining scapular protraction, the patient alternates tapping one hand with the opposite hand. This exercise is progressed in 15-s increments for up to a minute.

SLAP lesions. Initial muscular function goals should focus on improving scapular control as well as rotator cuff muscle strength with the elbow at the individual's side prior to progressing to more elevated humeral positions. As strength increases, the volume of resisted exercise must be increased to prepare the patient for the muscular endurance required for the repetitive demands of overhead sports. Once acceptable rotator cuff strength and scapular stability has been established, the treatment plan should advance to plyometric and closed kinetic chain activities that promote joint and core stability. The closed kinetic chain upper extremity stability test (CKCUEST) was initially developed as a field test to determine readiness for return to sport in upper extremity injuries.[57] However, this activity can also be used as a clinical treatment tool to enhance both core and scapular stability. Last, progressive sports-specific programs should be applied to safely prepare the athlete for the physical demands required by her activity. When the patient is completely asymptomatic and has demonstrated sufficient strength, endurance, and dynamic joint stability, she is ready to return to sport.

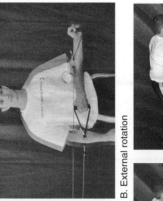

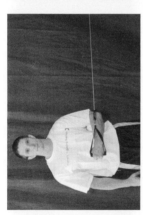

A. Internal rotation

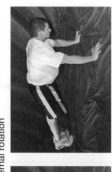
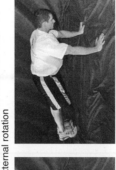
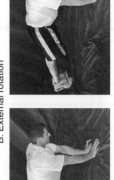
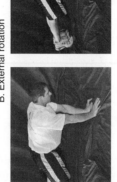
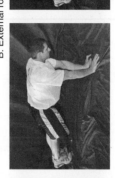

B. External rotation

C. Closed kinetic chain upper extremity stability test (CKCUEST)

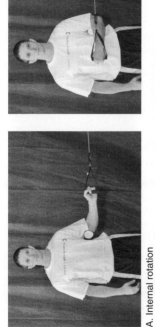

Figure 2-2. Strengthening interventions for individuals with SLAP lesions.

Evidence-Based Clinical Recommendations

SORT: Strength of Recommendation Taxonomy

A: Consistent, good-quality patient-oriented evidence
B: Inconsistent or limited-quality patient-oriented evidence
C: Consensus, disease-oriented evidence, usual practice, expert opinion, or case series

1. Nonoperative treatment is moderately effective for returning athletes with SLAP tears to sport. **Grade B**

2. Posterior shoulder stretching decreases pain in those overhead athletes who experience shoulder pain. **Grade B**

3. Rotator cuff and scapular stability strengthening improves function and decreases pain in overhead athletes with SLAP lesions. **Grade B**

COMPREHENSION QUESTIONS

2.1 A high school volleyball player presents with left shoulder pain during a "maximal cocking" mechanism of injury. What would *most* likely be the patient's classification of SLAP lesion?

A. Type I
B. Type II
C. Type III
D. Type IV

2.2 Which of the following concomitant pathologies is *most* likely to be present in younger overhead athletes with a type II SLAP lesion?

A. Rotator cuff tear
B. Avascular necrosis of the humeral head
C. Anterior shoulder instability
D. Spinoglenoid cysts

ANSWERS

2.1 **B.** Type II lesions are the most common form of SLAP tear within athletic populations. The eccentric load applied to the biceps during maximal cocking is thought to result in a peel-back lesion of the superior labrum and a type II defect. Type I lesions are associated with degeneration to the inner rim of the labrum and not common in younger populations (option A). Type III and IV SLAP lesions are bucket handle tears thought to be the result of fall on outstretched hand (FOOSH) mechanism of injury rather than traction to the biceps-labral complex (options C and D).

2.2 **C.** Excessive anterior joint instability or laxity and contracture of the posterior capsule is thought to be the result of repetitive overhead throwing activities. During maximal cocking, the humeral head translates anteriorly, stressing the anterior joint capsule. Due to the arthromechanics and repetitive nature of this activity, some authors maintain that anterior instability may result over time. The prevalence of rotator tears is low in younger overhead athletes (option A). Avascular necrosis is the result of severe vascular insufficiency associated with traumatic shoulder dislocations that can rupture the circumflex humeral arteries (option B). Spinoglenoid cysts are insidious in nature and result from suprascapular nerve palsy (option D).

REFERENCES

1. Costouras J, Warner J. Classification, clinical assessment, and imaging of glenohumeral instability. In: Galatz LM, ed. *Orthopedic Knowledge Update: Shoulder and Elbow, No. 3.* Rosemont, IL: American Academy of Orthopedic Surgeons; 2008:67-81.

2. Howell SM, Galinat BJ. The glenoid-labral socket. A constrained articular surface. *Clin Orthop Relat Res.* 1989;243:122-125.

3. Park M. Anatomy and function of the shoulder structures. In: Galatz LM, ed. *Orthopedic Knowledge Update: Shoulder and Elbow No. 3.* Rosemont, IL: American Academy of Orthopedic Surgeons; 2008.

4. Halder AM, Kuhl LG, Zorbitz ME, An KN. Effects of the glenoid labrum and glenohumeral abduction on stability of the shoulder joint through concavity-compression: an in vitro study. *J Bone Joint Surg Am.* 2001;83-A:1062-1069.

5. Andrews JR, Carson WG Jr, McLeod WD. Glenoid labrum tears related to the long head of the biceps. *Am J Sports Med.* 1985;13:337-341.

6. Snyder SJ, Karzel RP, Del Pizzo W, Ferkel RD, Friedman MJ. SLAP lesions of the shoulder. *Arthroscopy.* 1990;6:274-279.

7. Kampa RJ, Clasper J. Incidence of SLAP lesions in a military population. *J R Army Med Corps.* 2005;151:171-175.

8. Edwards SL, Lee JA, Bell JE, et al. Nonoperative treatment of superior labrum anterior posterior tears: improvements in pain, function, and quality of life. *Am J Sports Med.* 2010;38:1456-1461.

9. Handelberg F, Willems S, Shahabpour M, Huskin JP, Kuta J. SLAP lesions: a retrospective multicenter study. *Arthroscopy.* 1998;14:856-862.

10. Kim TK, Queale WS, Cosgarea AJ, McFarland EG. Clinical features of the different types of SLAP lesions: an analysis of one hundred and thirty-nine cases. *J Bone Joint Surg Am.* 2003;85-A:66-71.

11. Pagnani MJ, Deng XH, Warren RF, Torzilli PA, Altchek DW. Effect of lesions of the superior portion of the glenoid labrum on glenohumeral translation. *J Bone Joint Surg Am.* 1995;77:1003-1010.

12. Jobe CM. Posterior superior glenoid impingement: expanded spectrum. *Arthroscopy.* 1995;11: 530-536.

13. Burkhart SS, Morgan CD, Kibler WB. The disabled throwing shoulder: spectrum of pathology Part I: pathoanatomy and biomechanics. *Arthroscopy.* 2003;19:404-420.

14. Clavert P, Bonnomet F, Kempf JF, Boutemy P, Braun M, Kahn JL. Contribution to the study of th pathogenesis of type II superior labrum anterior-posterior lesions: a cadaveric model of a fall on t outstretched hand. *J Shoulder Elbow Surg.* 2004;13:45-50.

15. Maffet MW, Gartsman GM, Moseley B. Superior labrum-biceps tendon complex lesions o shoulder. *Am J Sports Med.* 1995;23:93-98.

16. Powell SE, Nord KD, Ryu RKN. The diagnosis, classification, and treatment of SLAP lesion *Tech Sports Med.* 2004;12:99-110.

17. Barber F. Superior labrum anterior and posterior injury. In: Galatz L, ed. *Orthopedic Knowledge Update: Shoulder and Elbow, No. 3*. Rosemont IL: American Academy of Orthopedic Surgeons; 2008:327-335.

18. Bey MJ, Elders GJ, Huston LJ, Kuhn JE, Blasier RB, Soslowsky LJ. The mechanism of creation of superior labrum, anterior, and posterior lesions in a dynamic biomechanical model of the shoulder: the role of inferior subluxation. *J Shoulder Elbow Surg*. 1998;7:397-401.

19. Nam EK, Snyder SJ. The diagnosis and treatment of superior labrum, anterior and posterior (SLAP) lesions. *Am J Sports Med*. 2003;31:798-810.

20. Snyder SJ, Banas MP, Karzel RP. An analysis of 140 injuries to the superior glenoid labrum. *J Shoulder Elbow Surg*. 1995;4:243-248.

21. Boileau P, Parratte S, Chuinard C, Roussanne Y, Shia D, Bicknell R. Arthroscopic treatment of isolated type II SLAP lesions: biceps tenodesis as an alternative to reinsertion. *Am J Sports Med*. 2009;37:929-936.

22. Burkhart SS, Morgan CD. The peel-back mechanism: its role in producing and extending posterior type II SLAP lesions and its effect on SLAP repair rehabilitation. *Arthroscopy*. 1998;14:637-640.

23. Dodson CC, Altchek DW. SLAP lesions: an update on recognition and treatment. *J Orthop Sports Phys Ther*. 2009;39:71-80.

24. Mileski RA, Snyder SJ. Superior labral lesions in the shoulder: pathoanatomy and surgical management. *J Am Acad Orthop Surg*. 1998;6:121-131.

25. Choi NH, Kim SJ. Avulsion of the superior labrum. *Arthroscopy*. 2004;20:872-874.

26. Kugler A, Kruger-Franke M, Reininger S, Trouillier HH, Rosemeyer B. Muscular imbalance and shoulder pain in volleyball athletes. *Br J Sports Med*. 1996;30:256-259.

27. Lajtai G, Pfirrmann CW, Aitzetmuller G, Pirkl C, Gerber C, Jost B. The shoulders of professional beach volleyball players: high prevalence of infraspinatus muscle atrophy. *Am J Sports Med*. 2009;37:1375-1383.

28. Verhagen EA, Van der Beek AJ, Bouter LM, Bahr RM, Van Mechelen W. A one season prospective cohort study of volleyball injuries. *Br J Sports Med*. 2004;38:477-481.

29. Reeser JC, Verhagen E, Briner WW, Askeland TI, Bahr R. Strategies for the prevention of volleyball related injuries. *Br J Sports Med*. 2006;40:594-600; discussion 599-600.

30. Taljanovic MS, Nisbet JK, Hunter TB, Cohen RP, Rogers LF. Humeral avulsion of the inferior glenohumeral ligament in college female volleyball players caused by repetitive microtrauma. *Am J Sports Med*. 2011;39:1067-1076.

31. Safran MR. Nerve injury about the shoulder in athletes, part 1: suprascapular nerve and axillary nerve. *Am J Sports Med*. 2004;32:803-819.

32. Andrews J, Carson W. The arthroscopic treatment of glenoid labrum tears in the throwing athlete. *Orthop Trans*. 1984;8:44.

'. Keener JD, Brophy RH. Superior labral tears of the shoulder: pathogenesis, evaluation, and treatment. *J Am Acad Orthop Surg*. 2009;17:627-637.

'higpen CA, Padua DA, Michener LA, et al. Head and shoulder posture affect scapular mechanics ' muscle activity in overhead tasks. *J Electromyogr Kinesiol*. 2010;20:701-709.

WB. The role of the scapula in athletic shoulder function. *Am J Sports Med*. 1998;26:325-337.

KG, Moline MT, Meister K. The relationship between forward scapular posture and poste-'er tightness among baseball players. *Am J Sports Med*. 2010;38:2106-2112.

'Jhl TL, Maddux JW, Brooks PV, Zeller B, McMullen J. Qualitative clinical evaluation of 'ction: a reliabililty study. *J Shouder Elbow Surg*. 2002;11:550-566.

'e P, Kareha S, Irwin D, Barbe MF. A clinical method for identifying scapular dyskinesis, 'hl Train. 2009;44:165-173.

'Kareha S, Irwin D, Zlupko E. A clinical method for identifying scapular dyskinesis, Train. 2009;44:160-164.

40. Schwab LM, Blanch P. Humeral torsion and passive shoulder range in elite volleyball players. *Phys Ther Sport*. 2009;10:51-56.

41. Shanley E, Rauh MJ, Michener LA, Ellenbecker TS, Garrison JC, Thigpen CA. Shoulder range of motion measures as risk factors for shoulder and elbow injuries in high school softball and baseball players. *Am J Sports Med*. 2011;39:1997-2006.

42. Wilk KE, Macrina LC, Fleisig GS, et al. Correlation of glenohumeral internal rotation deficit and total rotational motion to shoulder injuries in professional baseball pitchers. *Am J Sports Med*. 2011; 39:329-335.

43. Harryman DT II, Sidles JA, Clark JM, McQuade KJ, Gibb TD, Matsen FA III. Translation of the humeral head on the glenoid with passive glenohumeral motion. *J Bone Joint Surg Am*. 1990;72: 1334-1343.

44. Myers JB, Laudner KG, Pasquale MR, Bradley JP, Lephart SM. Glenohumeral range of motion deficits and posterior shoulder tightness in throwers with pathologic internal impingement. *Am J Sports Med*. 2006;34:385-391.

45. Yang JL, Lu TW, Chou FC, Chang CW, Lin JJ. Secondary motions of the shoulder during arm elevation in patients with shoulder tightness. *J Electromyogr Kinesiol*. 2009;19:1035-1042.

46. Lin JJ, Lim HK, Yang JL. Effect of shoulder tightness on glenohumeral translation, scapular kinematics, and scapulohumeral rhythm in subjects with stiff shoulders. *J Orthop Res*. 2006;24:1044-1051.

47. Cook C, Hegedus E. *Orthopedic Physical Examination Tests: An Evidence-Based Approach*. Upper Saddle River, NJ: Prentice Hall; 2008.

48. Richards RR, An K, Bigliani LU, et al. A standardized method for the assessment of shoulder function. *J Shoulder Elbow Surg*. 1994;3:347-352.

49. Hawkins RJ, Schutte JP, Janda DH, Huckell GH. Translation of the glenohumeral joint with the patient under anesthesia. *J Shoulder Elbow Surg*. 1996;5:286-292.

50. Pagnani MJ, Speer KP, Altchek DW, Warren RF, Dines DM. Arthroscopic fixation of superior labral lesions using a biodegradable implant: a preliminary report. *Arthroscopy*. 1995;11:194-198.

51. O'Brien SJ, Allen AA, Coleman SH, Drakos MC. The trans-rotator cuff approach to SLAP lesions: technical aspects for repair and a clinical follow-up of 31 patients at a minimum of 2 years. *Arthroscopy*. 2002;18:372-377.

52. Cohen DB, Coleman S, Drakos MC, et al. Outcomes of isolated type II SLAP lesions treated with arthroscopic fixation using a bioabsorbable tack. *Arthroscopy*. 2006;22:136-142.

53. Yoneda M, Hirooka A, Saito S, Yamamoto T, Ochi T, Shino K. Arthroscopic stapling for detached superior glenoid labrum. *J Bone Joint Surg Br*. 1991;73:746-750.

54. Laudner KG, Sipes RC, Wilson JT. The acute effects of sleeper stretches on shoulder range of motion. *J Athl Train*. 2008;43:359-363.

55. Tyler TF, Nicholas SJ, Lee SJ, Mullaney M, McHugh MP. Correction of posterior shoulder tightness is associated with symptom resolution in patients with internal impingement. *Am J Sports Med*. 2009;38:114-119.

56. Pappas AM, Zawacki RM, McCarthy CF. Rehabilitation of the pitching shoulder. *Am J Sports Med*. 1985;13:223-235.

57. Goldbeck TG, Davies GJ. Test-Retest reliability of the closed kinetic chain upper extremity stability test: a clinical field test. *J Sport Rehabil*. 2000;9:35-45.

Acute Shoulder Instability

Thomas J. Olson
Paul E. Westgard

CASE 3

A 22-year-old female snowboard instructor is referred to an outpatient physical therapy clinic from a medical center with a diagnosis of right shoulder pain. She fell while snowboarding 3 days ago and reports that her shoulder "popped out and went back in again." She attempted to teach today, but was unable to continue due to pain and a sense that her shoulder would "come out again" if she tried to help one of her fallen clients to stand up. Plain film images taken at the clinic showed no obvious bony abnormality; no additional imaging was performed. The patient's medical history is otherwise unremarkable. Signs and symptoms are consistent with anterior shoulder dislocation. The patient's goal is to continue snowboarding and teaching for the rest of the season.

▶ What examination signs may be associated with this diagnosis?
▶ What are the most appropriate examination tests?
▶ What precautions should be taken during physical therapy examination and interventions?
▶ What are the most appropriate physical therapy interventions?
▶ What referral may be appropriate based on her condition?
▶ What is her rehabilitation prognosis?

KEY DEFINITIONS

ALPSA LESION: Acronym for anterior labroligamentous periosteal sleeve avulsion; an anteroinferior labral detachment associated with a stripped, but continuous glenoid periosteum

BANKART LESION: Avulsion of the labrum and inferior glenohumeral ligament from the anteroinferior glenoid rim[1]

HAGL LESION: Acronym for humeral avulsion of the anterior glenohumeral ligament

HEMARTHROSIS: Bleeding into a joint

HILL-SACHS LESION: Impression fracture of the posterosuperior articular surface of the humeral head caused by translation of the humeral head over the glenoid rim[2]

SHOULDER DISLOCATION: Complete disruption of the humeral head from the glenoid fossa due to a force that overcomes the joint's static, capsulolabral, and dynamic restraints[3]

SHOULDER SUBLUXATION: Increased excursion of the humeral head on the glenoid fossa without complete displacement; also known as an incomplete or partial dislocation[3]

SLAP LESION: Tear of the superior labrum, anterior to posterior

Objectives

1. Describe the mechanism of injury and the resulting pathoanatomy associated with an anterior shoulder dislocation.

2. Identify the risk factors for primary and secondary dislocations.

3. Describe the benefits and risks related to conservative treatment and surgical intervention following a first-time anterior shoulder dislocation.

4. Prescribe an appropriate therapeutic exercise program for a patient who elects conservative treatment following a first-time anterior shoulder dislocation.

Physical Therapy Considerations

PT considerations during management of the individual with a diagnosis of acute anterior shoulder instability:

▶ **General physical therapy plan of care/goals:** Decrease pain; minimize loss of neuromuscular control and strength; restore functional joint stability

▶ **Physical therapy interventions:** Patient education regarding functional anatomy and injury pathomechanics; patient education regarding treatment options; sling for comfort; modalities and manual therapy to decrease pain; periscapular and rotator cuff neuromuscular retraining; resistance exercises to increase muscular endurance and strength; functional bracing for return to activity

▶ **Precautions during physical therapy:** Initial avoidance of shoulder abduction and external rotation to prevent continued anterior instability

▶ **Complications interfering with physical therapy:** Impaired neurovascular status; reoccurrence of dislocation

Understanding the Health Condition

The shoulder is designed to maximize mobility and, as a result, it possesses the greatest range of motion of any joint in the human body.[2] However, this freedom comes at a price. The glenohumeral joint is also the body's most commonly dislocated joint.[4,5] Approximately 70,000 shoulder dislocations present to hospital emergency departments annually, and many more are seen by primary care physicians and orthopaedic specialists.[6] Overall, shoulder dislocations occur in 1.7% of the general population[7] though the occurrence among athletes and military personnel is significantly higher.[8,9] Shoulder dislocations can be traumatic or atraumatic and can occur in either the anterior or posterior direction, but traumatic, anterior dislocations are the most common, occurring in 96% and 98% of all cases, respectively.[10]

Sports and recreation-related injuries account for nearly half of all shoulder dislocations in the United States.[6,7,11-14] Between one quarter and one-third of all reported upper extremity injuries occurring in football, soccer, basketball, and wrestling are shoulder dislocations.[6,15] Nontraditional sports like surfing, skiing, and snowboarding also demonstrate a significant number of shoulder dislocations annually.[16,17] Contact between competitors and contact with the playing surface are responsible for 75% of these dislocations with the classic mechanism of injury described as a forceful twisting of the arm into abduction and external rotation at or above shoulder level.[15] However, falls on an outstretched arm, forced end range flexion, or a direct blow to the shoulder are also causes of anterior dislocation in athletes.[3,9,11,13,18] Males are two to three times more likely to incur a shoulder dislocation than females[6,7,10] and younger athletes appear to be at the highest risk with 20% to 27% of dislocations occurring before 20 years of age.[10,13] College athletes are also at substantial risk: 47% of all shoulder dislocations occur among individuals 15 to 29 years of age.[6]

The glenohumeral joint's inherent instability is due to a lack of bony congruency and the disparity in size between the articulating surfaces of the large humeral head and the small, shallow glenoid fossa. Consequently, the joint is reliant on the support of both static and dynamic elements that function together to provide the shoulder stability necessary for function.[19]

The static stabilizers of the shoulder include the glenoid fossa, labrum, joint capsule, and ligaments. The glenoid labrum is a fibrocartilage ring that deepens the glenoid fossa and provides a vacuum seal to help center the head of the humerus on the glenoid fossa.[2,3] In addition, the labrum serves as the attachment site for the joint capsule and glenohumeral ligaments. The glenohumeral ligaments are thickenings of the joint capsule and are divided into separate superior, middle, and inferior entities, each with a slightly different stabilizing role.[20] The superior glenohumeral ligament originates from the superior glenoid tubercle, the upper part of the labrum, and the base of the coracoid process and inserts between the lesser tuberosity and anatomical neck of the humerus. It assists in preventing inferior displacement of the humeral head when the upper extremity is in a neutral position. The middle glenohumeral ligament is a wide ligament that lies under the tendon of the subscapularis muscle. It originates from the anterior glenoid rim and passes laterally to attach to the anatomic neck and lesser tuberosity of the humerus. The middle glenohumeral ligament works along with the subscapularis tendon to reinforce the anterior glenohumeral joint and limit external rotation of the humerus in mid-ranges of abduction. Finally, the inferior glenohumeral ligament, formed by anterior and posterior bands separated by a redundancy known as the axillary pouch, reinforces the anterior and inferior aspect of the joint capsule particularly in the upper ranges of abduction.[2,3] In addition to the aforementioned glenohumeral ligaments, the coracohumeral ligament adds stability to the joint. It originates from the coracoid process and passes inferolaterally to the humerus, blending with the supraspinatus muscle and joint capsule. It separates into two bands that attach to the greater and lesser tuberosities of the humerus, providing a tunnel through which the long head of the biceps tendon passes. It reinforces the superior joint capsule and stabilizes the tendon of the long head of the biceps brachii.[2,3]

Compressive forces generated during co-contraction of the rotator cuff muscles provide the dynamic stability of the glenohumeral joint. The force-couple created by co-contraction of supraspinatus, subscapularis, infraspinatus, and teres minor compresses the humeral head into the glenoid fossa, stabilizing the joint during activation of the shoulder's prime movers including the deltoid, pectoralis major, and latissimus dorsi muscles. Activation of a second force couple consisting of the upper, mid, and lower portions of the trapezius, along with the serratus anterior produces upward rotation of the scapulothoracic joint during upper extremity elevation. This activation also helps maintain humeral head centralization within the glenoid fossa, further increasing glenohumeral stability during functional movements above shoulder height.[21]

Acute anterior shoulder dislocations are caused by forceful disruptions of the joint's static and dynamic stabilizers resulting in several pathoanatomic findings observed either via diagnostic imaging or through arthroscopic evaluation. The aggressive anteroinferior translation of the humeral head associated with anterior dislocation may result in damage to the labrum, joint capsule, and ligaments, as well as to the bony surfaces of the humerus and glenoid fossa. When these injuries occur, a characteristic hemarthrosis develops more than 90% of the time and may interfere with healing.[11,22-25]

There are several common concomitant bony and soft tissue lesions associated with anterior shoulder dislocations. The most frequently observed lesion occurring in an acute anterior dislocation (68%-100% of cases) is called a Bankart lesion.[9,11,14,18,22-24,26] It is also considered the predominant pathology present in those who experience recurrent dislocation.[27] The ALPSA lesion involves the antero-inferior labrum and capsuloligamentous complex. In this injury, the anterior band of the inferior glenohumeral ligament, labrum, and the anterior scapular periosteum are stripped and displaced in a sleeve-type fashion, medially on the neck of the glenoid fossa. In a study by Antonio et al.,[28] this lesion was found in roughly 40% of all anteroinferior labral avulsions. The HAGL lesion is characterized by a lateral detachment of the anterior band of the inferior glenohumeral ligament from the humeral neck. In the late 1990s, Taylor et al.[23] reported that HAGL lesions occur infrequently—associated with only 1.6% of acute anterior shoulder dislocations. However, a more recent investigation performed by Liavaag and colleagues suggests the injury is more common, occurring in almost a quarter of individuals following anterior dislocation.[1] In addition to soft tissue injuries, bony lesions can also occur during anterior glenohumeral disruption. The "bony Bankart lesion" is an avulsion of the anterior inferior glenoid that occurs in 11.4% of traumatic anterior dislocations.[5] This injury can lead to a reduced resistance to anterior translation of the humeral head on the glenoid, much like a golf ball attempting to rest on a broken tee.[29] The most common bony lesion is the Hill-Sachs lesion. This is an impression fracture on the posterior humeral head resulting from a collision with the anterior glenoid rim as the humeral head comes to rest in the subcoracoid position following displacement. The incidence of Hill-Sachs lesions is between 38% and 100% for all traumatic anterior shoulder dislocations.[9-11,14,18,22-24,26] Despite being a near pathognomonic indicator of an anteroinferior glenohumeral dislocation, it is well-accepted that a Hill-Sachs lesion does not contribute significantly to the joint instability normally experienced following injury. Since this lesion usually occurs in the superior posterior aspect of the humeral head, it typically does not disrupt the articulation of the glenohumeral joint.

Other pathologies associated with acute anterior shoulder dislocation include SLAP lesions, which substantially increase glenohumeral instability in the presence of an anteroinferior labral lesion, glenoid rim fractures, greater tuberosity fractures, rotator cuff tears, long head of the biceps tears, capsular tears, and nerve injuries. These injuries are less common, presenting in less than a quarter of all cases.[10,11,14,18,22-24]

Physical Therapy Patient/Client Management

Recurrent instability is a typical consequence of anterior shoulder dislocation. The recurrence rate in patients without stabilization surgery is between 66% and 95% for those less than 20 years of age and between 40% and 74% for those between 20 and 40 years old.[7,8,10,13,14,18,22-24,26,27,30-34] Further, in those individuals less than 20 years of age whose initial dislocation occurred while participating in a sport, the recurrence rate can jump to greater than 80%.[35] These same individuals also demonstrate a shorter time period between the first and second dislocation compared to nonathletes.[5] **Age and activity level** are two of the most important factors that predict recurrence: athletes less than 30 years old at the time of their first dislocation are at greatest risk.[5,13,30,31] Clearly, the primary goal following anterior shoulder dislocation is to limit the chance for recurrence while allowing a return to normal activity with as few restrictions as possible.

Traditionally, conservative care following acute shoulder instability has involved dislocation reduction, sling immobilization, and physical therapy to restore range of motion and strength.[36,37] However, this approach has not been particularly successful as demonstrated by the aforementioned statistics regarding rates of recurrence.

As a result, **surgical intervention** is considered an appropriate alternative for first-time dislocators. Almost 30 years ago, Jobe and Jobe suggested that throwing athletes with a history of even one dislocation should undergo surgical repair to restore normal anatomy.[38] In a 2004 Cochrane review, Handoll et al.[39] examined five studies comparing surgical and conservative treatment for acute anterior shoulder dislocation and reported a relative risk reduction of 68% to 80% for recurrent instability in those treated surgically. Additionally, they noted that half of those initially treated nonoperatively eventually sought surgical intervention. They concluded that surgical stabilization is warranted for young, active individuals following first-time traumatic shoulder dislocation.[39] This conclusion is supported by a review published in 2009. Brophy and Marx describe that at 2-year follow-up, surgically treated patients showed a significantly lower rate of recurrent instability (7%) compared to those that received nonoperative care (46%).[40] This trend was also observed at a 10-year follow-up, with recurrence of 10% to 58%, respectively.[40] Based on these findings, a treatment algorithm has been proposed in which surgery is advocated for patients 15 to 25 years of age and a trial of physical therapy is recommended for patients 25 to 40 years of age with surgical intervention reserved to address recurrent dislocation. Finally, nonoperative care is endorsed for patients over 40 years of age secondary to low recurrence rates in this age group.[36]

Despite this evidence, the controversy regarding immediate surgical care for the first-time dislocator persists. Hovelius et al.[41] have shown that out of 229 anterior shoulder dislocations followed over 25 years, 49% of shoulders did not experience a second dislocation and 20% of those who were 12 to 22 years old at the time of primary dislocation had one or fewer subluxations or dislocations. This suggests that if the proposed algorithm were accepted, 30% to 50% of patients would endure unnecessary surgery. A frequently cited work by Aronen and Regan reports a 75% rate of stabilization at 3-year follow-up after patients completed a regimented conservative treatment protocol combining activity modification with focused strengthening of the shoulder internal rotators and adductors.[42]

Though the outcomes of the Aronen and Regan protocol have not been duplicated and recurrence rates seem to respond favorably to early surgical intervention, questions persist and the debate continues. As a result, providing education to the patient about the cost/benefit ratio for surgery versus conservative intervention is a large component of the physical therapist's role in managing a patient following an episode of acute anterior shoulder instability. Understanding the patient's lifestyle, including work responsibilities, recreational pursuits, and corresponding functional goals in the context of the risk factors and prognosis following shoulder dislocation, allows the physical therapist to accurately counsel a patient and create an appropriate, individualized plan of care.

Examination, Evaluation, and Diagnosis

The examination of a patient who has experienced an anterior glenohumeral dislocation depends on how recently the injury occurred. If a physical therapist is providing medical coverage for a sporting event and a competitor presents with significant pain and holding his arm in slight abduction and neutral rotation, the diagnosis is relatively apparent and the examination may be brief. On the sidelines, the mechanism of injury is likely to have been witnessed and an obvious deformity may be visible and palpable over the athlete's anterolateral chest just inferior to the coracoid process. Deformation or a "flattening/squaring off" of the deltoid musculature can also be appreciated as the acromion process becomes the most lateral structure of the shoulder. After an anterior dislocation, traction and compression of chest and shoulder soft tissue can compromise the neurovascular status of the upper extremity. A rapid, but thorough evaluation of sensation and motor function is imperative. Radial and brachial pulse identification,[43,44] dermatomal assessment of sensation to light touch or sharp/dull differentiation, with special attention given to the C5 region supplied by the often affected axillary nerve,[3,43,45] and a distal myotome strength evaluation of wrist and intrinsic finger strength should be performed and compared bilaterally. Joint reduction should then be attempted by a physician.[18] Restoration of normal anatomic alignment is advocated within an hour of dislocation to decrease the chance for neuropraxia or vascular trauma.[16] Following reduction, the neurovascular examination should be repeated,[43,44] the arm stabilized using a sling, and the patient referred to a physician for definitive care, including plain film imaging to assess for bony and capsulolabral injury. If reduction cannot be achieved easily at the event, the shoulder should be stabilized in the position found, and the patient should be rapidly transported to an emergency room for additional medical evaluation and treatment.

Occasionally, a dislocated shoulder spontaneously reduces and a patient may be unsure of exactly what happened. If a patient presents with a spontaneously relocated shoulder to the clinic several days after a traumatic event, a thorough subjective history and physical examination helps differentially diagnose an anterior shoulder dislocation or subluxation[1] versus a shoulder separation or acromioclavicular joint disruption. When patients describe the mechanism of injury involving the provocative position of abduction and external rotation, indirect forces applied to the distal upper extremity increasing torque at the shoulder joint,[3,16] and/or report a "dead-arm," generalized shoulder pain, and limitations in motion due to fear, the physical therapist should have an increased suspicion of anterior instability.[3,46] On physical examination, tenderness to palpation through the deltopectoral interval and over the bicipital groove, decreased active motion above 90° in flexion and abduction, plus pain and/or weakness with manual muscle testing of the shoulder rotators further suggests an anterior dislocation.

Several special tests can then be selected to help confirm the presence of anterior instability following dislocation or subluxation. First, the presence of a sulcus sign should be evaluated bilaterally with the upper extremity in a neutral position to assess general laxity and competency of the superior glenohumeral and coracohumeral ligaments (Fig. 3-1). The physical therapist should assess the integrity of the middle glenohumeral ligament, the rotator interval, and the glenoid rim by performing an anterior/posterior load and shift test.[47] Here, the therapist applies a force to centralize the humeral head in the glenoid fossa. Then, the therapist applies anteromedial and posterolateral directional stresses to the humeral head with the scapula stabilized. The amount of translation is noted and again compared

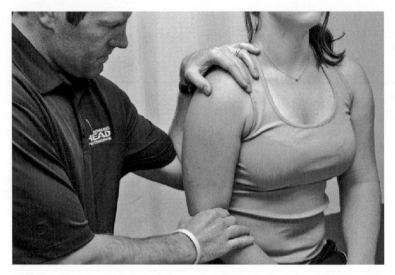

Figure 3-1. Sulcus sign to assess general laxity and competency of the superior glenohumeral and coracohumeral ligaments. Therapist grasps proximal to elbow and produces an inferior traction force. This assessment may also be performed in the supine position.

bilaterally. Patients with anterior shoulder instability may demonstrate increased anterior translation on the affected side.[48] Finally, apprehension, relocation, and anterior release tests may be performed on the involved upper extremity. Table 3-1 describes the three most common tests and their corresponding diagnostic accuracy statistics to help distinguish shoulder dislocation/subluxation versus impingement.

The psychometric properties described in Table 3-1 represent the test results when a positive test is operationally defined as apprehension. Apprehension can be identified by verbal acknowledgement of the shoulder "shifting, moving, dislocating,"[53] as well as through facial grimacing or a reluctance to assume the test position.[54] The presence or absence of pain alone does not accurately predict anterior shoulder instability.[49,50,53] Individually, the apprehension and anterior release tests appear to be most effective for ruling in the diagnosis of anterior shoulder dislocation or subluxation. The physical therapist should be careful because the anterior release test can dislocate the glenohumeral joint by replicating the original mechanism of injury. If the therapist chooses to perform the anterior release test, it should be performed after the apprehension and relocation tests so the therapist has an impression of the patient's shoulder instability and possibility for dislocation.[49] However, when the **apprehension and relocation tests** are performed consecutively and their results are clustered, the sensitivity is reported at 68% and specificity increases to 100% with a PPV of 100%.[53] Thus, the results of this test cluster make the additional inclusion of the anterior release test difficult to justify.

If the physical therapist suspects a diagnosis of posttraumatic anterior shoulder dislocation/subluxation, referral to a physician is warranted for imaging. Plain film images including three anteroposterior views: one in neutral (Grashey view), and

Table 3-1   DESCRIPTION OF SPECIAL TEST PERFORMANCE AND PSYCHOMETRIC PROPERTIES[a]

Test	Positioning	Findings	Psychometrics[49,50]
Apprehension (Fig. 3-2)	Patient is supine (or sitting) with scapula on treatment table for stabilization. Upper extremity is passively moved into 90° abduction and maximum external rotation. Therapist applies *anteriorly directed force* to posterior humeral head.[38,46,51]	*Apprehension:* positive for dislocation/subluxation[38] *Pain:* positive for impingement[38]	Sen: 53%-72% Spec: 96%-99% PPV: 98% NPV: 73% +LLR: 20.2
Relocation (Fig. 3-3)	Patient is supine with scapula on treatment table for stabilization. Upper extremity is passively moved into 90° abduction and maximum external rotation. Therapist applies *posteriorly directed force* to anterior humeral head.[51]	If the *apprehension* caused by increased external rotation is relieved by the posteriorly directed force, positive for dislocation/subluxation[51] If the *pain* caused by increased external rotation is relieved by the posteriorly directed force, positive for impingement[51]	Sen: 32%-81% Spec: 54%-100% PPV: 44% NPV: 56% +LLR: 10.4
Anterior release or "Surprise" (Fig. 3-4)	Patient is supine with scapula on treatment table for stabilization. Upper extremity is passively moved into 90° abduction and maximum external rotation. Therapist applies posteriorly directed force applied to anterior humeral head. External rotation is passively taken to end range and pressure is released from humeral head.[52]	*Return of apprehension:* positive for dislocation/subluxation[49]	Sen: 64% Spec: 99% PPV: 98% NPV: 78%

[a]Sen, sensitivity; Spec, specificity; PPV, positive predictive value; NPV, negative predictive value; LLR, likelihood ratio.

one each in internal and external rotation. In addition, a transscapular (scapular "Y" view) and an axillary view are commonly obtained. These images help confirm dislocation and identify the presence of bony abnormalities of the humeral head or glenoid rim.[2,55] A Striker Notch view can also be beneficial to specifically diagnose the Hill-Sachs lesion and the bony Bankart lesion that commonly accompany anterior dislocations.[55] Magnetic resonance imaging (MRI) is often performed to further explore the different anterior inferior labral lesions associated with 73% of

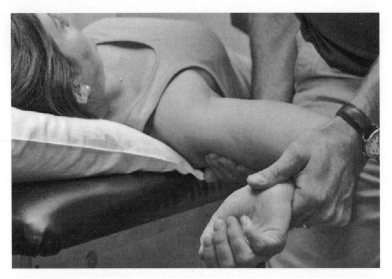

Figure 3-2. Apprehension test originally described with the application of an anterior force to the posterior humeral head. Care must be taken to protect a patient's shoulder from re-dislocation during performance of this test; therefore the therapist may forego the anterior force if apprehension is appreciated with the positioning alone.

glenohumeral dislocations.[1,28] These images also allow the inspection of the integrity of the rotator cuff musculature that is frequently compromised in individuals over 40 years of age who experience an anterior dislocation.[3,28] Reviewing these images and radiologist reports can help the physical therapist counsel the patient and establish an appropriate plan of care.

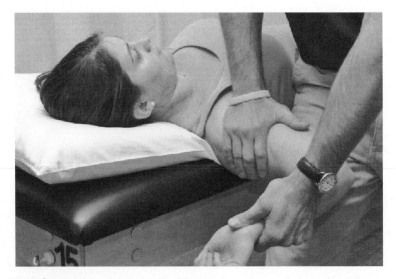

Figure 3-3. Relocation test.

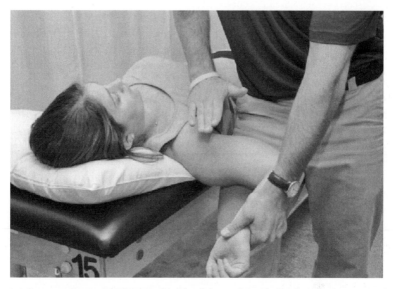

Figure 3-4. Anterior release test. This test should only be performed after the apprehension and relocation tests (if at all) secondary to potential for re-dislocation.

Plan of Care and Interventions

If a patient elects to pursue conservative treatment following an episode of acute anterior shoulder instability, the physical therapist's first goal is to protect the healing tissue. This is usually accomplished through sling immobilization, customarily with the shoulder positioned in internal rotation. However, currently there is no consensus regarding the proper duration or positioning for upper extremity immobilization following dislocation. A timeframe of 6 weeks is often proposed based on physiologic healing times of soft tissue, but evidence suggests this may be too long. Hovelius et al.[34] compared a group of first-time dislocators immobilized in internal rotation for 3 to 4 weeks with a group instructed to wear a sling as needed for up to 1 week. At 2- and 5-year follow-ups, there was no difference in recurrent dislocation between groups. A recent meta-analysis of level I and II evidence compared dislocation recurrence rates for individuals younger than 30 years old immobilized for one week or less with those immobilized for 3 weeks or more and concluded there was no benefit to conventional sling immobilization for longer than 1 week.[37]

As far as position of immobilization, shoulder internal rotation is typically selected secondary to issues of patient comfort and compliance. Nevertheless, a cadaveric study, several MRI studies, and a preliminary clinical trial suggest that **shoulder immobilization** with the shoulder in abduction and 10° of *external* rotation provides tension on anterior soft tissue structures, decreases hemarthrosis, and increases approximation of the labrum and capsule to the glenoid rim.[25,56-60] A clinical investigation by Finestone and colleagues contradicts this suggestion, reporting that those immobilized in external rotation experienced recurrence rates similar to those immobilized in internal rotation.[45] However, a meta-analysis and recent randomized controlled trial comparing internal and external immobilization indicate that immobilization in ER is superior to IR at reducing recurrence of dislocation.[37,61] Taskoparan et al.[61] reported patients who had been immobilized in ER for 3 weeks had significantly fewer recurrent dislocations (6.3%) during the subsequent two years than those who had been immobilized in IR (29.4%). Based on the best available evidence, a review published in the *Annals of Emergency Medicine* recommends that immobilization in external rotation be included in the standard of care for first-time traumatic anterior shoulder dislocations.[62]

Regardless of time and position selected for immobilization, the physical therapist must address the range of motion and strength impairments presented by the patient with anterior shoulder instability following immobilization. Reactivation of the **dynamic stabilizers of the glenohumeral joint**, including both the rotator cuff and periscapular musculature is essential.[3,42,51,63,64] Initially, isolated submaximal isometric exercises and closed chain activities that promote rotator cuff and periscapular muscle co-contraction performed below 90° of shoulder elevation are appropriate.[63,65] The therapist needs to closely monitor the patient's performance of these exercises. Until the patient has developed appropriate neuromuscular control, the therapist needs to provide verbal and tactile feedback to minimize the recruitment of prime movers (pectoralis major, latissimus dorsi, upper trapezius) that may contribute to further joint destabilization (Figs. 3-5 and 3-6). An early emphasis on posture and scapular positioning is also important to promote normal muscular firing patterns during upper extremity movement.

As range of motion normalizes, patients can be advanced to progressive isotonic resistance training. Some therapists may be tempted to focus on strengthening the subscapularis muscle at this time as a way to reinforce the anteroinferior

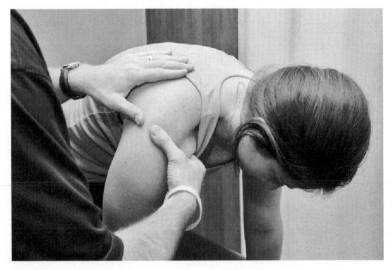

Figure 3-5. Isometric closed chain shoulder protraction for activating the serratus anterior in quadruped. Patient is cued to protract scapula while therapist provides tactile cueing to prevent compensatory pectoralis major contraction.

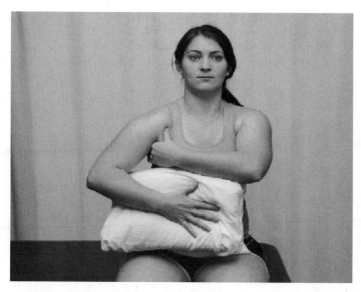

Figure 3-6. Isometric subscapularis activation. Patient performs isometric shoulder internal rotation while applying tactile cueing to prevent pectoralis major compensation.

glenohumeral capsulolabral complex and prevent recurrent dislocation. However, a cadaveric study by Werner et al.[66] demonstrated that although subscapularis primarily produces a stabilizing force by compressing the humeral head into the glenoid fossa, tension produced by the inferior segments of the muscle dislocated the joint in some specimens when the upper extremity was abducted and externally rotated. Consequently, a global approach to strengthening is warranted. Exercises that have demonstrated significant electromyographic activity for the key dynamic stabilizers of the shoulder are described in Table 3-2. Exercise prescription for this patient

Table 3-2	**EXERCISES FOR OPTIMUM ROTATOR CUFF AND PERISCAPULAR MUSCLE ACTIVATION**
Targeted Muscles	**Exercise**
Mid/lower trapezius	Prone position: horizontal abduction with external rotation[67,68] (Fig. 3-7)
Serratus anterior	Standing: band-resisted punch plus with shoulder ≥ 90° flexion[67,69] Push-up plus position: progression from vertical (*i.e.*, standing wall push-up position)→ horizontal (*i.e.*, traditional prone push-up position)[69]
Supraspinatus	Prone position: horizontal abduction with external rotation[70] Prone position: external rotation at 90° abduction[a] [70,71]
Infraspinatus/teres minor	Sidelying: shoulder external rotation[70]
Subscapularis	Sidelying shoulder IR. Progress to standing position with shoulder elevated to 90° in scapular plane performing IR against resistance with elastic band. Push-up plus position: progression from standing against vertical surface→horizontal surface[69]

[a]This exercise must be performed carefully during the later phases of rehabilitation due to the provocative abducted and externally rotated position required.

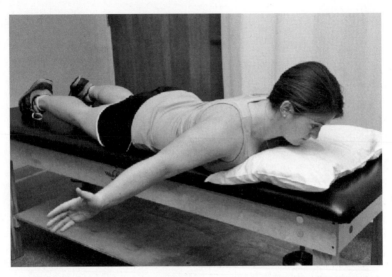

Figure 3-7. Prone horizontal abduction with shoulder external rotation to activate and strengthen middle and lower trapezius and supraspinatus muscles.

should emphasize high repetitions to build endurance of the stabilizing muscles and avoid compensation by prime movers in response to excessive loads.[63]

Proprioceptive training for muscular co-contraction should also be continued, not only to promote joint compression and stability, but also to address kinesthetic deficits associated with anterior shoulder instability. Smith and Brunoli demonstrated that joint position sense and joint movement perception are impaired following dislocation.[72] The cause of these impairments may be related to receptor damage in the muscles and capsule surrounding the joint, or to a decrease in afferent input from stretch receptors secondary to increased laxity. Regardless of the cause, the presence of these deficits may contribute to abnormal neuromuscular control and increased risk of recurrent instability.[72] Closed chain exercises performed with upper extremity weightbearing through an unstable surface challenge reflexive neuromuscular control and improve joint position sense.[63] Exercises performed in which the involved upper extremity is controlling an oscillating device (*e.g.*, Bodyblade, Thera-Band FlexBar) may also be valuable in stimulating receptors in both the dynamic and static stabilizers of the shoulder.[73] Exercises requiring shoulder hyperextension like full push-ups, dips, latissimus pull downs, and bench press should be avoided to limit stress on the anterior capsule and labrum.[51]

Sport-specific training can be initiated when symmetric motion and strength have been restored, and the patient can expect to return to sport 3 to 4 months following injury.[42] Athletes injured during the competitive season may not be willing or able to delay their return to competition for this duration, but combining physical therapy with the use of a functional brace that prevents upper extremity movement into the provocative position of abduction and external rotation can often allow them to complete their seasons. Buss et al.[74] used this approach and were able to return 87% of high school and college athletes to their sports in 0 to 30 days over a 2-year period. Despite this success, the risk of recurrent dislocation remained high and 37% of the athletes experienced at least one additional episode of instability during the remainder of their season. Almost half then underwent surgical stabilization during the off season.[74]

The methods for surgical repair of anterior glenohumeral instability fall into two categories: anatomic and nonanatomic reconstruction. Anatomic reconstruction focuses on restoring normal anatomy to the shoulder; nonanatomic reconstruction involves creating new structures to contain the humeral head.[75] The nonanatomic reconstruction procedures are typically not considered appropriate for first-time stabilization surgeries and are reserved for patients who require a second stabilization procedure. The anatomic reconstruction procedure most often selected for first time stabilization is the Bankart repair, which is designed to address the Bankart lesion common in patients with anterior instability. This repair restores tension to the anteroinferior capsule and inferior glenohumeral ligament complex by reattaching the anteroinferior labrum and capsuloligamentous tissue to the glenoid with suture anchors[76] (Fig. 3-8). Similar outcomes have been reported with open repairs and arthroscopic approaches.[40] In patients who demonstrate excessive capsular laxity, a capsular shift or rotator interval closure may also be performed in conjunction with the standard Bankart repair.

Postoperative care for a patient after a Bankart repair varies depending on the surgical technique used, the surgeon's preferences, and the patient's goals. A three-phase, 12-week postoperative protocol was described by Bottoni et al.[24] Phase I consisted of immobilization for 4 weeks with therapist-supervised pendulum and isometric exercises. Phase II emphasized progressive passive motion followed by active assisted motion. Phase III focused on full active motion and progressive resistance exercises. Contact sports, overhead, and heavy lifting were restricted until 4 months postoperatively. Wang et al.[77] described a slightly more conservative program with immobilization for six weeks. Active range of motion was emphasized during weeks 6 to 12.

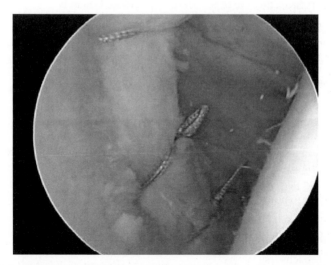

Figure 3-8. Arthroscopic Bankart repair using a 3 suture anchor technique. (Reproduced with permission from Dr. Peter Millett MD, MSc; The Steadman Clinic, Vail, Colorado.)

Resistance training was introduced about 12 weeks after surgery—after patients had achieved full, painless range of motion. Sport-specific exercises begin between weeks 16 to 20 and patients can expect to be cleared for return to contact sports between 20 and 24 weeks postoperatively.[77] These programs are similar to guidelines published by the American Society of Shoulder and Elbow Therapists (ASSET) that include a 4-week period of absolute immobilization, a staged recovery of full range of motion over a 3-month period, a strengthening progression beginning at week 6, and a functional progression for return to athletic activities between 4 and 6 months.[78]

Evidence-Based Clinical Recommendations

SORT: Strength of Recommendation Taxonomy

A: Consistent, good-quality patient-oriented evidence
B: Inconsistent or limited-quality patient-oriented evidence
C: Consensus, disease-oriented evidence, usual practice, expert opinion, or case series

1. Athletic males less than 30 years of age are at greatest risk of experiencing acute and recurrent anterior shoulder instability. **Grade A**

2. Surgical intervention for young active individuals following traumatic first-time anterior shoulder dislocation significantly reduces the rate of recurrent dislocation. **Grade A**

3. The apprehension and relocation tests have the best diagnostic accuracy to confirm a suspicion of acute anterior shoulder instability in patients with suggestive history and mechanism of injury. **Grade A**

4. Shoulder immobilization in external rotation after acute glenohumeral dislocation increases the approximation of the capsulolabral complex with the glenoid fossa and reduces the rate of recurrent dislocation. **Grade B**

5. Nonsurgical intervention focused on reestablishing neuromuscular control and strength of the shoulder's dynamic stabilizers provides patients with acute anterior shoulder instability the best chance to limit recurrent dislocation. **Grade C**

COMPREHENSION QUESTIONS

3.1 A physical therapist completed an examination of a young, active snowboard instructor who suffered an acute anterior shoulder dislocation three days ago. The therapist reviewed the radiograph and MRI reports to determine what underlying pathologies may be present. Which of the following pathologies is *most* likely to be seen in this patient?

    A. Rotator cuff lesion

    B. Bankart lesion

    C. Hill-Sachs lesion

    D. Bony Bankart lesion

3.2 A snowboard instructor decides she cannot undergo surgical intervention for an acute anterior shoulder dislocation due to financial constraints. She elects to pursue conservative treatment in an attempt to return to work as soon as possible. What is the *most* appropriate plan of care to assist her in achieving this goal?

A. Immobilization for 1 week, global rotator cuff and periscapular muscle strengthening below shoulder level, proprioceptive training in open and closed kinetic chain positions, functional bracing to prevent abduction and external rotation during work, education regarding prognosis in the event of recurrent dislocation

B. Immobilization for 1 week, joint mobilization to maximize range of motion, strength training to include dips, bench press, and behind the neck latissimus pull-downs, return to unrestricted activity

C. Immobilization for 3 weeks, isolated subscapularis muscle strengthening below shoulder level, proprioceptive training in open kinetic chain positions only, functional bracing to prevent abduction and external rotation during work, education regarding prognosis in the event of recurrent dislocation

D. Immobilization for 3 weeks, muscle strengthening in abduction and external rotation to increase stability and prevent recurrent dislocation, reassurance that dislocations are typically a single occurrence and should not be an issue in the future

ANSWERS

3.1 **B.** The Bankart lesion is considered the essential lesion of the acute anterior shoulder dislocation and can lead to recurrent anterior instability. This injury is characterized by separation of the anterior glenohumeral ligaments and glenoid labrum from the articular surface of the anterior inferior glenoid neck and can lead to increased anterior translation of the humeral head, particularly when the arm is in the abducted and externally rotated position.

3.2 **A.** Initial protection of the joint to minimize inflammation and pain is essential, but controversy persists regarding position and duration. If an internally rotated position is selected, Paterson et al.[37] suggest that there is no benefit to immobilization for longer than 1 week. However, if an externally rotated position is selected, 3 weeks appears to be more appropriate. Strength training focused only on the subscapularis muscle may actually destabilize the glenohumeral joint further in positions of abduction and external rotation (option C). Therefore, a balanced strength program addressing all the rotator cuff and periscapular musculature is recommended. Though open kinetic chain proprioceptive training is beneficial to restore kinesthetic awareness, closed chain exercises are also beneficial to promote joint stability through co-contraction of the glenohumeral dynamic stabilizers.

REFERENCES

1. Liavaag S, Stiris MG, Svenningsen S, Enger M, Pripp AH, Brox JI. Capsular lesions with glenohumeral ligament injuries in patients with primary shoulder dislocation: magnetic resonance imaging and magnetic resonance arthrography evaluation. *Scand J Med Sci Sports*. 2011;21:1-7.

2. Omoumi P, Teixeira P, Lecouvet F, Chung CB. Glenohumeral joint instability. *J Magn Reson Imaging*. 2011;33:2-16.

3. Glousman RE, Jobe FW. How to detect and manage the unstable shoulder. *J Musculoskel Med*. 1989;7:93-110.

4. Kazár B, Relovszky E. Prognosis of primary dislocation of the shoulder. *Acta Orthop Scand*. 1969;40:216-224.

5. Rhee YG, Cho NS, Cho SH. Traumatic anterior dislocation of the shoulder: factors affecting the progress of the traumatic anterior dislocation. *Clin Orthop Surg*. 2009;1:188-193.

6. Zacchilli MA, Owens BD. Epidemiology of shoulder dislocations presenting to emergency departments in the United States. *J Bone Joint Surg Am*. 2010;92:542-549.

7. Hovelius L. Incidence of shoulder dislocation in Sweden. *Clin Orthop Relat Res*.1982;166:127-131.

8. Hovelius L. Shoulder dislocation in Swedish ice hockey players. *Am J Sports Med*. 1978;6:373-377.

9. Owens BD, Duffey ML, Nelson BJ, DeBerardino TM, Taylor DC, Mountcastle SB. The incidence and characteristics of shoulder instability at the United States Military Academy. *Am J Sports Med*. 2007;35:1168-1173.

10. Rowe CR. Prognosis in dislocations of the shoulder. *J Bone Joint Surg*. 1956;38-A:957-977.

11. Baker CL, Uribe JW, Whitman C. Arthroscopic evaluation of acute intitial anterior shoulder dislocations. *Am J Sports Med*. 1990;18:25-28.

12. Hovelius L. Anterior dislocations of the shoulder in teen-agers and young adults. *J Bone Joint Surg*. 1987;69:393-399.

13. Simonet WT, Cofield RH. Prognosis in anterior shoulder dislocation. *Am J Sports Med*. 1984;12(1): 19-24.

14. Kirkley A, Griffin S, Richards C, Miniaci A, Mohtadi N. Prospective randomized clinical trial comparing the effectiveness of immediate arthroscopic stabilization versus immobilization and rehabilitation in first traumatic anterior dislocations of the shoulder. *Arthroscopy*.1999;15:507-514.

15. Bonza JE, Fields SK, Yard EE, Dawn Comstock R. Shoulder injuries among United States high school athletes during the 2005-2006 and 2006-2007 school years. *J Athl Train*. 2009;44:76-83.

16. McCall D, Safran MR. Injuries about the shoulder in skiing and snowboarding. *Br J Sports Med*. 2009;43:987-992.

17. Yamauchi K, Wakahara K, Fukuta M, et al. Characteristics of upper extremity injuries sustained by falling during snowboarding: a study of 1918 cases. *Am J Sports Med*. 2010;38:1468-1474.

18. Arciero RA, Wheeler JH, Ryan JB, McBride JT. Arthroscopic Bankart repair versus nonoperative treatment for acute, initial anterior shoulder dislocations. *Am J Sports Med*. 1994;22:589-594.

19. Abboud JA, Soslowsky LJ. Interplay of the static and dynamic restraints in glenohumeral instability. *Clin Orthop Rel Res*. 2002;400:48-57.

20. Burkart AC, Debski RE. Anatomy and function of the glenohumeral ligaments in anterior shoulder instability. *Clin Orthop Rel Res*. 2002;400:32-39.

21. Paine RM, Voight M. The role of the scapula. *J Orthop Sports Phys Ther*. 1993;18:386-391.

22. Wheeler JH, Ryan JB, Arciero RA, Molinari RN. Arthroscopic versus nonoperative treatment of acute shoulder dislocations in young athletes. *Arthroscopy*.1989;5:231-237.

23. Taylor DC, Arciero RA. Pathologic changes associated with shoulder dislocation: arthroscopic and physical examination findings in first-time, traumatic anterior dislocations. *Am J Sports Med*. 1997;25:306-311.

24. Bottoni CR, Wilckens JH, DeBerardino TM, et al. A prospective, randomized evaluation of arthroscopic stabilization versus nonoperative treatment in patients with acute, traumatic, first-time shoulder dislocations. *Am J Sports Med.* 2002;30:576-580.

25. Miller BS, Sonnabend DH, Hatrick C, et al. Should acute anterior dislocations of the shoulder be immobilized in external rotation? A cadaveric study. *J Shoulder Elbow Surg.* 2004;13:589-592.

26. Henry JH, Genung JA. Natural history of glenohumeral dislocation—revisited. *Am J Sports Med.* 1982;10:135-137.

27. Larrain MV, Botto GJ, Montenegro HJ, Mauas DM. Arthroscopic repair of acute traumatic anterior shoulder dislocation in young athletes. *Arthroscopy.* 2001;17:373-377.

28. Antonio GE, Griffith JF, Yu AB, Yung PS, Chan KM, Ahuja AT. First-time shoulder dislocation: high prevalence of labral injury and age-related differences revelaed by MR arthrography. *J Magn Reson Imaging.* 2007;26:983-991.

29. Bushnell BD, Creighton RA, Herring MM. Bony instability of the shoulder. *Arthroscopy.* 2008;24:1061-1073.

30. Sachs RA, Lin D, Stone ML, Paxton E, Kuney M. Can the need for future surgery for acute traumatic anterior shoulder dislocation be predicted? *J Bone Joint Surg.* 2007;89:1665-1674.

31. Rowe CR, Sakellarides HT. Factors related to recurrences of anterior dislocations of the shoulder. *Clin Orthop.*1961;20:40-48.

32. McLaughlin HL, MacLellan DI. Recurrent anterior dislocation of the shoulder. II. A comparative study. *J Trauma.* 1967;7:191-201.

33. McLaughlin HL, Cavallaro WU. Primary anterior dislocation of the shoulder. *Am J Surg.* 1950;80:615-621.

34. Hovelius L, Eriksson K, Fredin H, et al. Recurrences after initial dislocation of the shoulder. Results of a prospective study of treatment. *J Bone Joint Surg Am.* 1983;65:343-349.

35. Deitch J, Mehlman CT, Foad SL, Obbehat A, Mallory M. Traumatic anterior shoulder dislocation in adolescents. *Am J Sports Med.* 2003;31:758-763.

36. Boone JL, Arciero RA. First-time anterior shoulder dislocations: has the standard changed? *Br J Sports Med.* 2010;44:355-360.

37. Paterson WH, Throckmorton TW, Koester M, Azar FM, Kuhn JE. Position and duration of immobilization after primary anterior shoulder dislocation: a systematic review and meta-analysis of the literature. *J Bone Joint Surg Am.* 2010;92:2924-2933.

38. Jobe FW, Jobe CM. Painful athletic injuries of the shoulder. *Clin Orthop Relat Res.* 1983;173:117-124.

39. Handoll HH, Almaiyah MA, Rangan A. Surgical versus non-surgical treatment for acute anterior shoulder dislocation. *Cochrane Database Syst Rev.* 2004;(1):CD004325.

40. Brophy RH, Marx RG. The treatment of traumatic anterior instability of the shoulder: nonoperative and surgical treatment. *Arthroscopy.* 2009;25:298-304.

41. Hovelius L, Olofsson A, Sandström B, et al. Nonoperative treatment of primary anterior shoulder dislocation in patients forty years of age and younger: a prospective twenty-five-year follow-up. *J Bone Joint Surg Am.* 2008;90:945-952.

42. Aronen JG, Regan K. Decreasing the incidence of recurrence of first time anterior shoulder dislocations with rehabilitation. *Am J Sports Med.* 1984;12:283-291.

43. Caudevilla Polo S, Estébanez de Miguel E, Lucha López O, Tricás Moreno JM, Pérez Guillén S. Humerus axial traction with acromial fixation reduction maneuver for anterior shoulder dislocation. *J Emerg Med.* 2011;41:282-284.

44. Şahin N, Oztürk A, Özkan Y, Atici T, Özkaya G. A comparison of the scapular manipulation and Kocher's technique for acute anterior dislocation of the shoulder. *Eklem Hastalik Cerrahisi.* 2011;22:28-32.

45. Finestone A, Milgrom C, Radeva-Petrova DR, et al. Bracing in external rotation for traumatic anterior dislocation of the shoulder. *J Bone Joint Surg Br.* 2009;91:918-921.

46. Rowe CR, Zarins B. Recurrent transient subluxation of the shoulder. *J Bone Joint Surg Am.* 1981;63:863-872.

47. Hawkins RJ, Schutte JP, Janda DH, Huckell GH. Translation of the glenohumeral joint with the patient under anesthesia. *J Shoulder Elbow Surg.* 1996;5:286-292.

48. Faber KJ, Homa K, Hawkins RJ. Translation of the glenohumeral joint in patients with anterior instability: awake examination versus examination with the patient under anesthesia. *J Shoulder Elbow Surg.* 1999;8:320-323.

49. Lo IK, Nonweiler B, Woolfrey M, Litchfield R, Kirkley A. An evaluation of the apprehension, relocation, and surprise tests for anterior shoulder instability. *Am J Sports Med.* 2004;32:301-307.

50. Farber AJ, Castillo R, Clough M, Bahk M, McFarland EG. Clinical assessment of three common tests for traumatic anterior shoulder instability. *J Bone Joint Surg Am.* 2006;88:1467-1474.

51. Jobe FW, Kvitne RS, Giangarra CE. Shoulder pain in the overhand or throwing athlete. The relationship of anterior instability and rotator cuff impingement. *Orthop Rev.* 1989;18:963-975.

52. Gross ML, Distefano MC. Anterior release test. A new test for occult shoulder instability. *Clin Orthop Relat Res.* 1997;339:105-108.

53. Speer KP, Hannafin JA, Altchek DW, Warren RF. An evaluation of the shoulder relocation test. *Am J Sports Med.* 1994;22:177-183.

54. Rowe CR. Dislocations of the shoulder. In: Rowe CR, ed. *The Shoulder.* New York: Churchill Livingstone; 1988:165-292.

55. Sanders TG, Zlatkin M, Montgomery J. Imaging of glenohumeral instability. *Semin Roentgenol.* 2010;45:160-179.

56. Itoi E, Hatakeyama Y, Urayama M, Pradhan RL, Kido T, Sato K. Position of immobilization after dislocation of the shoulder. A cadaveric study. *J Bone Joint Surg Am.* 1999;81:385-390.

57. Itoi E, Sashi R, Minagawa H, Shimizu T, Wakabayashi I, Sato K. Position of immobilization after dislocation of the glenohumeral joint. A study with use of magnetic resonance imaging. *J Bone Joint Surg Am.* 2001;83-A:661-667.

58. Itoi E, Hatakeyama Y, Kido T, et al. A new method of immobilization after traumatic anterior dislocation of the shoulder: a preliminary study. *J Shoulder Elbow Surg.* 2003;12:413-415.

59. Siegler J, Proust J, Marcheix PS, Charissoux JL, Mabit C, Arnaud JP. Is external rotation the correct immobilisation for acute shoulder dislocation? An MRI study. *Orthop Traumatol Surg Res.* 2010;96:329-333.

60. Scheibel M, Kuke A, Nikulka C, Magosch P, Ziesler O, Schroeder RJ. How long should acute anterior dislocations of the shoulder be immobilized in external rotation? *Am J Sports Med.* 2009;37: 1309-1316.

61. Taşkoparan H, Kilinçoğlu V, Tunay S, Bilgiç S, Yurttaş Y, Kömürcü M. Immobilization of the shoulder in external rotation for prevention of recurrence in acute anterior dislocation. *Acta Orthop Traumatol Turc.* 2010;44:278-284.

62. McNeil NJ. Postreduction management of first-time traumatic anterior shoulder dislocations. *Ann Emerg Med.* 2009;53:811-813.

63. Jaggi A, Lambert S. Rehabilitation for shoulder instability. *Br J Sports Med.* 2010;44:333-340.

64. Burkhead WZ Jr, Rockwood CA Jr. Treatment of instability of the shoulder with an exercise program. *J Bone Joint Surg Am.* 1992;74:890-896.

65. Kibler WB. The role of the scapula in athletic shoulder function. *Am J Sports Med.* 1998;26:325-337.

66. Werner CM, Favre P, Gerber C. The role of the subscapularis in preventing anterior glenohumeral subluxation in the abducted, externally rotated position of the arm. *Clin Biomech.* 2007;22:495-501.

67. Ekstrom RA, Donatelli RA, Soderberg GL. Surface electromyographic analysis of exercises for the trapezius and serratus anterior muscles. *J Orthop Sports Phys Ther.* 2003;33:247-258.

68. Cools AM, Dewitte V, Lanszweert F, et al. Rehabilitation of scapular muscle balance: which exercises to prescribe? *Am J Sports Med.* 2007;35:1744-1751.

69. Decker MJ, Hintermeister RA, Faber KJ, Hawkins RJ. Serratus anterior muscle activity during selected rehabilitation exercises. *Am J Sports Med.* 1999;27:784-791.

70. Reinold MM, Wilk KE, Fleisig GS, et al. Electromyographic analysis of the rotator cuff and deltoid musculature during common shoulder external rotation exercises. *J Orthop Sports Phys Ther.* 2004;34:385-394.

71. Boettcher CE, Ginn KA, Cathers I. Which is the optimal exercise to strengthen supraspinatus? *Med Sci Sports Exerc.* 2009;41:1979-1983.

72. Smith RL, Brunolli J. Shoulder kinesthesia after anterior glenohumeral joint dislocation. *J Orthop Sports Phys Ther.* 1990;11:507-513.

73. Buteau JL, Eriksrud O, Hasson SM. Rehabilitation of a glenohumeral instability utilizing the body blade. *Physiother Theory Pract.* 2007;23:333-349.

74. Buss DD, Lynch GP, Meyer CP, Huber SM, Freehill MQ. Nonoperative management for in-season athletes with anterior shoulder instability. *Am J Sports Med.* 2004;32:1430-1433.

75. Wilk KE, Reinold MM, Andrews JR. *The Athlete's Shoulder.* 2nd ed. Philadelphia, PA: Churchill Livingston Elsevier; 2009.

76. Romeo AA, Cohen BS, Carreira DS. Traumatic anterior shoulder instability. *Orthop Clin North Am.* 2001;32:399-409.

77. Wang RY, Arciero RA, Mazzocca AD. The recognition and treatment of first-time shoulder dislocation in active individuals. *J Orthop Sports Phys Ther.* 2009;39:118-123.

78. Gaunt BW, Shaffer MA, Sauers EL, Michener LA, McCluskey GM, Thigpen C; American Society of Shoulder and Elbow Therapists. The American Society of Shoulder and Elbow Therapists' Consensus Rehabilitation Guideline for Arthroscopic Anterior Capsulolabral Repair of the Shoulder. *J Orthop Sport Phys Ther.* 2010;40:155-168.

Surgical Stabilization for Shoulder Instability: Return-to-Sport Rehabilitation

Laura Stanley
Ellen Shanley

CASE 4

Four months ago, a 16-year-old high school multisport athlete (football quarterback/ defensive back and baseball shortstop/relief pitcher) was injured in a football game against his team's rival. He sustained a glenohumeral dislocation when a defensive lineman contacted his arm at maximal cocking (90° of abduction and external rotation). He was unable to continue the game and needed reduction of his dislocation in the emergency room. This was his second instability episode. He was diagnosed with a Bankart and Hill-Sachs lesion of his right (dominant) shoulder. Ten days after the dislocation, he had arthroscopic fixation of the Bankart lesion, anterior capsule plication, and remplissage. The patient was referred to physical therapy on postoperative day one (POD 1) by his orthopaedic surgeon. The patient is the starting shortstop and relief pitcher (throws right-handed and is a switch hitter) for the varsity baseball team. The patient hopes to be ready for baseball season; however, his primary goal is to earn the starting role at quarterback for the upcoming football season. The patient is now 4 months postsurgery and able to begin return-to-sport rehabilitation.

► Based on the patient's diagnosis and surgical intervention, what do you anticipate may be the special considerations for the timeframe to return to sport?
► What criteria are critical for progression to the return-to-sport program for baseball?
► What examination techniques could be used to clarify the athlete's readiness for the tasks of the sport?
► What are the most appropriate interventions at this stage of the rehabilitation program?
► What are possible complications that may limit or delay the athlete's return to full participation?

KEY DEFINITIONS

BANKART LESION: Described as the "essential lesion" of the shoulder by Bankart in 1923[1]; includes an avulsion of the anteroinferior labrum from its glenoid attachment, generally resulting from an anterior shoulder dislocation

CRITICAL INSTANTS OF FORCE PRODUCTION: The moment during a throwing motion at which peak force is required of the dynamic muscular stabilizers to resist glenohumeral distraction

HILL-SACHS LESION: Impact fractures of the posterolateral aspect of the humeral head usually caused by anterior dislocation of the glenohumeral joint; this fracture may contribute to recurrent shoulder instability[2]

PLICATION: Surgical tightening of soft tissue structures of the shoulder joint; purpose is to reduce the joint volume and looseness to make the joint tighter

REMPLISSAGE: Surgical technique involving transfer of the posterior capsule and infraspinatus tendon into the Hill-Sachs lesion to prevent engagement of the lesion with the glenoid fossa when the arm is abducted and externally rotated to 90°[3]

Objectives

1. Identify risk factors for shoulder dislocation related to sport participation and recurrent instability episodes.

2. Prescribe appropriate interventions to restore the athlete's upper extremity motion, strength, endurance, and joint proprioception by the end of traditional rehabilitation, but prior to returning to sport.

3. Determine appropriate criteria for advancement into a return-to-sport progression based on the imposed demands of each sport in which the athlete participates.

Physical Therapy Considerations

PT considerations during management of the athlete following surgical shoulder stabilization:

▸ **General physical therapy plan of care/goals:** Restore pain-free range of motion; increase dynamic shoulder girdle muscular strength and endurance; sport-related functional biomechanical assessment; return athlete to sport

▸ **Physical therapy interventions:** Patient education related to involved anatomy and surgical procedure; manual therapy to restore range of motion and joint mobility; muscular flexibility exercises; resistance training to increase rotator cuff and scapular strength to provide dynamic stability; core and lower extremity strength and endurance training to provide stability and power

▶ **Precautions during physical therapy:** Consideration of postsurgical timeline regarding tissue healing properties and appropriate selection and dosage of therapeutic exercise

▶ **Complications interfering with physical therapy:** Patient noncompliance, premature phase progression, poor tissue healing, psychosocial challenges

Understanding the Health Condition

The anatomical structure of the shoulder girdle (clavicle, scapula, and humerus) permits multiplanar range of motion. As a result, it requires a balance of stability and mobility to allow functional activities, which is achieved through coordinated activity of both passive and active structures (Table 4-1). Glenohumeral instability is traditionally classified into two categories: traumatic and multidirectional. Instability is a term used to describe a pathological condition involving unwanted and uncontrolled translation within the joint, often following trauma to the shoulder. Laxity is a nonpathological, objective finding of capsuloligamentous integrity, concerning the degree of passive translation without associated symptoms.[4,5]

Traumatic shoulder injury can result in damage to multiple structures about the shoulder girdle, including soft tissue (muscle-tendon unit) rupture, capsular tearing, and glenoid and/or humeral head fracture (Fig. 4-1). An individual's age plays

Table 4-1 ANATOMICAL COMPONENTS OF SHOULDER STABILITY	
Static/Passive	**Dynamic/Active**
Bony structures	Rotator cuff
Glenoid labrum	Long head of biceps
Capsular structures	Scapular positioning
Negative intra-articular pressure	Concavity compression
Coefficient of friction	Neuromuscular control

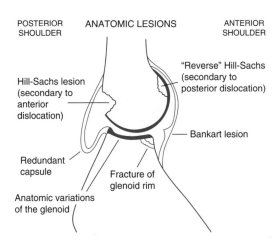

Figure 4-1. Anatomic lesions producing shoulder instability. (Reproduced with permission from Skinner HB. *Current Diagnosis & Treatment in Orthopedics.* 4th ed. New York: McGraw-Hill; 2006. Figure 4-31.

a profound role in **risk of recurrent instability**, with recurrence rates upward of 85% to 95% in individuals younger than 25 years old.[6-8] Activity level has been hypothesized to be an additional risk factor. Simonet et al.[9] showed that 82% of young athletes had recurrent dislocation compared to only 30% of nonathletes of similar age.

Acute traumatic anterior shoulder dislocations are more common than traumatic posterior dislocations.[4,10] When associated bony injury to the humeral head (Hill-Sachs lesion) is present in conjunction with anteroinferior capsulolabral disruption, immediate surgical intervention is indicated to restore anatomical alignment and glenohumeral joint arthrokinematics.

Physical Therapy Patient/Client Management

Following arthroscopic anterior stabilization of the shoulder as was performed in this case, rehabilitation with return-to-sport goals must include intentional planning and thorough communication of appropriate timelines and criteria for advancement. The physical therapist should consider involved tissues, healing time, and specific imposed demands of the desired sport in forming the treatment plan. Table 4-2 outlines the sports-specific considerations for each position that this athlete plays.

Evidence-based recommendations for necessary shoulder range of motion (ROM) and strength have been established in the athletic population. For the postsurgical athlete, obtaining and maintaining the proper shoulder girdle kinematics should be a focus throughout the rehabilitation process. In football players, arthroscopic treatment of anterior shoulder instability has allowed athletes to return to play within 1 year of their surgery.[11] In this study, none of the athletes returning to football lost more than 15° of external rotation on side-to-side comparison and the average external rotation loss was only 5°.[11]

Critical instants of force production during pitching have been demonstrated to occur just before maximal external rotation during the late cocking phase and immediately after ball release.[12] External rotation (ER) at maximum cocking in adult pitchers has been reported to reach 165°-180° of motion.[13] The total arc of approximately 180° is necessary to move from maximum external rotation to maximal internal rotation (IR).[14] Loss of glenohumeral IR in pitchers has been related to posterior-inferior capsular thickening and potential pathomechanical compromise

Table 4-2 SPORT-SPECIFIC CONSIDERATIONS DURING REHABILITATION	
Sport (Position)	Specific Considerations
Football (quarterback)	Throwing Contact Protection: bracing
Baseball (starting shortstop, relief pitcher)	Throwing Pitching Hitting

of rotator cuff, biceps tendon, and labral integrity.[15] One of the primary roles of the physical therapist is to help the athlete successfully return to sport, which may be dependent on restoration of functional shoulder rotational ROM.

Examination, Evaluation, and Diagnosis

Considering the extent of surgical stabilization required for this athlete, a conservative return-to-activity program is recommended. For the first 4 months postsurgery, the athlete is guided through the first two phases of rehabilitation. The first phase emphasizes pain control, protection of surgical repair to promote tissue healing, and normalization of ROM and neuromuscular control. The second phase progresses the athlete to activities focused on re-establishing coordinated upper extremity movement and muscular endurance.

At 4 months postsurgical stabilization, the physical therapist would expect this athlete to present with full, pain-free active ROM without compensation patterns, good scapular control during motion and strengthening activities, and the ability to perform all prescribed strengthening exercises with little to no pain ($\leq 2/10$ on the visual analog scale).[16] The next phase of rehabilitation should emphasize enhancing glenohumeral and scapular muscular endurance, as well as overall neuromuscular control of the shoulder girdle during sport-specific movement patterns and positions. It is essential that the physical therapist carefully considers, modifies, and monitors the stresses placed on each reconstructed tissue to ensure protection of the surgical repair while promoting progression in functional ability. Following anterior stabilization, the anteroinferior capsule is most notably stressed when the shoulder is placed in ER above 90° of abduction.[16] Therefore, ER motion must be obtained systematically following an *intentional* progression, particularly for an overhead athlete who requires this mobility for his sport. In the earlier rehabilitation phases, the athlete demonstrated the necessary physical performance, including functional motion, muscular strength and endurance, and appropriate body control. Now, as the athlete is preparing for return to his sports, it is appropriate to begin stressing these tissues in overhead ranges of motion.

When designing a return-to-play program for this athlete, utilization of objective tests and measures is necessary to assess his physical readiness to handle the demands of each of his sports and minimize risk of future injury. The selective use of special tests during the return-to-sport phase of rehabilitation is warranted to compare to presurgical findings and assess resolution of instability. Table 4-3 describes three common tests to determine shoulder instability.[17]

Passive shoulder range of motion, including ER, IR, and horizontal adduction, should also be evaluated when making return-to-play decisions. Myers et al.[19] demonstrated better overall clinical accuracy, including superior reliability and validity, when measuring shoulder ROM in the supine versus the sidelying position. The supine position was also shown to be more sensitive in identifying changes in overhead athletes who tend to demonstrate greater posterior shoulder tightness than non-overhead athletes.

Table 4-3	SPECIAL TESTS ASSOCIATED WITH SHOULDER INSTABILITY		
Test	Type of Instability	Patient Position	Findings
Apprehension	Anterior	Patient lies supine on edge of table; therapist stands at the involved side. Therapist positions shoulder at 90° abduction, grasps forearm and wrist, and externally rotates the humerus.	Positive test is defined as patient report of apprehension and/or pain.
Relocation	Anterior	Performed following a *positive* apprehension test. If patient indicates apprehension or pain with humeral ER, the therapist applies a posterior force at proximal humerus.	Positive test is defined as a decrease in apprehension and/or pain when posterior force is applied.
Sulcus	Anterior, posterior, or inferior	Patient is seated; therapist stands beside patient. Therapist applies an inferior long traction force at the patient's elbow, measuring the distance (cm) between the inferior acromion and superior humeral head. Rowe modification: Patient stands and bends forward slightly with arm relaxed by side. Therapist reassesses translation.	Distance of humeral head translation[18] Grade 1: < 1.5 cm Grade 2: 1.5-2 cm Grade 3: > 2 cm

The therapist should utilize objective performance-based tests for determining readiness for returning to sport. For a pitcher and quarterback, **performance testing** is geared towards assessing shoulder function, including rotator cuff endurance and scapular stability in dynamic overhead positions (Table 4-4).

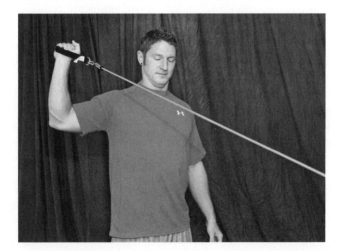

Figure 4-2. Exercise to assess right posterior rotator cuff endurance. Patient holds band with involved shoulder in 90° abduction and rotates band to end-range external rotation while maintaining the abducted position.

Table 4-4 SAMPLE PERFORMANCE TESTS FOR ROTATOR CUFF AND SCAPULAR ENDURANCE TO HELP DETERMINE READINESS FOR SPORT PARTICIPATION

Test	Goal of Test	Technique	Return-to-Play Performance Criteria
ER > 90°	Assess posterior rotator cuff endurance before and after sport-specific training.	Patient stands facing wall. Anchor resistance band to wall at patient's head height. Patient holds band with involved arm in 90° abduction. Patient rotates band to end-range ER while maintaining abducted position (Fig. 4-2).	Pre-throwing session: 1 min of repetitions with medium-resistance elastic band Post-throwing session: 30 s of repetitions with, medium-resistance elastic There should be no loss in timing or control during repetitions.
Closed kinetic chain upper extremity stability test (CKCUE; hand tap test)[20]	Assess glenohumeral, scapular, and core stability through endurance-based closed-chain dynamic movement.	Place two lines on floor at distance of 3 ft apart. Patient assumes push-up position and moves hands alternately back and forth between lines as fast as possible. Number of taps recorded at 15 and 30 s (Fig. 4-3).	*15 s:* 18 taps (male) 20 taps (female) *60 s:* 90 taps
Scapular dyskinesis Test[21,22]	Assess scapular position during overhead motion	Patient holds 5-lb dumbbell in each hand and performs 10 repetitions of overhead elevation in scapular plane.	Normal or only subtle dyskinesis following throwing session

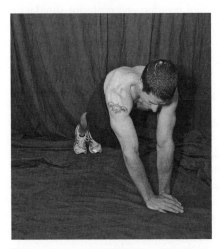

Figure 4-3. Closed Kinetic Chain Upper Extremity (CKCUE) Stability Test to assess glenohumeral, scapular, and core stability in an endurance task. Place two lines on floor at distance of 3 ft apart. Patient assumes push-up position and moves hands alternately back and forth between lines that are approximately 3 ft apart. The therapist records the number of taps at 15 and 30 seconds.

Plan of Care and Interventions

A strengthening program should work on acquiring dynamic stability of the rotator cuff muscles. There are three main biomechanical functions of the rotator cuff: compression of the humeral head in the glenoid fossa, rotation of the humeral head, and provision of muscular balance to limit stress placed on static joint stabilizers. The primary shoulder internal and external rotators act in concert as a muscular force couple to provide compression and centering of the humeral head within the glenoid fossa. Placing a towel roll between the patient's trunk and humerus when performing strengthening activities close to the plane of the body maximizes rotator cuff activation and subacromial space to avoid impingement and minimize hypovascularity at the muscle-tendon junction.[23] Reinold et al.[24] demonstrated a 10% increase in maximum voluntary muscle contraction of the infraspinatus/teres minor force couple when healthy subjects used a towel roll during shoulder external rotation at 0° abduction. As the athlete advances, the rotator cuff should be trained in greater planes of elevation and abduction to simulate sport-specific positions in which the athlete must demonstrate excellent dynamic stability.

When progressing upper extremity resistance band exercises, the therapist can alter the demand of the activity by altering numerous variables, including resistance level, repetitions, speed, and type of muscle contraction (isometric, concentric, eccentric). Strengthening exercises for the overhead athlete should primarily address rotator cuff and scapular stability, as well as lumbopelvic or "core" strength. Ellenbecker and Davies recommended increasing the isokinetic shoulder external rotation (ER) to internal rotation (IR) strength ratio to 66% to 76% to bias the ER strength for patients with shoulder pathology.[25] This ER bias would help create a "posterior dominant" shoulder to increase dynamic stability and aid in preventing reinjury in throwing and racquet-sport athletes.[25]

The benefits of **internal rotation and posterior shoulder stretching programs** for individuals with posterior shoulder tightness and postural deficits have been well documented. These include improved posture and scapular kinematics, decreased pain, and fewer days missed from sport participation.[26-28] In 2003, Kibler et al.[29] demonstrated a decrease in risk of injury following an IR stretching program. This is consistent with the findings by Shanley et al.[30] which showed that baseball players with a decrease of ≥25° of IR in the dominant shoulder (as compared to the nondominant shoulder) were at four times greater risk for upper extremity injury than those who lost < 25° over the course of one season.[30,31] Resolution of impingement symptoms has been demonstrated in those enrolled in a posterior shoulder stretching program.[32]

Finally, the overhead athlete needs to progress through an interval throwing program (ITP). A separate program for baseball and football should be designed and implemented at the appropriate time. The goal of an interval-throwing program is to return the athlete to preinjury status through a stepwise progression, taking care to prevent overtraining. Although little evidence is available for the specific design of such programs, several themes should be present and consistent.[33-37] First, athletes must be educated on the importance of following the prescribed program, with the risks of poor compliance outlined in understandable terms. Athletes should understand the implication of pain during or following throwing. Soreness rules should be implemented; each athlete's subjective report defines the modification of the ITP progression.[36] For example, the athlete should rest 1-2 days and not move to the next step of his ITP if there is specific or generalized arm soreness noted during warm-up, throws, or soreness that lasts longer than one hour following workout. An ITP should include a specific and consistent warm-up routine and emphasize technique over quantity. The parameters (number of pitches, sets, and outings/week) should be defined based on the individual's specific pitching role (*e.g.*, starter vs. reliever) and age.[36] Each outing should be defined based on effort level, distance, and duration of throws.[38] In Table 4-5, suggested return-to-play criteria are outlined based on documented clinical norms and rehabilitation progressions previously cited in peer-reviewed literature.[16,20-22,30,33,34]

The physical therapist should be prepared to counsel the athlete if he encounters obstacles as he returns to sport. Many athletes experience muscle soreness after being removed from a live athletic environment for extended recovery and rehabilitation. Progression through each stage of rehabilitation and continued participation following return to sport should be guided by subjective report of pain. The athlete must be informed that concordant shoulder pain is a flag for reassessment and that progression should be paused. However, the athlete should expect muscle soreness as the physical demand of sport increases. The therapist should educate the athlete on the use of appropriate modalities to address soreness. Yanagisawa et al.[39,40] showed that using ice after pitching reduced shoulder muscle soreness both immediately and 24 hours postpitching. The athlete may also experience psychological challenges as he reintegrates into sport. A potential referral to a sports psychologist may be warranted and valuable to provide mental training regarding the athlete's perception of performance, expectation, and outcomes.

Table 4-5 RETURN-TO-PLAY CRITERIA	
Dimension	Expected Outcome
Pain	No pain at rest
Range of motion	Full, pain-free rotational range of motion
Muscle strength	Manual muscle testing 5/5 in all planes Hand-held dynamometry: ≥ 90% of uninvolved UE following throwing session
Muscle performance	ER/IR ratio 2:3 (measured in pounds of force) (Strength of shoulder external rotators should be at least two-thirds of the strength of shoulder internal rotators of same upper extremity.) ER/IR at 90-90 position, repetitions for 1 min with medium band
Scapular stability	Open chain: normal or subtle scapular dyskinesis during shoulder elevation with 3-lb dumbbells for 10 repetitions Closed chain: 90 repetitions in 1 min on CKCUE stability test
Subjective outcome measures	Disability of the arm, shoulder, and hand (DASH) outcome Measure: < 5% disability DASH-sport: < 10% disability

Consideration of the athlete's complete physical and mental readiness to meet the demands of athletics following a traumatic injury and surgical repair is essential to successful participation and decreasing risk of future injury.

Evidence-Based Clinical Recommendations

SORT: Strength of Recommendation Taxonomy

A: Consistent, good-quality patient-oriented evidence
B: Inconsistent or limited-quality patient-oriented evidence
C: Consensus, disease-oriented evidence, usual practice, expert opinion, or case series

1. Age (< 25 years) and increased activity level are positively correlated with increased risk of recurrent shoulder instability. **Grade B**

2. Both open and closed kinetic chain performance tests provide the most comprehensive assessment of an overhead athlete's functional performance after injury. **Grade C**

3. Internal rotation and posterior shoulder stretching for overhead athletes improves posture and scapular kinematics, decreases pain and risk of injury, and results in fewer days missed from sport participation. **Grade A**

COMPREHENSION QUESTIONS

4.1 A sports physical therapist is treating an overhead athlete 4 months following surgical anterior shoulder stabilization. Which of the following positions should *only* be incorporated during the *final* phase of the rehabilitation program?

   A. Internal rotation at 0° abduction

   B. Shoulder elevation in scapular plane

   C. External rotation at 90° abduction

   D. Horizontal adduction at 90° abduction

4.2 Which of the following combinations of tests provides the therapist with the *most* complete assessment of the athlete's readiness to resume a full return to overhead sports?

   A. Number of repetitions of shoulder external and internal rotation performed in 0° abduction with medium resistance in 60 seconds

   B. Completion of interval throwing program without pain and with safe technique; CKCUE stability test

   C. Number of push-ups and pull-ups performed after a throwing session

   D. Manual muscle testing score of 5/5 for all shoulder girdle musculature following throwing session

ANSWERS

4.1 **C.** Coupling shoulder external rotation and abduction places the greatest stress across the inferior glenohumeral ligament complex. This capsuloligamentous structure was repaired surgically and therefore must be protected by avoiding positions that would increase tension across the tissue for at least 12 weeks. Therefore, this therapeutic intervention should be reserved for later stages of rehabilitation.

4.2 **B.** An interval throwing program and the CKCUE stability test provide the best evidence-based information for the therapist to make an objective decision on returning to sport. These two tests are also most relevant to the athlete's sports of baseball and football as they directly assess throwing biomechanics as well as global upper quarter strength, stability, and endurance.

REFERENCES

1. Bankart ASB. The pathology and treatment of recurrent shoulder dislocation of the shoulder. *Br J Surg*. 1939;26:23-29.

2. Cho SH, Cho NS, Rhee YG. Preoperative analysis of the Hill-Sachs lesion in anterior shoulder instability: how to predict engagement of the lesion. *Am J Sports Med*. 2011;39:2389-95.

3. Purchase RJ, Wolf EM, Hobgood ER, Pollock ME, Smalley CC. Hill-Sachs "remplissage": an arthroscopic solution for the engaging Hill-Sachs lesion. *Arthroscopy*. 2008;24:723-726.

4. Park M. Anatomy and function of the shoulder structures. In: Galatz LM, ed. *Orthopedic Knowledge Update: Shoulder and Elbow, No. 3*. Rosemont, IL: American Academy of Orthopaedic Surgeons; 2009.

5. Jia X, Ji JH, Petersen SA, Freehill MT, McFarland EG. An analysis of shoulder laxity in patients undergoing shoulder surgery. *J Bone Joint Surg Am*. 2009;91:2144-2150.

6. Rowe CR, Sakellarides HT. Factors related to recurrences of anterior dislocations of the shoulder. *Clin Orthop*. 1961;20:40-48.

7. Arciero RA, Wheeler JH, Ryan JB, McBride JT. Arthroscopic Bankart repair versus nonoperative treatment for acute, initial anterior shoulder dislocations. *Am J Sports Med*. 1994;22:589-594.

8. McLaughlin HL, MacLellan DI. Recurrent anterior dislocation of the shoulder. II. A comparative study. *J Trauma*. 1967;7:191-201.

9. Simonet WT, Cofield RH. Prognosis in anterior shoulder dislocation. *Am J Sports Med*. 1984;12:19-24.

10. Rowe CR. Prognosis in dislocations of the shoulder. *J Bone Joint Surg Am*. 1956;38-A: 957-977.

11. Pagnani MJ, Dome DC. Surgical treatment of traumatic anterior shoulder instability in American football players. *J Bone Joint Surg Am*. 2002;84-A:711-715.

12. Fleisig GS, Andrews JR, Dillman CJ, Escamilla RF. Kinetics of baseball pitching with implications about injury mechanism. *Am J Sports Med*. 1995;23:233-239.

13. Fleisig GS, Dillman CJ, Andrews JA. Proper mechanics for baseball pitching. *Clin Sports Med*. 1989;1:151-170.

14. Wilk KE, Meister K, Andrews JR. Current concepts in the rehabilitation of the overhead throwing athlete. *Am J Sports Med*. 2002;30:136-151.

15. Burkhart SS, Morgan CD, Kibler WB. The disabled throwing shoulder: spectrum of pathology, part II: evaluation and treatment of SLAP lesions in throwers. *Arthroscopy*. 2003;19:531-539.

16. Gaunt BW, Shaffer MA, Sauers EL, Michener LA, McCluskey GM, Thigpen C, American Society of Shoulder and Elbow Therapists. The American Society of Shoulder and Elbow Therapists' consensus

rehabilitation guideline for arthroscopic anterior capsulolabral repair of the shoulder. *J Orthop Sports Phys Ther.* 2010;40:155-168.

17. Cook C, Hegedus EJ. *Orthopedic Physcial Examination Tests: An Evidence-Based Approach.* Upper Saddle River, NJ: Pearson Prentice Hall; 2008.

18. Silliman JF, Hawkins RJ. Classification and physical diagnosis of instability of the shoulder. *Clin Orthop Relat Res.* 1993;(291):7-19.

19. Myers JB, Oyama S, Wassinger CA, et al. Reliability, precision, accuracy, and validity of posterior shoulder tightness assessment in overhead athletes. *Am J Sports Med.* 2007;35:1922-1930.

20. Goldbeck TG, Davies GJ. Test-retest reliability of the closed kinetic chain upper extremity stability test: a clinical field test. *J Sport Rehabil.* 2000;9:35-45.

21. Tate AR, McClure P, Kareha S, Irwin D, Barbe MF. A clinical method for identifying scapular dyskinesis, part 2: validity. *J Ath Train.* 2009;44:165-173.

22. McClure P, Tate AR, Kareha S, Irwin D, Zlupko E. A clinical method for identifying scapular dyskinesis, part 1: reliability. *J Ath Train.* 2009;44:160-164.

23. Reinold MM, Wilk KE, Hooks TR, Dugas JR, Andrews JR. Thermal-assisted capsular shrinkage of the glenohumeral joint in overhead athletes: a 15- to 47-month follow-up. *J Orthop Sports Phys Ther.* 2003;33:455-467.

24. Reinold MM, Wilk KE, Fleisig GS, et al. Electromyographic analysis of the rotator cuff and deltoid musculature during common shoulder external rotation exercises. *J Orthop Sports Phys Ther.* 2004;34:385-394.

25. Ellenbecker TS, Roetert EP, Bailie DS, Davies GJ, Brown SW. Glenohumeral joint total rotation range of motion in elite tennis players and baseball pitchers. *Med Sci Sports Exerc.* 2002;34: 2052-2056.

26. Thigpen CA, Padua DA, Michener LA, et al. Head and shoulder posture affect scapular mechanics and muscle activity in overhead tasks. *J Electromyogr Kinesiol.* 2010;20:701-709.

27. Lynch SS, Thigpen CA, Mihalik JP, Prentice WE, Padua D. The effects of an exercise intervention on forward head and rounded shoulder postures in elite swimmers. *Br J Sports Med.* 2010;44:376-381.

28. Wang CH, McClure P, Pratt NE, Nobilini R. Stretching and strengthening exercises: their effect on three-dimensional scapular kinematics. *Arch Phys Med Rehabil.* 1999;80:923-929.

29. Kibler WB, Chandler TJ. Range of motion in junior tennis players participating in an injury risk modification program. *J Sci Med Sport.* 2003;6:51-62.

30. Shanley E, Rauh MJ, Michener LA, Ellenbecker TS, Garrison JC, Thigpen CA. Shoulder range of motion measures as risk factors for shoulder and elbow injuries in high school softball and baseball players. *Am J Sports Med.* 2011;39:1997-2006.

31. Keeley DW, Hackett T, Keirns M, Sabick MB, Torry MR. A biomechanical analysis of youth pitching mechanics. *J Pediatr Orthop.* 2008;28:452-459.

32. Tyler TF, Nicholas SJ, Lee SJ, Mullaney M, McHugh MP. Correction of posterior shoulder tightness is associated with symptom resolution in patients with internal impingement. *Am J Sports Med.* 2010;38:114-119.

33. Axe MJ, Snyder-Mackler L, Konin JG, Strube MJ. Development of a distance-based interval throwing program for Little League-aged athletes. *Am J Sports Med.* 1996;24:594-602.

34. Axe MJ, Windley TC, Snyder-Mackler L. Data-based interval throwing programs for collegiate softball players. *J Ath Train.* 2002;37:194-203.

35. Coleman AE, Axe MJ, Andrews JR. Performance profile-directed simulated game: an objective functional evaluation for baseball pitchers. *J Orthop Sports Phys Ther.* 1987;9:101-105.

36. Axe MJ, Wickham R, Snyder-Mackler L. Data-based interval throwing programs for Little League, high school, college, and professional baseball pitchers. *Sports Med Arthrosc Rev.* 2001;9:24-34.

37. Love S, Aytar A, Bush H, Uhl TL. Descriptive analysis of pitch volume in southeastern conference baseball pitchers. *N Am J Sports Phys Ther.* 2010;5:194-200.

38. Olsen SJ II, Fleisig GS, Dun S, Loftice J, Andrews JR. Risk factors for shoulder and elbow injuries in adolescent baseball pitchers. *Am J Sports Med.* 2006;34:905-912.

39. Yanagisawa O, Miyanaga Y, Shiraki H, et al. The effects of various therapeutic measures on shoulder strength and muscle soreness after baseball pitching. *J Sports Med Phys Fitness.* 2003;43:189-201.

40. Yanagisawa O, Miyanaga Y, Shiraki H, et al. The effects of various therapeutic measures on shoulder range of motion and cross-sectional areas of rotator cuff muscles after baseball pitching. *J Sports Med Phys Fitness.* 2003;43:356-366.

Rotator Cuff Repair: Rehabilitation Weeks 1-4

Todd S. Ellenbecker
David S. Bailie

CASE 5

A 55-year-old male is referred to physical therapy following arthroscopic rotator cuff repair performed 2 weeks prior. The patient's injury occurred 3 months ago when he hit a series of repetitive serves during a tennis match while experiencing gradually progressive shoulder pain. The pain did not subside after the match. The pain escalated to the point where it was present at rest, during sleep, and with all activities of daily living. The patient consulted the referring orthopaedic surgeon who evaluated his shoulder and found significant weakness in the right (dominant) shoulder in external rotation and elevation and pain along the anterior and lateral margins of the acromion. An MRI scan with contrast enhancement showed a 2-cm full-thickness tear in the supraspinatus tendon extending posteriorly into the infra-spinatus without a concomitant labral tear. The patient was found to have a type II acromion. The patient successfully underwent an arthroscopic rotator cuff repair using suture anchors and a modest acromioplasty to address the type II acromion. He was given immediate postoperative instructions including: Codman pendulum exercises, shoulder shrugs and scapular retractions, grip-strengthening exercises, and instructions to use a sling to protect the shoulder. Two weeks after the surgery, the patient had his incisions inspected, external sutures removed, and he was referred with the order of "evaluate and treat" to physical therapy. The patient presents with the right shoulder immobilized in a sling with a pillow that places the shoulder in approximately 20° of abduction in the scapular plane. He has no complaints of radiation of symptoms into the distal right upper extremity and he rates his pain on the visual analog scale as 2/10 at rest and 5/10 with movement of the right shoulder. The patient's medical history is otherwise unremarkable.

► Based on the patient's diagnosis and surgery, what do you anticipate may be the contributors to his activity limitations?

► What are the most appropriate physical therapy interventions?

► What is his rehabilitation prognosis?

KEY DEFINITIONS

ACROMIOPLASTY: Surgical procedure whereby the surgeon removes the anterior-inferior portion of a type II acromion to more closely resemble a flat type I acromion

ROTATOR CUFF TEAR: Tearing and failure of the tendon of the supraspinatus and infraspinatus rotator cuff muscles; tears can be full thickness (involving entire thickness of the rotator cuff) or partial thickness. Partial-thickness tears can involve the superior (bursal) surface or inferior (articular) side of the tendon. Superior partial rotator cuff tears result from abrasion and impingement of the rotator cuff tendon against the coracoacromial arch, whereas articular side partial-thickness rotator cuff tears most often result from tensile overload of the muscle tendon unit.

TYPE II ACROMION: Acromion with a curved shape from an anterior to posterior (sagittal plane) orientation. A type I acromion is flat, allowing for maximal room in the subacromial space.

Objectives

1. Describe and apply key range of motion and glenohumeral joint mobilization interventions that can be safely applied to the patient following arthroscopic rotator cuff repair.

2. Describe important initial scapular stabilization interventions that can safely be prescribed for the patient following rotator cuff repair.

3. Identify evidence-based physical therapy interventions for early stage rehabilitation after rotator cuff repair.

4. List initial precautions for rehabilitation following rotator cuff repair.

Physical Therapy Considerations

PT considerations during early postoperative management (1-4 weeks) of the individual with a surgically repaired rotator cuff tear:

▶ **General physical therapy plan of care/goals:** Decrease pain; increase active and passive range of motion; increase upper extremity rotator cuff and scapular strength

▶ **Physical therapy interventions:** Patient education regarding functional anatomy and injury pathomechanics and general precautions regarding protection of healing tendons; modalities and manual therapy to decrease pain; mobilization and passive stretching to improve joint mobility and prevent/minimize capsular restriction; submaximal resistance exercises to increase muscular strength and endurance of the rotator cuff and scapular stabilizers, home exercise instruction

▶ **Precautions during physical therapy:** Monitor neural signs and symptoms; address precautions or contraindications for exercise based on patient's pre-existing condition(s)

▶ **Complications interfering with physical therapy:** Tear size; tissue quality; medical or lifestyle issues that interfere with optimal tissue healing (*e.g.*, smoking); health complications that limit the patient's ability to be positioned for range of motion or attend physical therapy sessions

Understanding the Health Condition

The etiology of rotator cuff pathologic conditions can be described along a continuum, ranging from overuse microtraumatic tendinosis to either degenerative or macrotraumatic full-thickness rotator cuff tears. A second continuum of rotator cuff etiology consists of glenohumeral joint instability and primary impingement or compressive disease.[1] The clinical challenge of treating the patient with a rotator cuff injury begins with a specific evaluation and clear understanding of the underlying stability and integrity of not only the components of the glenohumeral joint, but also of the entire upper extremity kinetic chain.

Full-thickness rotator cuff tears can be caused by degeneration of the rotator cuff over time, as well as by repetitive loading of the tendon (*e.g.*, as occurs in an overhead athlete). Forces encountered during a traumatic event are greater than the normal tendon can tolerate. Full-thickness tears of the rotator cuff, with bony avulsions of the greater tuberosity, can occur from single traumatic episodes. According to Cofield,[2] injuries to normal tendons do not occur easily because 30% or more of the tendon must be damaged to produce a substantial reduction in strength. Although a single traumatic event resulting in tendon failure is often reported by the patient in the subjective examination, repeated microtraumatic insults and degeneration over time may have created a substantially weakened tendon. The tendon *ultimately* failed under the heavy load described by the patient. Full-thickness rotator cuff tears require surgical treatment and aggressive rehabilitation to achieve a positive functional outcome.[3,4]

Several etiologic factors are important to consider with respect to rotator cuff tears. The vascularity of the rotator cuff, specifically the supraspinatus, has been extensively studied beginning in 1934 by Codman.[5] In his classic monograph on ruptures of the supraspinatus tendon, Codman described a critical zone of hypovascularity that appeared anemic and infarcted and was located 0.5 inches proximal to the insertion on the greater tuberosity. The biceps long head tendon was found to have a similar region of hypovascularity in its deep surface 2 cm from its insertion.[6] Rathbun and MacNab[7] reported the effects of position on the microvascularity of the rotator cuff. With the glenohumeral joint in a position of adduction, a constant area of hypovascularity was found near the insertion of the supraspinatus tendon. This consistent pattern was not observed with the arm in a position of abduction. These investigators termed this observation the "wringing out phenomenon" and also noticed a similar response in the long head tendon of the biceps. This positional relationship has clinical ramifications for both exercise positioning and immobilization. Brooks et al.[8] found no significant vascular differences between the tendinous insertions of the supraspinatus and infraspinatus tendons; both were hypovascular when studied by quantitative histologic analysis. In contrast, research published by Swiontowski et al.[9] does not support this region of hypovascularity or critical zone. Blood flow (as measured by Doppler flowmetry) was greatest in the critical zone compared with other parts of the tendon in patients with rotator cuff tendinitis from subacromial impingement.

Several primary types of rotator cuff tears are commonly described in the literature. Full-thickness tears consist of tears that comprise the entire thickness (from top to bottom) of the rotator cuff tendon or tendons. Full-thickness tears are often initiated in the critical zone of the supraspinatus tendon and can extend to include the infraspinatus, teres minor, and subscapularis tendons.[10] A tear in the subscapularis tendon is often associated with a subluxation of the biceps long head tendon from the intertubercular groove, or either a partial or complete tear of the biceps tendon. Histologically, full-thickness rotator cuff tears show various findings ranging from almost entirely acellular and avascular margins to neovascularization with cellular infiltrate.[10]

The effects of a full-thickness rotator cuff tear on glenohumeral joint stability were studied by Loehr et al.[11] Changes in stability of the glenohumeral joint were assessed by selective division of the supraspinatus or infraspinatus tendons. Findings indicated that a one-tendon lesion of either the supraspinatus or infraspinatus did not influence the movement patterns of the glenohumeral joint, whereas a two-tendon lesion induced notable changes compatible with instability of the glenohumeral joint.[11] Therefore, patients with full-thickness rotator cuff tears may have additional stress and dependence placed on the dynamic stabilizing function of the remaining rotator cuff tendons because of increased humeral head translation and the ensuing instability.

Additional research on full-thickness rotator cuff tears has notable clinical ramifications. Miller and Savoie examined 100 consecutive patients with full-thickness tears of the rotator cuff to determine the incidence of associated intra-articular injuries.[12] Seventy-four of these 100 patients had one or more coexisting intra-articular abnormalities: anterior labral tears occurred in 62 patients and biceps tendon tears were noted in 16 patients. The results of this study clearly indicate the importance of a thorough clinical examination of the patient with a rotator cuff injury.

Physical Therapy Patient/Client Management

Patients presenting for physical therapy following arthroscopic rotator cuff repair can benefit from interventions consisting of modalities such as electrical stimulation and ultrasound, as well as the use of heat and ice. Additional manual therapy, outlined in this case, in addition to submaximal therapeutic exercise is of tremendous benefit to these patients to restore range of motion, muscular strength, and ultimately shoulder function following repair. Information regarding the tissue stresses following rotator cuff repair helps the physical therapist to optimize the initial range of motion of the shoulder without jeopardizing tissue healing.

Examination, Evaluation, and Diagnosis

Key highlights for examination of the postoperative shoulder consist of neurologic screening and passive range of motion (PROM) measurement of the involved extremity and measurement of active ROM of the uninvolved extremity.

The physical therapist should view the patient from the posterior aspect to inspect for atrophy of the scapular and rotator cuff muscles, which is often seen more easily when the patient places his hands on his hips.[13] When inspecting the resting position of the scapula, the therapist should assess for prominence of the inferior or medial borders of the scapula, which indicates the need for scapular stabilization interventions.[14,15]

Examination of the stability of the glenohumeral joint is very important. Tests like the load and shift[16] (see Case 2, Table 2-1) and multidirectional instability (MDI) sulcus sign[17] (see Case 2, Table 2-1) should be performed bilaterally and compared. Identification of excessive hypermobility or excessive capsular tightness at this initial stage has critical ramifications for the formulation of a plan of care. The patient in this case has significant atrophy of the infraspinatus muscle evident by atrophy in the infraspinous fossa as well as inferior angle prominence of the right scapula at rest and in the hands-on-hips position. There is no evidence of instability with grade I anterior-posterior translation noted during the load and shift test. The MDI sulcus test is negative bilaterally.

Plan of Care and Interventions

Initial postsurgical rehabilitation focuses on shoulder ROM to prevent capsular adhesions while protecting the surgically repaired tissues. Some postsurgical rehabilitation protocols specify ROM limitations to be applied during the first 6 weeks of rehabilitation. Several basic science studies have provided rationale for the safe application of glenohumeral joint ROM and the movements that allow joint excursion and capsular lengthening, yet provide safe and protective inherent tensions produced in the repaired tendon.

In human cadavers, Hatakeyama et al.[18] repaired 1 × 2 cm supraspinatus tears and studied the effects of humeral rotation on the tension in the supraspinatus in 30° of arm elevation in the coronal, scapular, and sagittal planes. Compared to tension in a position of neutral rotation, 30° and 60° of external rotation *decreased* the tension within the supraspinatus muscle tendon unit. In contrast, 30° and 60° of internal rotation *increased* tension within the supraspinatus tendon. This study provides important insight into the safety of performing early PROM into external rotation following rotator cuff repair. Most patients are placed in positions of internal rotation during the period of postsurgical immobilization. This study suggests that postsurgical immobilization positioning provides increased tension onto the repaired supraspinatus tendon. Based on the study by Hatakeyama et al.,[18] physical therapists should understand that moving the shoulder up to 60° of external rotation in 30° of elevation in the scapular or coronal plane provides *less* tissue tension than the position of typical immobilization (30°-60° of internal rotation). Controlled tension in the repair is advocated to improve tendon strength and healing without jeopardizing healing or tendon-bone congruity.

Another aspect of clinical relevance that can be derived from the study by Hatakeyama et al.[18] was the comparison of the intrinsic tensile load in the repaired supraspinatus tendon between the coronal, scapular, and sagittal planes during humeral rotation. Significantly higher loading was present in the supraspinatus tendon during humeral rotation in the sagittal plane compared to both the coronal

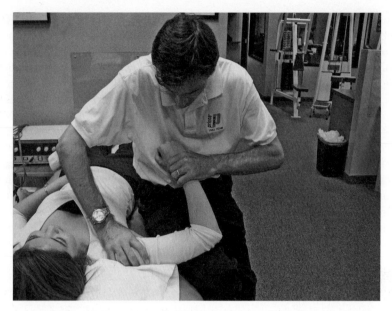

Figure 5-1. Right humeral rotation ROM with the glenohumeral joint in the scapular plane.

and scapular planes. Therefore, based on this study, early PROM should be performed into the directions of both external and internal humeral rotation using the *scapular plane* position to minimize tensile loading in the repaired tendon.[18] Figure 5-1 shows a technique used to perform humeral rotation ROM with the glenohumeral joint placed in the scapular plane. The use of a platform or the therapist's leg provides a supported position in the scapular plane allowing the therapist's hands to be free to provide support to mobilize the humeral head.

Another cadaveric study provides guidance for ROM application in the early postoperative phase. Muraki et al.[19] studied the effects of passive upper extremity motion on tensile loading of the supraspinatus tendon in human cadavers. They found no significant increases in strain in either the supraspinatus or infraspinatus tendons at 60° of shoulder flexion during the movement of horizontal adduction. However, internal rotation performed at 30° and 60° of flexion increased tension in the inferior-most portion of the infraspinatus tendon compared to the resting or neutral position. This study provides additional guidance to therapists for selecting safe ROM positions following surgery: the use of internal rotation and cross arm adduction ranges of motion can be performed while putting minimal strain in the repaired supraspinatus tendon. This study also illustrated the importance of knowing the degree of tendon involvement and repair because posteriorly based rotator cuff repairs (those involving the infraspinatus and teres minor) may be subjected to increased tensile loads if early internal rotation is applied during postoperative rehabilitation. Therefore, communication between the surgeon and treating physical therapist is of vital importance to ensure that optimal range of motion is performed following repair.

One area of initial concern in the rehabilitation process following rotator cuff repair is the progression from PROM to active assisted range of motion (AAROM) and active range of motion (AROM). Some disagreement regarding the degree of muscular activation occurring during these commonly used rehabilitation activities can be clarified by a review of the appropriate literature. Research by McCann et al.[20] provided clear delineation of the degree of muscular activation of the supraspinatus during supine assisted flexion range of motion and seated elevation with the use of a pulley. While both activities arguably produce low levels of inherent muscular activation in the supraspinatus, the seated upright pulley activity produced significantly more muscular activity compared to the similar supine activities. This study clearly demonstrated the effect of patient positioning on muscular activation and provides **therapeutic rationale for the use of supine, gravity-neutral elevation exercise in the early phase** following rotator cuff repair to protect the healing tendon.

Ellsworth et al.[21] have quantified levels of muscular activation during **Codman pendulum exercise**. Their study showed minimal levels of muscular activation in the rotator cuff musculature during Codman pendulum exercise. However, this exercise cannot be considered passive because the musculature is still activated, especially in individuals with shoulder pathology. While many therapists (including the authors of this case) do not recommend the use of weight application in the hand during pendulum exercises due to the potential for unwanted anterior glenohumeral translation, Ellsworth et al.[21] found that muscular activity in the rotator cuff musculature was unchanged with and without weight application during the performance of pendulum exercises. Pendulum exercises (with or without weight) still activate rotator cuff musculature, which calls into question their prescription in the early postsurgery phase in cases when only passive movements may be indicated.

These studies give objective guidance for the early application of active assisted ROM activities that can be applied safely in the early postsurgical rehabilitation following rotator cuff repair. As further research becomes available, physical therapists will be able to make evidence-based decisions regarding the appropriateness of specific rehabilitation exercises based on their inherent muscular activation. Rehabilitation in the first 2 to 4 weeks following rotator cuff repair typically consists of the use of truly passive, as well as several minimally active or active assisted exercises for the rotator cuff such as active assisted flexion using overhead pulleys and pendulum exercises. To recruit rotator cuff and scapular muscular activity, the patient can use the "balance point" position (90° of shoulder flexion) in supine; the patient is cued to perform small active motions of flexion/extension from the 90° starting position. These exercises should be coupled with early scapular stabilization via manual resistance techniques emphasizing direct hand contacts on the scapula to bypass force application to the rotator cuff and optimize trapezius, rhomboid, and serratus anterior muscular activation (Fig. 5-2). Kibler et al.[22] quantified the muscular activity (via electromyography) during low-level closed chain exercises such as weight shifting on a rocker board (patient in a standing position with upper extremity resting on a rocker board sitting on a table top). They showed that this activity produced low levels of activation of the rotator cuff and scapular musculature (<10%).

New research has explored the effects of simulated shoulder AROM on the integrity of a cadaveric supraspinatus repair performed using either transosseous tunnels or suture anchors.[23] The results showed no difference between repair constructs following repetitive loading, indicating the ability of an arthroscopically based suture

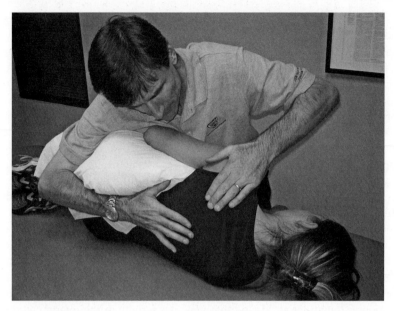

Figure 5-2. Therapist applying manual resistance on patient's scapula to facilitate trapezius, rhomboid, and serratus anterior muscular activation.

anchor fixation model to withstand active loading in a similar fashion to transosseous repair used during mini-open and open rotator cuff repair. Future research will help to identify the effects of simulated submaximal loads on rotator cuff repair constructs to allow for optimal application of resistive exercise sequences for patients following rotator cuff repair.

In the initial phase of rehabilitation (1-4 weeks postsurgical repair), care must be taken regarding strengthening because the priority in this phase is to optimize shoulder ROM, protect the repair, and initiate scapular stabilization. The use of AROM exercises such as sidelying external rotation against gravity with little or no weight application can be prescribed to begin activating the posterior rotator cuff musculature (Fig. 5-3). This exercise has been shown to produce levels of muscular activation of the infraspinatus and teres minor muscles in experimental electromyographic research studies.[24,25] As the patient progresses, emphasis shifts to strengthening of the entire rotator cuff complex. In this early phase, exercises are also applied with elastic resistance to provide an isometric contraction of the internal and external humeral rotators (rotator cuff) through the use of an exercise commonly called "dynamic isometrics" or step-outs (Fig. 5-4). A small towel roll is placed under the axilla during the exercise to place the shoulder in the scapular plane.[7] The use of elastic resistance allows the physical therapist to ensure that the patient is not exercising with loads that exceed his present tolerance due to standardized elongation parameters of the Thera-Band colored tubing progression (Hygenic Corp, Akron OH). Elastic resistance is preferred over other methods of isometric exercise using a wall or pillow in which the physical therapist has less ability to control or monitor the patient's exercise intensity.

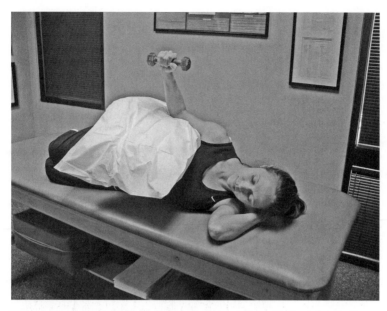

Figure 5-3. Sidelying external rotation against gravity with small dumbbell weight to begin activating posterior rotator cuff musculature.

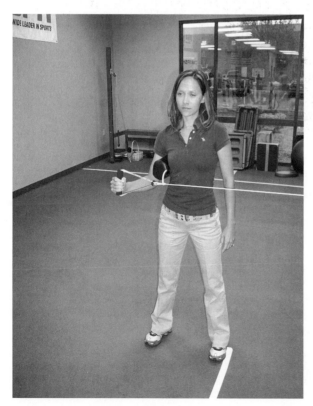

Figure 5-4. Resistance exercise for right humeral rotator cuff complex. Roll under the axilla keeps the shoulder in the scapular plane. The exercise is performed by taking a step away ("step-out") from the band's attachment site while maintaining the same upper extremity position.

Key components of rehabilitation in the first month following rotator cuff repair include the use of early shoulder ROM, glenohumeral joint mobilization, submaximal rotator cuff and scapular active movement, and subtle resistance. Basic science research can be applied during this initial stage to ensure that appropriate loading parameters are encountered by the postsurgical tissue to produce successful ROM and strength outcomes following rehabilitation. Future research will further elucidate optimal loading and immobilization periods following surgical repair of the rotator cuff.

Evidence-Based Clinical Recommendations

SORT: Strength of Recommendation Taxonomy

A: Consistent, good-quality patient-oriented evidence
B: Inconsistent or limited-quality patient-oriented evidence
C: Consensus, disease-oriented evidence, usual practice, expert opinion, or case series

1. Supine, gravity-neutral elevation exercise is advocated to protect the healing tendon in the first 4 weeks after surgical rotator cuff repair. **Grade B**

2. Codman pendulum exercises (with or without weight) in the early postsurgery phase when only passive movements may be indicated may not be appropriate since this exercise still activates rotator cuff musculature. **Grade B**

3. In the first 4 weeks after surgical repair of the rotator cuff, a rehabilitation program emphasizing early shoulder ROM, glenohumeral joint mobilization, submaximal rotator cuff and scapular active movement, and subtle resistance produces good patient outcomes for range of motion, muscular strength, and shoulder function. **Grade C**

COMPREHENSION QUESTIONS

5.1 In the first 4 weeks following rotator cuff repair, the application of humeral rotation range of motion should be done in which of the following planes to minimize loading and tension on the repair?

A. Sagittal plane

B. Scapular plane

C. Coronal plane

D. Transverse plane

5.2 Which of the following is *not* a component of early rehabilitation following rotator cuff repair?

A. Scapular stabilization exercise

B. Glenohumeral joint mobilization

C. Aggressive strengthening of the supraspinatus

D. Submaximal activation of the posterior rotator cuff

ANSWERS

5.1 **B.** Hatakeyama et al.[18] have shown in cadaveric research that humeral rotation exercise performed in the scapular plane produces less tensile loading than similar ranges of motion performed in the sagittal plane.

5.2 **C.** Aggressive loading of the rotator cuff has been shown to produce failures in both traditional transosseous repair constructs as well as single and double row suture anchor fixation methods. Care must be taken when implementing loading strategies to the repaired rotator cuff following surgical repair in the early postoperative period.[23]

REFERENCES

1. Jobe FW, Kvitne RS, Giangarra CE. Shoulder pain in the overhand or throwing athlete. The relationship of anterior instability and rotator cuff impingement. *Orthop Rev.* 1989;28:963-975.

2. Cofield RH. Current concepts review of rotator cuff disease of the shoulder. *J Bone Joint Surg Am.* 1985;67:974-979.

3. Andrews JR, Alexander EJ. Rotator cuff injury in throwing and racquet sports. *Sports Med Arthroscop Rev.* 1995;3:30-38.

4. Neer CS II. Impingement lesions. *Clin Orthop Relat Res.*1983;173:70-77.

5. Codman EA. *The Shoulder.* 2nd ed. Brooklyn, NY: Miller & Medical; 1934.

6. Chansky HA, Iannotti JP. The vascularity of the rotator cuff. *Clin Sports Med.* 1991;10:807-822.

7. Rathbun JB, Macnab I. The microvascular pattern of the rotator cuff. *J Bone Joint Surg Br.* 1970;52:540-553.

8. Brooks CH, Revell WJ, Heatley FW. A quantitative histological study of the vascularity of the rotator cuff tendon. *J Bone Joint Surg Br.* 1992;74:151-153.

9. Swiontowski MF, Iannotti JP, Boulas HJ, et al. Intraoperative assessment of rotator cuff vascularity using laser Doppler flowmetry. In: Post M, Morrey BF, Hawkins RJ, eds. *Surgery of the Shoulder.* St. Louis, MO: Mosby Year Book; 1990:208-212.

10. Iannotti JP. Lesions of the rotator cuff: pathology and pathogenesis. In: Matsen FA, Fu FH, Hawkins RJ, eds. *The Shoulder: A Balance of Mobility and Stability.* Rosemont, IL: American Academy of Orthopaedic Surgeons; 1993.

11. Loehr JF, Helmig P, Sojbjerg JO, Jung A. Shoulder instability caused by rotator cuff lesions. An in vitro study. *Clin Orthop Relat Res.* 1994;304:84-90.

12. Miller C, Savoie FH. Glenohumeral abnormalities associated with full-thickness tears of the rotator cuff. *Orthop Rev.*1994;23:159-162.

13. Ellenbecker TS. *Clinical Examination of the Shoulder.* St. Louis, MO: W.B. Saunders; 2004.

14. Kibler WB. Role of the scapula in the overhead throwing motion. *Contemp Orthop.* 1991;22: 525-532.

15. Kibler WB, Uhl TL, Maddux JW, Brooks PV, Zeller B, McMullen J. Qualitative clinical evaluation of scapular dysfunction: a reliability study. *J Shoulder Elbow Surg.* 2002;11:550-556.

16. Gerber C, Ganz R. Clinical assessment of instability of the shoulder. With special reference to anterior and posterior drawer tests. *J Bone Joint Surgery.* 1984;66:551-556.

17. McFarland EG, Torpey BM, Curl LA. Evaluation of shoulder laxity. *Sports Med.* 1996;22:264-272.

18. Hatakeyama Y, Itoi E, Urayama M, Pradham RL, Sato K. Effect of superior capsule and coracohumeral ligament release on strain in the repaired rotator cuff tendon. A cadaveric study. *Am J Sports Med.* 2001;29:633-640.

19. Muraki T, Aoki M, Uchiyama E, Murakami G, Miyamoto S. The effect of arm position on stretching of the supraspinatus, infraspinatus, and posterior portion of deltoid muscles: a cadaveric study. *Clin Biomech*. 2006;21:474-480.

20. McCann PD, Wooten ME, Kadaba MP, Bigliani LU. A kinematic and electromyographic study of shoulder rehabilitation exercises. *Clin Orthop Rel Res*. 1993;288:178-188.

21. Ellsworth AA, Mullaney M, Tyler TF, McHugh M, Nicholas S. Electromyography of selected shoulder musculature during un-weighted and weighted pendulum exercises. *N Am J Sports Phys Ther*. 2006;1:73-79.

22. Kibler WB, Livingston B, Bruce R. Current concepts in shoulder rehabilitation. In: Stauffer RN, Erlich MG. *Advances in Operative Orthopaedics*. Vol 3. St Louis, MO: Mosby; 1995:249-297.

23. Tashjian RZ, Levanthal E, Spenciner DB, Green A, Fleming BC. Initial fixation strength of massive rotator cuff tears: in vitro comparison of single-row suture anchor and transosseous tunnel constructs. *Arthroscopy*. 2007;23:710-716.

24. Townsend H, Jobe FW, Pink M, Perry W. Electromyographic analysis of the glenohumeral muscles during a baseball rehabilitation program. *Am J Sports Med*. 1991;19:264-272.

25. Reinold MM, Macrina LC, Wilk KE, et al. Electromyographic analysis of the supraspinatus and deltoid muscles during 3 common rehabilitation exercises. *J Athl Train*. 2007;42:464-469.

Adhesive Capsulitis—Diagnosis

Jason Brumitt

CASE 6

A 36-year-old female self-referred to an outpatient physical therapy clinic with a 2-month history of right (dominant) shoulder pain. She reports first experiencing pain while fastening her bra. The patient denies any trauma; this is the first time she has sought care for a shoulder injury. Pain intensity has increased since onset and regularly affects her ability to sleep on her right side. In addition to pain, she reports an inability to clean her house, reach overhead, or reach behind her back. The patient's presenting signs and symptoms are consistent with primary adhesive capsulitis of the right shoulder.

► Based on the patient's suspected diagnosis, what do you anticipate may be the contributing factors to her condition?
► What symptoms are associated with this diagnosis?
► What are the most appropriate examination tests?

KEY DEFINITIONS

AXILLARY FOLD: Region of the armpit consisting of a portion of the pectoralis major muscle forming the anterior border and portions of the latissimus dorsi and teres major muscles forming the posterior border

IDIOPATHIC: An unknown cause

PRIMARY ADHESIVE CAPSULITIS: Musculoskeletal condition of the shoulder of unknown etiology marked by significant restriction in shoulder active and passive range of motion[1,2]

ROTATOR INTERVAL: Triangular region of the anterior shoulder that contains the coracoid process, supraspinatus and subscapularis tendons, long head of the biceps tendon, and the superior glenohumeral and coracohumeral ligaments

Objectives

1. Describe the differences between primary (idiopathic) and secondary adhesive capsulitis.
2. Describe the pathophysiology associated with primary adhesive capsulitis.
3. Describe symptoms associated with adhesive capsulitis.
4. Describe appropriate clinical examination tests that help rule in primary adhesive capsulitis.

Physical Therapy Considerations

PT considerations during examination of the individual with suspected primary adhesive capsulitis:

▶ **General physical therapy plan of care/goals:** Decrease pain; increase muscular flexibility; increase or prevent loss of shoulder range of motion; increase upper quadrant strength; prevent or minimize loss of aerobic fitness capacity

▶ **Physical therapy tests and measures:** Observation of the upper quadrant, active and passive range of motion testing, passive accessory joint motion testing, coracoid pain test, palpation

▶ **Differential diagnoses:** Rotator cuff strain, rotator cuff tendinosis, subacromial impingement, osteoarthritis, tumor, fracture

Understanding the Health Condition

Adhesive capsulitis (also known as frozen shoulder) affects up to 5% of the general population and upward of 30% of those with diabetes.[2,3] Adhesive capsulitis (AC) primarily affects women between the ages of 40 and 60.[4] It is considered

Table 6-1 THREE STAGES OF PRIMARY ADHESIVE CAPSULITIS		
Stage	Duration	Clinical Features
1. Freezing	2.5-9 mo[5,6]	Constant pain; worse at night Gradual loss of motion
2. Frozen	4-12 mo[5,6]	Joint stiffness (loss of motion) Pain may decrease, but intensifies at end ranges of motion
3. Thawing	5-26 mo[5] 12-42 mo[6]	Restoration of motion and function

a self-limiting condition with some patients experiencing a gradual resolution of symptoms without treatment.

There are two types of AC: primary (idiopathic) and secondary. Patients experiencing pain and stiffness with no history of trauma or surgery are diagnosed with primary AC. Those with shoulder stiffness due to a history of trauma or surgery in the shoulder region are diagnosed with secondary AC. It is currently believed that the two types are unique entities sharing only the similarities in pain and loss of shoulder range of motion.[2]

There are three stages associated with primary AC; each stage varies in length and can overlap other stages (Table 6-1). The first stage is associated with an insidious, gradual onset of pain and stiffness in the shoulder. The patient may describe increased pain at night, especially when attempting to sleep on the involved shoulder. The second stage is associated with reduced shoulder pain, except for an increase in pain intensity at the end ranges of available motion. During the final stage, a patient may experience a gradual and spontaneous restoration of pain-free motion.

Our understanding of the pathophysiology associated with primary AC has evolved from Neviaser's initial description in 1945.[7] Based on surgical findings, the loss of shoulder motion associated with AC was thought to be the result of the axillary fold adhering to itself and to the humerus at the anatomic neck.[2,7] However, AC is now believed to be the result of abnormal production of **cytokines**.[8,9] Excessive cytokine activity has been shown to increase the activity of fibroblasts, which may cause thickening and contracture of the anterior shoulder capsule.[10] The loss of motion associated with AC is the result of contracture of the following shoulder structures: coracohumeral ligament, rotator interval, and the anterior and inferior capsules.[2] Adhesive capsulitis in individuals with diabetes mellitus results from a unique biochemical pathogenesis; however, further studies are needed.[2]

Examination, Evaluation, and Diagnosis

Diagnosis is based on patient history and motion testing of the shoulder. Observation of the patient may reveal disuse atrophy of the deltoid muscle. The patient may hold her arm in a position of comfort against the side of the body.[6]

Patients with AC present with significant loss of active and passive shoulder range of motion. The glenohumeral **loss of motion pattern** historically associated

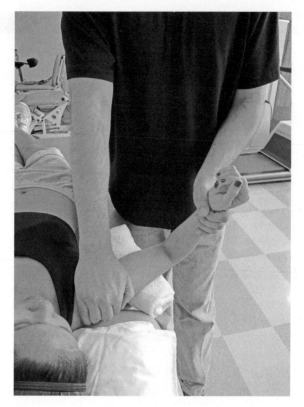

Figure 6-1. Physical therapist assessing glenohumeral external rotation passive range of motion.

with AC is external rotation presenting the greatest loss of motion (as a percentage of the contralateral uninvolved shoulder), followed by loss of abduction, and finally loss of internal rotation.[11,12] However, recent reports suggest that there is *not* a consistent order of motion loss; the loss of external rotation motion is the primary restriction observed in all patients with AC.[12-14] Assessment of glenohumeral (GH) passive range of motion is performed with the patient lying supine. The physical therapist supports the involved upper extremity to assess passive external rotation of the GH joint (Fig. 6-1). The end feel associated with AC is a firm (capsular) end point that is reproducible. Passive motion testing and goniometry should be performed for all cardinal motions.

Carbone et al.[15] have proposed a clinical test to diagnose AC. The **coracoid pain test** (CPT) is performed by applying digital pressure to the coracoid process (Fig. 6-2). A positive test is associated with pain at the coracoid process that is greater than pain (by ≥3 points on a visual analog scale) experienced when applying digital pressure to the ipsilateral acromioclavicular joint and to the anterolateral subacromial region. When compared against asymptomatic adults, the CPT had a sensitivity of 0.99 (95% CI = 0.99-1.00) and a specificity of 0.98 (95% CI = 0.97-0.99). When the test was performed on clients with other common shoulder

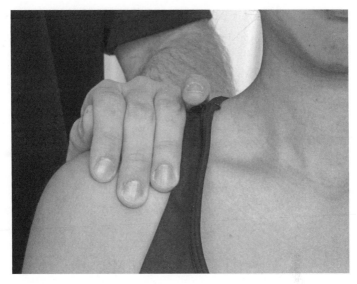

Figure 6-2. Coracoid pain test.

conditions (*e.g.*, calcific tendonitis, rotator cuff tear, acromioclavicular arthritis, GH arthritis), the CPT had a sensitivity of 96% and a specificity of 87% to 89%.[15]

Plan of Care and Interventions

The physical therapy plan of care and interventions are discussed in Case 7. The patient should be referred to an orthopaedic physician while physical therapy treatment is continued.

Concurrent, nonoperative treatments may include glucocorticoid injection(s) into the joint and/or oral administration of nonsteroidal anti-inflammatory drugs and/or glucocorticoids.[16,17]

Evidence-Based Clinical Recommendations

SORT: Strength of Recommendation Taxonomy
A: Consistent, good-quality patient-oriented evidence
B: Inconsistent or limited-quality patient-oriented evidence
C: Consensus, disease-oriented evidence, usual practice, expert opinion, or case series

1. Abnormal excessive cytokine activity increases fibroblastic activity that is associated with fibrosis and contracture of the anterior shoulder capsule. **Grade B**

2. There is a consistent order of glenohumeral joint range of motion loss associated with adhesive capsulitis. **Grade C**

3. The coracoid pain test accurately identifies patients with adhesive capsulitis. **Grade B**

COMPREHENSION QUESTIONS

6.1 Which of the cardinal motions experiences the greatest loss of passive motion (as a percentage of the contralateral shoulder) in adhesive capsulitis?

A. Shoulder abduction

B. Shoulder external rotation

C. Shoulder internal rotation

D. Shoulder flexion

6.2 Which of the following statements correctly identifies the differences between primary and secondary adhesive capsulitis (AC)?

A. Primary AC is due to trauma whereas secondary AC is due to surgery.

B. In general, the pain experienced by those with a diagnosis of secondary AC is greater than the pain intensity experienced by those with primary AC.

C. Primary AC is idiopathic and secondary AC is due to either surgery or trauma.

D. External rotation range of motion is significantly decreased in those with secondary AC, but not in those with primary AC.

ANSWERS

6.1 **B.** In AC, the greatest overall loss of motion is in shoulder external rotation due to contracture of the anterior and inferior shoulder structures (coracohumeral ligament, rotator interval, and anterior and inferior capsules). Arthroscopic surgical release of the rotator interval may help to rapidly restore external rotation range of motion.

6.2 **C.** Primary AC is idiopathic in nature; there is no known trauma related to the onset of the condition.

REFERENCES

1. Zuckerman J, Rokito S. Frozen shoulder: a consensus approach. *J Shoulder Elbow Surg.* 2011;20:322-325.

2. Hsu JE, Anakwenze OA, Warrender WJ, Abboud JA. Current review of adhesive capsulitis. *J Shoulder Elbow Surg.* 2011;20:502-514.

3. Balci N, Balci MK, Tuzuner S. Shoulder adhesive capsulitis and shoulder range of motion in type II diabetes mellitus: association with diabetic complications. *J Diabetes Complications.* 1999;13:135-140.

4. Hand C, Clipsham K, Rees JL, Carr AJ. Long-term outcome of frozen shoulder. *J Shoulder Elbow Surgery.* 2008;17:231-236.

5. Rizk TE, Pinals RS. Frozen shoulder. *Semin Arthritis Rheum.* 1982;11:440-452.

6. Dias R, Cutts S, Massoud S. Frozen shoulder. *BMJ.* 2005;331:1453-1456.

7. Neviaser JS. Adhesive capsulitis of the shoulder: a study of pathological findings in periarthritis of the shoulder. *J Bone Joint Surg Am.* 1945;27:211-222.

8. Rodeo SA, Hannafin JA, Tom J, Warren RF, Wickiewicz TL. Immunolocalization of cytokines and their receptors in adhesive capsulitis of the shoulder. *J Orthop Res.* 1997;15:427-436.

9. Bunker TD, Reilly J, Baird KS, Hamblen DL. Expression of growth factors, cytokines and matrix metalloproteinases in frozen shoulder. *J Bone Joint Surg Br.* 2000;82:768-773.

10. Gharaee-Kermani M, Phan SH. Role of cytokines and cytokine therapy in wound healing and fibrotic diseases. *Curr Pharm Des.* 2001;7:1083-1103.

11. Neviaser RJ, Neviaser TJ. The frozen shoulder. Diagnosis and management. *Clin Orthop Relat Res.* 1987;223:59-64.

12. Mitsch J, Casey J, McKinnis R, Kegerreis S, Stikeleather J. Investigation of a consistent pattern of motion restriction in patients with adhesive capsulitis. *J Man Manip Ther.* 2004;12: 153-159.

13. Rundquist PJ, Anderson DD, Guanche CA, Ludewig PM. Shoulder kinematics in subjects with frozen shoulder. *Arch Phys Med Rehabil.* 2003;84:1473-1479.

14. Rundquist PJ, Ludewig PM. Patterns of motion loss in subjects with idiopathic loss of shoulder range of motion. *Clin Biomech.* 2004;19:810-18.

15. Carbone S, Gumina S, Vestri AR, Postacchini R. Coracoid pain test: a new clinical sign of shoulder adhesive capsulitis. *Int Orthop.* 2010;34:385-388.

16. Buchbinder R, Hoving JL, Green S, Hall S, Forbes A, Nash P. Short course prednisolone for adhesive capsulitis (frozen shoulder or stiff painful shoulder): a randomised, double blind, placebo controlled trial. *Ann Rheum Dis.* 2004;63:1460-1469.

17. Lorbach O, Anagnostakos K, Scherf C, Seil R, Kohn D, Pape D. Nonoperative management of adhesive capsulitis of the shoulder: oral cortisone application versus intra-articular cortisone injections. *J Shoulder Elbow Surg.* 2010;19:172-179.

Adhesive Capsulitis—Treatment

Jason Brumitt

The patient's history, symptoms, and examination findings are consistent with a diagnosis of primary adhesive capsulitis (Case 6). Her right shoulder passive range of motion (PROM) is limited to 100° of flexion, 40° of extension, 85° of abduction, 10° of external rotation (ER), and 50° of internal rotation (IR). The PROM of her left (uninvolved) shoulder presents with: flexion 170°, extension 40°, abduction 170°, ER 90°, and IR 70°. Palpation of the right shoulder reveals tenderness at the greater tubercle (rotator cuff insertion site), intertubercular groove, and the coracoid (positive coracoid pain test).

► Describe a physical therapy plan of care based on each stage of the health condition.
► Based on the patient's diagnosis, what are appropriate physical therapy interventions?

KEY DEFINITIONS

ARTHOGRAPHY: Injection of a contrast medium (*e.g.*, Hexabrix and 2% Xylocaine; 1:1 ratio) into a joint (*i.e.*, glenohumeral) performed during fluoroscopy; shoulder arthrogram is performed to assess joint capacity; results may aid in the diagnosis of adhesive capsulitis.

CONSTANT SCORE: Valid and reliable outcome measure for patients with shoulder pathology

KALTENBORN MOBILIZATION GRADING SCALE: I to III graded mobilization scale; grade I technique is a traction mobilization performed to decrease pain. Grade II is a glide or traction mobilization performed to increase joint play and decrease pain. Grade III is performed to increase joint play at end range.[1]

MAITLAND MOBILIZATION GRADING SCALE: I to V graded mobilization scale; oscillatory mobilizations are performed with grades I to IV; a high-velocity low-amplitude thrust is performed with grade V; purpose of grades I and II mobilizations is to decrease pain, whereas purpose of grades III to V mobilizations is to increase joint mobility.[2]

MOBILIZATION: Skilled, passive movement of a synovial joint performed by a therapist for the purpose of decreasing pain and/or improving joint range of motion

MULLIGAN MOBILIZATIONS WITH MOVEMENT: Joint mobilization technique that consists of active movement performed by the patient when a mobilization force is provided by the physical therapist

PRIMARY ADHESIVE CAPSULITIS (AC): Musculoskeletal shoulder condition of unknown etiology marked by significant restriction in active and passive range of motion

Objectives

1. Describe appropriate physical therapy interventions for patients with primary AC.
2. Compare outcomes between treatment approaches reported in the literature.
3. Describe treatments that may be prescribed or performed by orthopaedic physicians.

Physical Therapy Considerations

PT considerations during treatment of the individual with a diagnosis of primary adhesive capsulitis:

▶ **General physical therapy plan of care/goals:** Decrease pain; increase muscular flexibility, range of motion, accessory joint movement, and upper quadrant strength; prevent or minimize loss of aerobic fitness capacity

▶ **Physical therapy interventions:** Patient education regarding functional anatomy and injury pathomechanics; modalities and manual therapy to decrease pain;

muscular flexibility exercises; self-mobilization exercises to increase range of motion; resistance exercises to increase muscular endurance of the scapular stabilizers and to increase strength of the upper extremity muscles; aerobic exercise program

▶ **Precautions during physical therapy:** Monitor vital signs; adhere to postsurgical contraindications if patient has surgical release or manipulation under anesthesia; monitor patient response to therapist-performed stretching and/or manual therapy

Plan of Care and Interventions

Nonoperative treatments for primary AC include physical therapy (exercise, manual therapy, modalities), nonsteroidal anti-inflammatory drugs, oral glucocorticoids, sodium hyaluronate injections, and glucocorticoid injections.[3-15] Some patients may be receiving two or more nonoperative treatments at any one time. If a patient fails to improve with conservative measures, an orthopaedic physician may consider a surgical release or a manipulation under anesthesia.[16,17]

Therapeutic modalities (e.g., ultrasound, moist heat, cryotherapy, electrical stimulation) are frequently utilized when treating patients with AC. However, their primary use is as an adjunct to therapeutic exercise and manual therapy techniques.[18] Thermal agents may be used at the start of a treatment session to increase collagen extensibility prior to manual therapy or performance of therapeutic exercise.[19,20] Cryotherapy and electrical modalities may help decrease pain at the end of a treatment session.[7]

Joint mobilization techniques have traditionally been included in the plan of care for the patient with AC. It is thought that mobilization techniques help mobilize the adhered capsule. Certain **manual therapy techniques** have been shown to improve shoulder range of motion (ROM) in patients with AC (Table 7-1).

The manual therapy techniques that have been studied on patients with AC are low-grade and high-grade glenohumeral mobilizations (Maitland grades I-IV), sustained end-range mobilizations (Kaltenborn grade III), mobilizations with movement (Mulligan), effleurage, and other soft tissue mobilization techniques.[19,21-24] Johnson et al.[19] randomized adults with primary AC into two groups: a group receiving anterior glide mobilizations to the glenohumeral (GH) joint ($n = 10$) and a group receiving posterior glide mobilizations to the GH joint ($n = 8$). The protocol consisted of thermal ultrasound to the shoulder capsule, followed by shoulder mobilizations, and 3 minutes of upper body ergometry (UBE). Stretch mobilizations (Kaltenborn grade III) were performed in either an anterior (Fig. 7-1) or posterior (Fig. 7-2) direction (with the shoulder positioned into end-range abduction and external rotation). Each sustained mobilization was held for 1 minute. A total of 15 mobilization repetitions were performed during each of the 6 treatment sessions. Although anterior glide mobilizations might have been expected to provide superior ROM gains because a sustained mobilization force in an anterior direction should have had a greater effect on the fibrotic anterior capsule, the subjects in the *posterior* glide mobilization group experienced statistically significant mean improvement in

Table 7-1 SUMMARY OF MANUAL THERAPY-BASED STUDIES FOR THE TREATMENT OF PRIMARY AC

Author(s) (Year)	Study Design	Participants (symptom duration)	Manual Techniques (and additional treatments)	Outcomes
Vermeulen et al. (2000)	Case series	7 patients (3 women; mean age 50.2 ± 6.0 y) with AC diagnosed by orthopaedic surgeon Symptom duration: mean 8.4 mo; range 3-12 mo	End-range glenohumeral mobilization techniques: grades III and IV	Improvements in glenohumeral AROM and PROM
Wies (2005)	Case series	8 patients (6 women) with AC diagnosed by a rheumatologist Symptom duration ≥ 3 mo	Soft tissue mobilization: effleurage, prolonged soft-tissue approximation, cross-friction, sustained pressure, home exercise program consisting of stretching and strengthening exercises	Significant improvement in AROM (flexion, abduction, ER, and composite total)
Vermeulen et al. (2006)	Randomized controlled trial	100 patients: high-grade mobilization techniques (HGMT; $n = 49$; mean age 51.6 ± 7.6 y) and LGMT (n = 51; 51.7 ± 8.6 y) Symptom duration: HGMT 8 mo (range 5-14.5 mo); LGMT 8 mo (range 6-14 mo)	HGMT (grades III and IV) and low-grade mobilization techniques (LGMT, grades I and II) to the glenohumeral joint	HGMT: significant improvement in passive abduction range and active and passive external rotation
Johnson et al. (2007)	Randomized controlled trial	18 patients (14 women) with AC diagnosed by orthopaedic physicians Symptom duration (median and range): group 1: 8.4 mo (2-12 mo); group 2: 10.9 mo (4-60 mo)	Group 1: anterior glenohumeral mobilization; group 2: posterior glenohumeral mobilization (Both groups received ultrasound prior to mobilization and 3 min UBE after mobilization)	Group 2 (posterior mobilization) experienced significant increase in shoulder ER
Yang et al. (2007)	Randomized controlled multiple-treatment trial	28 patients with primary AC; group 1: mean age 53.3 ± 6.5 y; group 2: mean age 58 ± 10.1 y Symptom duration: SD: group 1: 18 ± 8 mo; group 2: 22 ± 10 mo)	End range mobilization (ERM), mid-range mobilization (MRM), and mobilization with movement (MWM)	ROM gains were statistically greater with use of ERM and MWM techniques

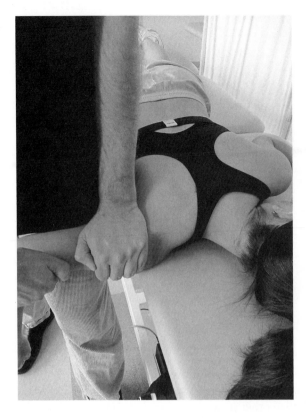

Figure 7-1. Anterior glenohumeral mobilization.

shoulder ER (31°) whereas those in the anterior glide mobilization did not experience significant mean improvement in shoulder ER (3°).

The use of oscillation mobilization techniques has also been reported to improve ROM in patients with AC. Vermeulen et al.[21] performed grades III and IV (Maitland) mobilizations to the GH joint for 30 minutes, twice per week for 3 months. Improvements in active range of motion (AROM), PROM, and GH joint capacity (measured by arthrography) occurred at the end of the 3-month treatment period. A subsequent study compared outcomes between groups based on mobilization intensity.[22] One group was treated with high-grade mobilization techniques (HGMT; or Maitland grades III and IV) and the other group was treated with low-grade mobilization techniques (LGMT; or Maitland grades I and II). Patients were treated for 30 minutes, twice per week, for up to 12 weeks. Subjects in the HGMT group had significant improvements in shoulder active and passive ER and passive abduction. Although the HGMT group had greater ROM improvements compared to the LGMT group in these motions, the authors suggested that for patients who wish to avoid the pain that may be associated with HGMT, they may still be able to make improvements with a LGMT approach.[22]

Based on the aforementioned studies, it appears that manual therapy techniques should be included as part of a physical therapy treatment program for patients with primary AC. However, there are two major limitations to these

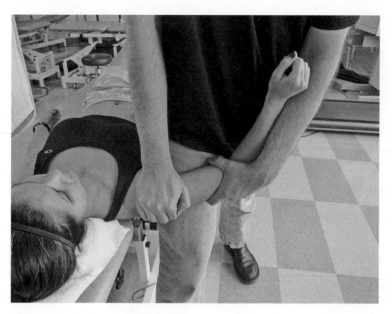

Figure 7-2. Posterior glenohumeral mobilization.

studies.[25] First, subjects were not homogeneous based on their symptom duration. There are three stages of primary AC: freezing, frozen, and thawing. Each stage varies in length and can overlap other stages. These studies do not allow conclusions to be drawn about the effect of manual therapy on subjects in each stage of AC. It is possible that some subjects in the freezing or frozen stages failed to experience changes in AROM or PROM with treatment, whereas subjects in the thawing phase may have experienced increases in ROM due to the natural history of the condition and not due to the manual techniques performed. The second limitation to these investigations is the lack of either a nonmanual therapy comparison group or a control group. The lack of a nonmanual therapy comparison group limits the ability to determine the efficacy of these treatments as part of a comprehensive therapy program. The lack of a control group comparison limits the ability to determine the efficacy of these treatments against the natural history of this condition.

Therapeutic **exercises, specifically stretching and self-mobilization exercises** are frequently prescribed to patients with AC.[5,10,13,14,16,20,26,27] Miller et al.[20] reported that a two-phase conservative treatment program successfully restored ROM in most patients with AC. Phase I consisted of rest, use of a sling, moist heat, and the use of prescription anti-inflammatory and/or opiate medications. The purpose of phase I was to decrease pain prior to initiating the exercises in phase II. Passive range of motion and active assisted ROM exercises (*i.e.*, wall climb, posterior capsule stretch, pendulum, overhead pulley, and cane exercises for flexion, extension, internal rotation, and external rotation) were prescribed. Griggs et al.[26] assessed the benefits of a four-exercise stretching program in patients who were diagnosed with stage II AC (frozen stage). Seventy-five adults (58 females) with a mean duration of 9.2 months (range, 1.3-47 months) of pain were prescribed the following exercises: supine passive forward-elevation stretch, supine passive external rotation stretch, passive horizontal adduction stretch, and a passive behind-the-back internal rotation stretch. The majority of patients reported satisfactory outcomes (90%) with only five requiring arthroscopic capsular release or manipulation under anesthesia. Patients with self-reported satisfactory outcomes experienced significant improvements in AROM and PROM.

These two studies demonstrated the potential value of prescribing stretching exercises to patients with AC; however, they shared similar internal validity threats to those in the manual therapy studies. To date, only one investigation has compared a stretching program against a more "aggressive" physical therapy routine. Diercks et al.[27] compared the effects of a "supervised neglect" program and a "standardized treatment protocol." Subjects in the supervised neglect group were educated about the natural course of the condition, prescribed pendulum and active exercises within a pain-free range, and advised to continue participation in all other activities as tolerated. The subjects in the standardized treatment group were passively stretched and the affected GH joint was manipulated by a physical therapist. In addition, all subjects were prescribed an exercise program consisting of active exercises to be performed *above* their pain threshold. The authors concluded that a program of supervised neglect was superior to the standard treatment program. After 1 year, 64% of subjects in the supervised neglect group had achieved a good outcome (a score of 80 on the Constant Score test), whereas none of the subjects in the standardized treatment group had reached this goal. At 2 years, 89% in the supervised neglect group and 63% in the standardized treatment group achieved this goal. This study appears to be the first to compare a pain-free self-stretching program to an intensive, pain-provoking physical therapy program. Despite the strengths of this study (*e.g.*, longitudinal, comparison between groups), various threats to internal validity may have introduced bias. First, this was a quasi-experimental study of successive cohorts instead of a randomized controlled trial. Second, the authors did not provide details regarding the mobilization techniques or grades that were employed. In addition, they failed to adequately describe the prescribed exercises. Third, the number of treatment sessions was not reported for the groups. Finally, the authors prescribed anti-inflammatory medication and/or analgesics to patients in each group as needed; however, details regarding how many subjects were prescribed medications or dosages taken were not provided.

Additional investigations are warranted to identify the best treatment or combination of treatments for patients with primary AC. In addition, a major question to be answered is whether there are specific treatment strategies based on the stage of the condition. Kelley et al.[10] have proposed a treatment strategy based on the irritability (high, moderate, or low) of the joint. They recommended that a highly irritable joint should be treated with modalities, pain-free PROM, and active assisted ROM exercises (Table 7-2), and low-grade (grades I and II) mobilizations. As the tissue

Table 7-2   STRETCHING/ROM EXERCISES FREQUENTLY PRESCRIBED TO PATIENTS WITH PRIMARY AC

Exercise	Alternate Positions
Pendulum exercises	Pendulum exercise with hand of involved shoulder weightbearing on Physioball
Supine overhead stretch using opposite arm (Fig. 7-3)	1. Sitting with arm supported on table (Fig. 7-4) 2. Standing shoulder forward flexion with arms placed on Physioball
Supine external rotation stretch with wand (Fig. 7-5)	Sitting with arm supported on table and using wand to assist shoulder external rotation
Overhead pulleys	Wall walks
Sleeper stretch (Fig. 7-6)	1. Cross arm adduction stretch 2. Arm behind back stretch

becomes less irritable (moderate stage), the intensity of ROM/stretching exercises may be progressed along with the progression from low-grade to high-grade (Maitland grades III and IV) mobilizations. Finally, at the low irritability stage, high-grade mobilizations (Maitland) and sustained holds (Kaltenborn) can be added.[10] This strategy incorporates the successful treatment programs that utilized either pain-free ROM exercises or manual therapy techniques. To determine the efficacy of a stage-specific therapeutic program, researchers will need to progress patients based on specific diagnostic criteria instead of therapist impression.

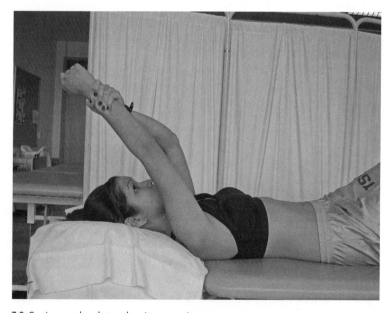

Figure 7-3. Supine overhead stretch using opposite arm.

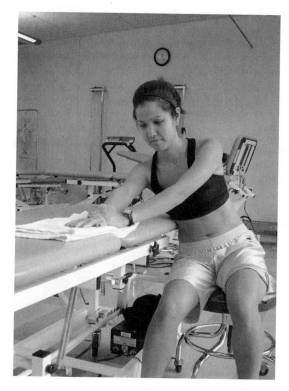

Figure 7-4. Sitting with arm supported on table.

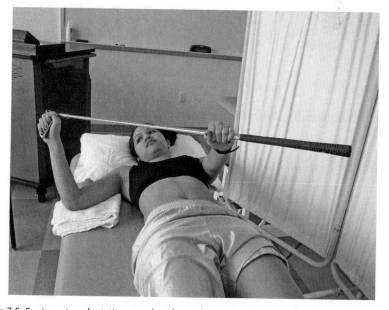

Figure 7-5. Supine external rotation stretch with wand.

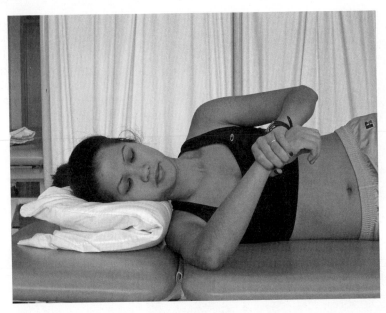

Figure 7-6. Sleeper stretch.

Evidence-Based Clinical Recommendations

SORT: Strength of Recommendation Taxonomy
A: Consistent, good-quality patient-oriented evidence
B: Inconsistent or limited-quality patient-oriented evidence
C: Consensus, disease-oriented evidence, usual practice, expert opinion, or case series

1. Modalities increase shoulder ROM and/or decrease pain in patients with adhesive capsulitis. **Grade C**

2. Sustained stretch or oscillatory mobilization techniques increase shoulder ROM in patients with AC. **Grade B**

3. Stretching exercises (self-mobilization) are superior to manual therapy techniques in increasing shoulder ROM and improving function in patients with AC. **Grade B**

COMPREHENSION QUESTIONS

7.1 Joint mobilization techniques are used to increase shoulder PROM and AROM in patients with AC. Which technique used by Johnson et al. significantly increased shoulder ER?

    A.   Anterior glide end-range mobilizations (Kaltenborn grade III)

    B.   Posterior glide low-grade mobilizations (Maitland grades I and II)

    C.   Anterior glide low-grade mobilizations (Maitland grades I and II)

    D.   Posterior glide end-range mobilizations (Kaltenborn grade III)

7.2 Patients with primary AC present with significant loss of ROM, especially shoulder ER. During the first treatment session, the physical therapist wants to prescribe a stretch to increase shoulder ER. The patient is unable to assume a supine position secondary to a pre-existing low back injury. Of the following four exercises, which one would be *most* appropriate to address shoulder ER deficits?

A. Sitting with involved extremity supported on table (elbow at 90°) using a wand to passively mobilize the shoulder into ER

B. Overhead pulleys

C. Sleeper stretch

D. Wall walks

ANSWERS

7.1 **D.**

7.2 **A.** The other positions are performed to increase shoulder elevation/flexion (options B and D) or internal rotation (option C).

REFERENCES

1. Kaltenborn FM, Evjenth O, Kaltenborn TB, Vollowitz E. *The Spine. Basic Evaluation and Mobilization Techniques.* 2nd ed. Oslo, Norway: Olaf Norlis Bokhandel; 1993.

2. Hengeveld E, Banks K, Maitland GD. *Maitland's Peripheral Manipulation.* 4th ed. Edinburgh, United Kingdom: Butterworths Heinemann; 2005.

3. Bal A, Eksioglu E, Gulec B, Aydog E, Gurcay E, Cakci A. Effectiveness of corticosteroid injection in adhesive capsulitis. *Clin Rehabil.* 2008;22:503-512.

4. Bell AD, Conaway D. Corticosteroid injections for painful shoulders. *Int J Clin Pract.* 2005;59:1178-1186.

5. Blanchard V, Barr S, Cerisola FL. The effectiveness of corticosteroid injections compared with physiotherapeutic interventions for adhesive capsulitis: a systematic review. *Physiotherapy.* 2010;96:95-107.

6. Calis M, Demir H, Ulker S, Kirnap M, Duygulu F, Calis HT. Is intraarticular sodium hyaluronate injection an alternative treatment in patients with adhesive capsulitis? *Rheumatol Int.* 2006;26:536-540.

7. Cheing GL, So EM, Chao CY. Effectiveness of electroacupuncture and interferential electrotherapy in the management of frozen shoulder. *J Rehabil Med.* 2008;40:166-170.

8. Dias R, Cutts S, Massoud S. Frozen shoulder. *BMJ.* 2005;331:1453-1456.

9. Gulick DT, Borger A, McNamee L. Effect of analgesic nerve block electrical stimulation in a patient with adhesive capsulitis. *Physiother Theory Pract.* 2007;23:57-63.

10. Kelley MJ, McClure PW, Leggin BG. Frozen shoulder: evidence and a proposed model guiding rehabilitation. *J Orthop Sports Phys Ther.* 2009;39:135-148.

11. Levine WN, Kashyap CP, Bak SF, Ahmad CS, Blaine TA, Bigliani LU. Nonoperative management of idiopathic adhesive capsulitis. *J Shoulder Elbow Surg.* 2007;16:569-573.

12. Lorbach O, Anagnostakos K, Scherf C, Seil R, Kohn D, Pape D. Nonoperative management of adhesive capsulitis of the shoulder: oral cortisone application versus intra-articular cortisone injections. *J Shoulder Elbow Surg.* 2010;19:172-179.

13. Harrast MA, Rao AG. The stiff shoulder. *Phys Med Rehabil Clin N Am*. 2004;15:557-573.

14. Neviaser AS, Hannafin JA. Adhesive capsulitis: a review of current treatment. *Am J Sports Med*. 2010;38:2346-2356.

15. Yilmazlar A, Turker G, Atici T, Bilgen S, Bilgen OF. Functional results of conservative therapy accompanied by interscalene brachial plexus block and patient-controlled analgesia in cases with frozen shoulder. *Acta Orthop Traumatol Turc*. 2010;44:105-110.

16. Hsu JE, Anakwenze OA, Warrender WJ, Abboud JA. Current review of adhesive capsulitis. *J Shoulder Elbow Surg*. 2011;20:502-514.

17. Tasto JP, Elias DW. Adhesive capsulitis. *Sports Med Arthrosc*. 2007;15:216-221.

18. Jewell DV, Riddle DL, Thacker LR. Increased or decreased likelihood of pain reduction and improved function in patients with adhesive capsulitis: a retrospective cohort study. *Phys Ther*. 2009;89: 419-429.

19. Johnson AJ, Godges JJ, Zimmerman GJ, Ounanian LL. The effect of anterior versus posterior glide joint mobilization on external rotation range of motion in patients with shoulder adhesive capsulitis. *J Orthop Sports Phys Ther*. 2007;37:88-99.

20. Miller MD, Wirth MA, Rockwood CA Jr. Thawing the frozen shoulder: the "patient" patient. *Orthopedics*. 1996;19:849-853.

21. Vermeulen HM, Obermann WR, Burger BJ, Kok GJ, Rozing PM, van Den Ende CH. End-range mobilization techniques in adhesive capsulitis of the shoulder joint: a multiple-subject case report. *Phys Ther*. 2000;80:1204-1213.

22. Vermeulen HM, Rozing PM, Obermann WR, le Cessie S, Vliet Vlieland TP. Comparison of high-grade and low-grade mobilization techniques in the management of adhesive capsulitis of the shoulder: randomized controlled trial. *Phys Ther*. 2006;86:355-368.

23. Wies J. Treatment of eight patients with frozen shoulder: a case study series. *J Bodyw Mov Ther*. 2005;9:58-64.

24. Yang JL, Chang CW, Chen SY, Wang SF, Lin JJ. Mobilization techniques in subjects with frozen shoulder syndrome: randomized multiple-treatment trial. *Phys Ther*. 2007;87:1307-1315.

25. Brumitt J. [Commentary on] The effect of anterior versus posterior glide joint mobilization on external rotation range of motion in patients with shoulder adhesive capsulitis. *NZ J Physiother*. 2008;36:29-30.

26. Griggs SM, Ahn A, Green A. Idiopathic adhesive capsulitis. A prospective functional outcome study of nonoperative treatment. *J Bone J Surg*. 2000;82-A:1398-1407.

27. Diercks RL, Stevens M. Gentle thawing of the frozen shoulder: a prospective study of supervised neglect versus intensive physical therapy in seventy-seven patients with frozen shoulder syndrome followed up for two years. *J Shoulder Elbow Surg*. 2004;13:499-502.

Chronic Cervical Spine Pain

Jake Bleacher

A 43-year-old female was referred to outpatient physical therapy for chronic neck pain by her family physician. The patient has worked as an administrative assistant for the past 20 years. Her initial onset of neck pain was 2 years ago with a significant increase in pain in the past 6 months. On the visual analog scale, she reports a pain score of 2/10 at the beginning of the day, which worsens to 10/10 by the end of the day. She describes her symptoms as "tightness" and "aching" extending from the superior scapula and shoulder up toward her neck and occipital area. She reports recently having headaches and an "aching" pain radiating into her dominant right arm by the end of the day. Her day consists of sitting at a computer 75% of the time and using the computer mouse 50% of that time. Her workload has increased 2 to 3 hours per day (overtime) due to staffing shortages over the past 6 months. She denies any significant medical history or trauma to the cervical spine and her cervical x-rays are unremarkable. She reports a small improvement in her symptoms over the last week since she started taking a nonsteroidal anti-inflammatory medication and a muscle relaxant prescribed by her family physician. She states that her physical activity level (*e.g.*, exercising or participating in recreational sports) has declined the past 2 years due to her busy schedule.

▶ Based on the patient's diagnosis, what do you anticipate may be the contributing factors to her condition?
▶ What are the most appropriate physical therapy outcome measures for neck pain?
▶ What are the most appropriate physical therapy interventions?
▶ What are possible complications interfering with physical therapy?
▶ What are the concerns regarding the pain radiating into her arm and shoulder?

KEY DEFINITIONS

ELONGATED MUSCLE: Lengthening of a muscle secondary to being in a sustained elongated position for prolonged period of time

ERGONOMIC INTERVENTION: Workstation assessment performed to determine risk of injury and/or symptoms, followed by implementation of workstation modifications to decrease musculoskeletal symptoms

FORWARD HEAD POSTURE: Position of the head is markedly anterior to an imaginary line bisecting the glenohumeral joint in which the mid- and lower-cervical spine are flexed and the upper cervical spine is extended

MYOFASCIAL TRIGGER POINT: Knots or nodes that form within a taut band of muscle or at myotendinous junctions

NEUROMUSCULAR CONTROL: Integration of peripheral sensations relative to joint position and processing this information into an effective efferent motor response

POSTURAL NECK PAIN: Pain associated with sustained static loading of the cervical spine and shoulder girdle during occupational or leisure activities

POSTURE: Segmental alignment of the body at rest or in equilibrium and the forces acting upon the body

Objectives

1. Describe postural neck pain and its contributing factors.
2. Describe components of the musculoskeletal examination that would assist in ruling in postural neck pain and ruling out cervical and/or shoulder conditions.
3. Prescribe appropriate treatment interventions for the patient with postural neck pain.
4. Identify factors complicating the treatment of patients with postural neck pain.
5. Describe key elements in designing a work style intervention for a patient with postural neck pain.
6. List risk factors for the development of postural neck pain.

Physical Therapy Considerations

PT considerations during management of the individual with postural cervical pain:

▶ **General physical therapy plan of care/goals:** Decrease pain; increase muscular flexibility and strength; improve postural awareness and correction strategies

▶ **Physical therapy interventions:** Manual therapy to decrease pain, decrease circulatory stasis and improve muscle and joint flexibility; patient education regarding symptoms and cause and effect of chronic sustained postures; postural and movement correction strategies to minimize postural stress; exercises to improve muscular strength and endurance in cervical and shoulder girdle stabilizing muscles; stress management; work and computer station modifications to minimize postural strain

▶ **Precautions during physical therapy:** Rule out possibility of significant cervical pathology including cervical disc herniation, spondylosis, thoracic outlet syndrome, cervical stenosis, and nonmusculoskeletal causes of pain; monitor vital signs; address precautions or contraindications for exercise

▶ **Complications interfering with physical therapy:** Failure to break the pain cycle due to patient's inability to minimize continuous hours at the computer or take substantial rest periods

Understanding the Health Condition

Postural neck pain (PNP) is associated with activities that cause prolonged low-level static exertions of the cervical spine and shoulder girdle.[1] Postural neck pain is common in individuals who work primarily on computers or at video display terminals. Based on studies in Australia and Sweden, prevalence ranges from 20% to 63% with a higher rate in female office workers.[2] Epidemiologic studies examining risks associated with musculoskeletal disorders of the neck and shoulder have found strong correlations between longer duration of computer usage and higher prevalence rates of neck and arm symptoms.[3-5] In a study of more than a thousand high school computer users, frequent computer exposure was the one consistent predictor of developing neck pain.[5] Additional risk factors for the development of PNP are psychosocial stress, wearing bifocal lenses, using a computer mouse for extended periods of time, and prolonged bouts of computer use without a rest period.[4] The physical demands of computer work impose low-level static exertions in which there is little to no relaxation phase for the muscles involved. Muscles that are commonly painful in individuals with PNP include splenius capitis and cervicis, upper trapezius, levator scapulae, sternocleidomastoid, and the scalenes. The head and neck postures typically adopted with prolonged computer use affect these muscles because they span the shoulder girdle and cervical and thoracic spinal regions. The effects of sustained low-load forces can cause creep—the time-dependent deformation to soft tissues.[5,6] This low-level mechanical tissue deformation may result in an inflammatory process, stimulation of nociceptors in symptomatic tissues, and the development of myofascial trigger points.[1] When these low-level stresses are applied over a long period of time, it can cause excessive wear to the articular surfaces, stretching of the ligaments, and the development of osteophytes and bone spurs.[7]

Symptom chronicity may promote altered neuromuscular recruitment and activation patterns in muscles that are frequently symptomatic in patients with PNP. Szeto et al.[8] found that individuals with neck pain related to computer use had aberrant muscle activation patterns in the upper trapezius as well as frequent movement into scapular protraction compared to an asymptomatic control group. In fact, postural muscles of symptomatic individuals work harder and longer when using a computer mouse. Szeto et al.[9] used electromyography (EMG) to measure the contraction frequency and amplitude of the upper trapezius and erector spinae. They found that individuals with PNP had significantly higher levels of muscle contraction and fewer periods of rest in their upper trapezius and erector spinae compared to asymptomatic individuals with similar exposure working at a computer. In a study of individuals with chronic neck pain, Falla et al.[9,10] showed altered motor strategies in the deep cervical flexors (longus colli and longus capitis) during a functional reach test. The subjects with chronic PNP demonstrated increased latency in the feed-forward contraction of the deep cervical flexors necessary for joint support and control. In addition, the superficial muscles (scalene and sternocleidomastoid) of those with PNP exhibited increased activity and fatigability along with a lack of coordinated activation with the deep cervical flexors.[10]

Individuals with chronic PNP also exhibit poor postural and kinesthetic awareness. In a study by Edmondston et al.[11], individuals with chronic PNP had a different perception of "good posture" than asymptomatic individuals. Symptomatic individuals demonstrated a protracted head position and more upper cervical extension than the asymptomatic group. Falla et al.[12] demonstrated similar findings: individuals with PNP had a reduced ability to maintain an erect neutral spine posture when performing a typing task. Key **intrinsic factors** contributing to the perpetuation of chronic postural cervical pain include differences in neuromuscular control and decreased postural awareness.[13] **Extrinsic factors** contributing to PNP include the workstation setup (*e.g.*, seating, keyboard, monitor, mouse), frequency and duration of time spent working at the computer, and psychosocial factors such as stress involved with high work demands and decreased rest periods.[14,15]

Physical Therapy Patient/Client Management

Physical therapy management of patients with chronic PNP is multifaceted, and may include the use of modalities, soft tissue and joint mobilization, therapeutic exercises, postural correction strategies, and ergonomic interventions.[2,4,6,14-16] The patient should also be taught behavioral modifications to reduce stress and to monitor total time working on the computer.[10,15-18] At the beginning of treatment sessions, modalities and passive treatments (*e.g.*, electrical stimulation, ultrasound, soft tissue and joint mobilization) are often used to decrease pain and muscle guarding. Initially, the prescription of therapeutic exercises should focus on re-educating the deep cervical flexors and postural muscles; later, general strengthening exercises should be introduced.[12] This treatment approach is similar to that used when treating a patient with low back pain in which the initial focus is on activating the local stabilizing muscles (transversus abdominis and multifidi), followed by the prescription of general and functional strengthening exercises.[13] To prevent recurrence of PNP, appropriate management strategies need to be implemented into the treatment program. These include teaching proper ergonomic workstation setup and implementing rest periods and preventative exercises.[13]

Examination, Evaluation, and Diagnosis

Individuals presenting with PNP tend to have symptoms of low to moderate intensity that do not preclude them from completing their functional and work-related tasks. Symptoms of PNP are generally chronic in nature, lacking a history of acute onset or significant trauma. Due to the insidious onset of symptoms, the physical therapist must rule out systemic pathology through a thorough medical history, including any recent health status changes (*e.g.*, unexplained weight loss), nonmechanical pain, and/or a history of cancer.[19] A mechanical source of symptoms has predictable pain patterns and symptoms should be intermittent and mitigated when the underlying stressors are decreased or eliminated. Symptoms of PNP should be worse during sustained activities or postures at computer workstations, and diminished when not performing these activities.[19]

When PNP symptoms radiate into the arm, it is important to rule out more serious pathology including, but not limited to cervical disc herniation, degenerative joint disease, or foraminal stenosis. A neurologic examination including testing of deep tendon reflexes, manual muscle testing of the cervical myotomes, and sensory testing for dermatomal changes must be performed. One of the differential diagnoses that the physical therapist must rule *out* in the patient with PNP is cervical radiculopathy (Table 8-1). A clinical prediction rule for assisting in diagnosis of cervical radiculopathy has been established and found to be reliable.[20] The clinical prediction rule for diagnosis of cervical radiculopathy consists of positive findings on several tests: positive Upper Limb Tension Test (ULTT I), ipsilateral cervical rotation less than 60°, positive cervical spine compression and distraction, and positive Spurling test. These tests are typically *negative* for reproducing peripheral symptoms in individuals presenting with chronic PNP because the source of the pain is myofascial and not neurovascular.[20,21]

Table 8-1	SPECIAL TESTS FOR CERVICAL RADICULOPATHY	
Tests	Patient Position	Findings
Cervical compression	Patient is seated. Therapist stands behind patient with hands folded and resting on crown of head. Therapist gently applies axial load downward. (Fig. 8-1)	Reproduction of pain in the arm or shoulder constitutes a positive test.
Cervical distraction	Patient is seated. Therapist stands behind patient. With the heels of hands under mandible, therapist applies upward vertical distraction force on head on neck. (Fig. 8-2)	Relief of shoulder or upper extremity pain constitutes a positive test.
Spurling test	Patient is seated. Therapist stands behind patient. Patient actively side bends head *toward* affected side. Therapist then applies an axial load on the head in the side bent position. (Fig. 8-3)	Reproduction of arm or neck pain on same side of compression constitutes a positive test.
Upper limb tension test I	Patient is supine. Therapist stands facing patient at shoulder level. Therapist depresses shoulder girdle, abducts the glenohumeral joint to approximately 110°. With patient's elbow flexed at 90°, forearm in neutral rotation and wrist slightly extended, the therapist gently extends elbow wrist and fingers at same time while supinating the forearm. (Fig. 8-4)	Reproduction of upper extremity symptoms constitutes a positive test.

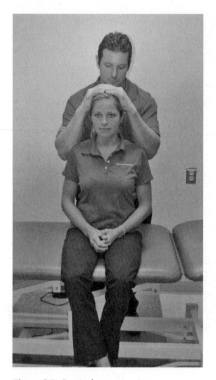

Figure 8-1. Cervical compression.

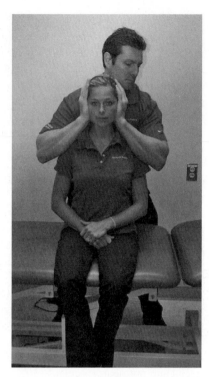

Figure 8-2. Cervical distraction.

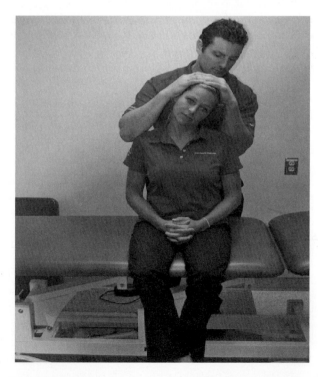

Figure 8-3. Spurling test.

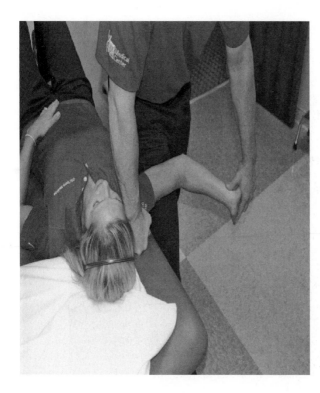

Figure 8-4. Upper limb tension test.

It is critical to observe the patient in her natural posture to be able to gather information on her postural awareness and habits. Valuable information can be gathered by observing the patient in her most relaxed position in the waiting area as well as during the subjective history, when she is less aware that her posture is being assessed.

A detailed standing postural assessment should be performed from anterior, posterior, and lateral views observing for postural deviations and muscular asymmetries.[7] In the *ideal* posture, the ear bisects the acromion and the bodies of the cervical vertebrae. A common posture observed in the patient with PNP is a forward head posture in which the head is anterior to the acromion, shoulders are rounded anteriorly, scapulae are protracted, and the mid- and lower-cervical spine are flexed with compensatory upper cervical extension (Fig. 8-5). Active range of motion (ROM) of the cervical spine should be measured in all directions, noting any limitations and painful responses. The cervical range of motion device (CROM; Performance Attainment Associates, St. Paul, MN) has been found to be reliable in measuring cervical ROM.[20] The CROM is a device that is worn by the patient as a head and spectacle frame with a shoulder-mounted piece. It consists of three gravity-driven dial meters to measure cervical ROM in three axes of movement.[20]

The muscles that typically present with decreased flexibility (adaptive shortening to prolonged poor posture) due to a chronic forward head posture are levator scapulae, sternocleidomastoids, scalenes, suboccipitals, upper trapezius, and pectoralis major and minor. Muscle length or flexibility tests, as well as palpation tests, should be performed to confirm adaptively shortened or lengthened muscles and to

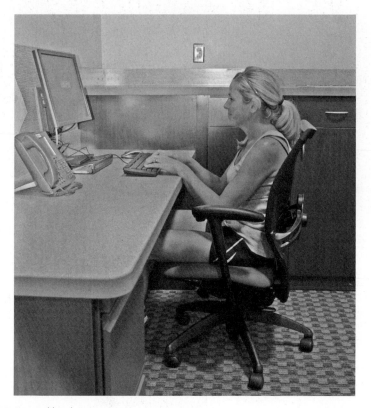

Figure 8-5. Forward head sitting posture.

identify trigger points. Chronic forward head posture typically lengthens lower cervical and thoracic erector spinae, middle and lower trapezius, rhomboids, and deep cervical flexors. The muscles that are lengthened by a chronic forward head posture are typically weaker due to the altered relationship of the contractile elements (actin and myosin) when the muscles are in sustained stretched positions.[22] This pattern of opposing muscle tightness and weakness has been referred to as "upper crossed syndrome." The habitual "poking" chin of the forward head posture causes tightness in upper cervical region and weakness in deep neck flexors, tightness in the anterior chest and shoulders, and weakness in the scapular stabilizers (Fig. 8-5).[7,9,20]

Manual muscle testing must be performed to confirm weakness in the muscles commonly lengthened (middle and lower trapezius, rhomboids, and deep neck flexors) in patients presenting with chronic forward head posture. Due to the importance of the deep cervical flexors in maintaining ideal cervical posture, an assessment of the strength and endurance of the deep cervical flexors should be performed. The supine capital flexion test is performed by having the patient lie supine and raise her head approximately two inches off the table while keeping the chin tucked. The physical therapist records the time she is able to maintain the chin in a tucked position.[17,23] Jull et al.[24] have modified the test by placing a pressure sensor (stabilizer or blood pressure cuff) in the suboccipital region while the patient performs a head

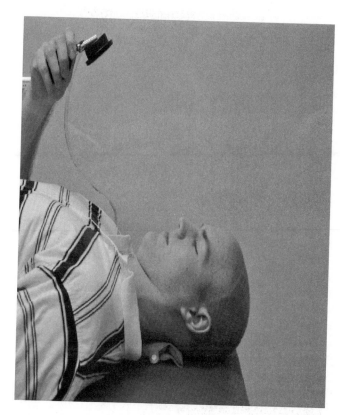

Figure 8-6. Test position for the craniocervical flexion test. The exercise for the deep neck flexors is also performed in this position.

nod, and holds this position for 5 to 10 seconds in five incremental stages starting at a baseline of 20 mm Hg and working to a final level of 30 mm Hg (craniocervical flexion test, Fig. 8-6). If the patient is unable to perform neck flexion with incremental increases in pressure and maintain the position for the allotted time without compensation of the superficial neck flexors (resorting to retraction), this indicates decreased neuromuscular control and endurance of the deep neck flexors.

Joint mobility assessment should be performed to determine areas of cervical and thoracic spine hypomobility. In patients with chronic forward head posture, mobility restrictions are common in the upper cervical and upper- and mid-thoracic regions.[25,26] Fernandez-de-las-Penas et al.[25] found a significant correlation between decreased cervical mobility and patients with forward head posture. Subjects with forward head posture had a significantly decreased mean craniovertebral angle and significant limitations with cervical ROM in almost all directions when compared to a control group. Typically, palpation and spring tests to the involved joint segments are hypomobile and elicit a painful response with accessory motion testing. Jull et al.[27] found excellent inter-examiner reliability between experienced manual therapists in identifying dysfunctional symptomatic joints in the cervical spine.

Last, the physical therapist should assess how the patient performs her occupation. A work style assessment includes looking at the interaction of ergonomic and psychosocial risk factors affecting the development and maintenance of shoulder and neck pain in office workers. There is a complex interaction between biomechanical stressors from poor ergonomics as well as psychosocial stressors involved with high-volume workloads. In a study aimed to address ergonomic issues and psychosocial issues, Bernaards et al.[14,15] found that when ergonomic interventions were coupled with counseling for behavioral modifications to cope with high work demands, office workers had long-term improvements in neck and shoulder pain.

Plan of Care and Interventions

A standardized program of 12 physical therapy sessions over 4 to 6 weeks is recommended to address musculoskeletal impairments, correct faulty posture, and implement appropriate ergonomic interventions.[27-31]

Restoring pain-free ROM through the use of modalities, active range of motion (AROM) exercises, and joint mobilizations to the cervical spine and thoracic spine may alleviate pain, muscle guarding, and circulatory stasis.[30] Loss of cervical AROM, especially cervical retraction and cervical rotation, is common in patients with PNP. Loss of these motions is due to chronic forward head posture and muscular tightness in the superficial cervical and axial skeletal muscles. The performance of frequent gentle cervical retraction and cervical rotation (up to 5 times per day) in a neutral spine position helps restore cervical AROM.[18] If excessive pain or muscle guarding prevents the patient from being able to perform the exercises in a weightbearing position, exercises may be initiated in supine and progress to sitting. To regain normal postural control and alignment, muscles that have become adaptively shortened in the axial skeleton and upper cervical spine need to have adequate muscle flexibility. This can be achieved through static stretching of the muscles, and typically should be performed for 30 seconds each for 2 repetitions, performed 3 times per day (Table 8-2).

Patients with PNP demonstrate impaired activation patterns and endurance in the deep cervical flexors, similar to the dysfunctional activation patterns of the transversus abdominis displayed by patients with low back pain. Jull et al.[24] demonstrated the importance of **improving neuromuscular control and endurance in the deep cervical flexors** in maintaining cervical posture and stabilizing the cervical spine when performing reaching and upper extremity tasks. The training program consisted of low-load activation of the deep flexors using a pressure gauge (Stabilometer, Chattanooga Group Inc, Hixson, TN). Each repetition was held for up to 10 seconds to increase muscular endurance and to avoid activating the superficial cervical muscles. The gauge was set at 20 mm Hg pressure with 10-second holds and increased by incremental steps of 2 mm Hg using color-coded stripes for visual feedback[32] (Fig. 8-6).

Strengthening exercises to improve scapular orientation and muscle recruitment patterns should be prescribed to individuals with PNP. Chronic forward head posture decreases activation in the scapular stabilizers due to aberrant positioning of the scapula from midline.[31] Frequently, the middle and lower trapezius, rhomboids, and serratus anterior have decreased activation patterns in patients experiencing cervical and shoulder pain.[8,31] Similar to training the deep cervical flexors, the stabilizing muscles of the scapulae can be adequately trained with low-load exercises and

Table 8-2   POSTURAL EXERCISES FOR THE PATIENT WITH POSTURAL NECK PAIN

Exercise	Starting Position	Exercise Technique
Cervical retraction	Sitting with fingertips placed on chin (Fig. 8-7)	Push head straight backward until stretch is felt in neck and upper thoracic region. Hold 5-10 s.
Cervical rotation	Sitting with head in a neutral position (not in forward head posture)	Rotate head as far as possible in one direction without pain and apply slight overpressure with your hand in a pain-free range. Hold 5 s. Repeat to other side.
Suboccipital stretch	Supine with 2-3 inch towel roll placed at base of occiput (Fig. 8-8)	Slide occiput superiorly, maintaining contact of head on table. Hold position 10 s.
Pectoralis stretch	Standing in a corner with elbows at shoulder height (Fig. 8-9)	Lean toward corner slowly until stretch is felt in anterior chest. Hold 30 s.
Upper trapezius stretch	Sitting with one arm behind back, slightly depressing shoulder, rest opposite hand on side of head (Fig. 8-10)	Using hand on top of head, gently pull head laterally while depressing opposite shoulder until stretch is felt in the upper trapezius. Hold for 30 s.
Levator scapulae stretch	Sitting with one arm behind back and the contralateral hand on occipital area (Fig. 8-11)	Gently pull head down toward axilla until stretch is felt in levator scapulae. Hold for 30 s.
Upper extremity wall slides	Standing with back against wall (arms close to a 90°/90° position) (Fig. 8-12)	Slide arms upward as far as possible, while maintaining contact of arms against wall. This exercise facilitates postural control of the scapular stabilizers.

the use of visual or verbal cues for scapular positioning (Table 8-3). Using EMG recordings, Wegner et al.[31] showed that patients with chronic PNP who demonstrated altered scapular activation patterns during a typing task showed significant improvements in activating the middle trapezius following simple instructions and feedback to position their scapulae in midline. For example, patients presenting with a downwardly rotated scapula were instructed to "gently lift the tip of your shoulder" to improve scapular orientation and muscle activation.

Research has also demonstrated the efficacy of joint mobilizations to the cervical spine and manipulation to the thoracic spine to improve cervical ROM and decrease pain in patients with PNP.[17,25,29,33] A systematic Cochrane review comparing manipulation versus mobilization for patients with neck pain showed moderate quality evidence that both treatments produced similar effects on pain, function, and patient satisfaction at a 6-month follow-up.[33]

Identifying and addressing risk factors contributing to chronic PNP is an important component to achieving long-term success. Once discharged from physical therapy, most patients return to the same employment or personal pursuits, likely spending a significant amount of work and leisure time at video display terminals in sustained postures.[4,15] An ergonomic assessment and intervention should be performed to address improper workstation setup. An adjustable chair is a key component for a workstation: a properly fitting chair can significantly reduce shoulder and

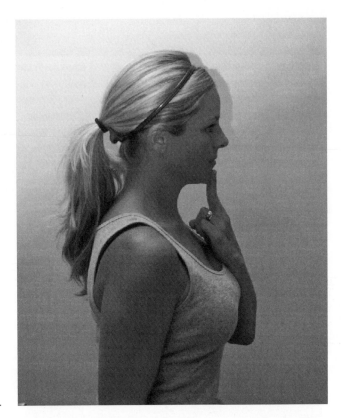

Figure 8-7. Cervical retraction (chin tuck).

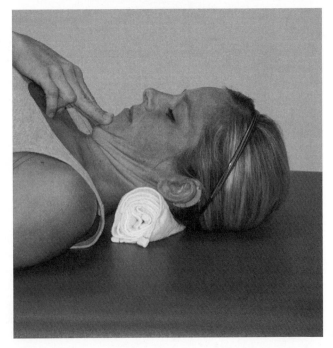

Figure 8-8. Suboccipital stretch.

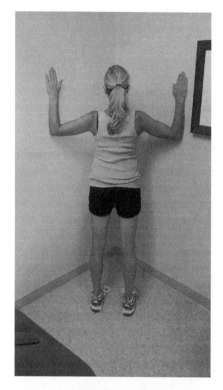

Figure 8-9. Corner pectoralis stretch.

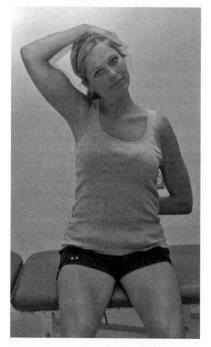

Figure 8-10. Upper trapezius stretch.

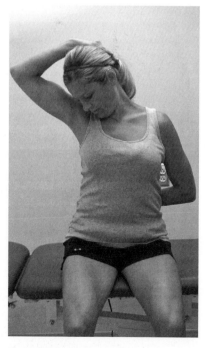

Figure 8-11. Levator scapulae stretch.

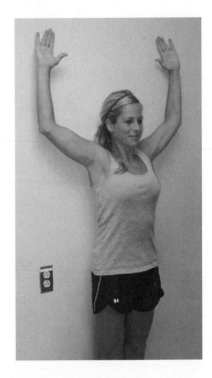

Figure 8-12. Upper extremity wall slides.

Table 8-3 SCAPULAR STABILIZATION STRENGTHENING EXERCISES		
Scapular Exercise	**Starting Position**	**Exercise Technique**
Prone retraction	Lying prone with small towel roll under forehead, arms at side with palms facing down	Initiate movement by squeezing shoulder blades together, then externally rotate and slightly extend shoulders. Hold for 5-10 s. (Fig. 8-13)
Prone middle trapezius	Lying prone with small towel roll under forehead, arms at a 90° angle ("T" position), thumbs pointed up	Initiate movement by squeezing shoulder blades together, then raise both arms parallel to body position. Hold for 5-10 s. (Fig. 8-14)
Prone lower trapezius	Lying prone with small towel roll under forehead, arms at a 135° angle ("Y" position), thumbs pointing up	Initiate movement by squeezing shoulder blades together, then raise arms to parallel to body position. Hold for 5-10 s. (Fig. 8-15)
Seated row	Seated position and holding resistance band with arms close to body	Allow arms to extend out in front to chest level. Initiate movement by squeezing shoulder blades together, then pull arms to sides.
Serratus wall slide	Standing with forearms in neutral rotation, resting on foam roll at chest level against the wall	Shift weight forward. Using scapular muscles, slide roll to overhead position. (Fig. 8-16)

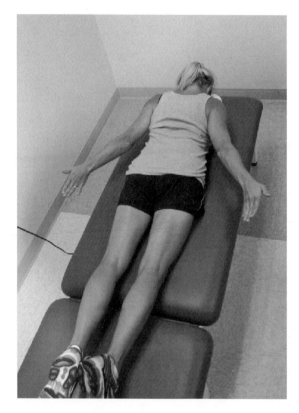

Figure 8-13. Prone scapular retraction.

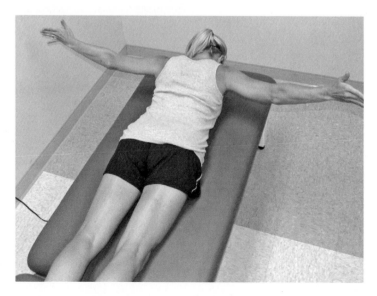

Figure 8-14. Prone middle trapezius.

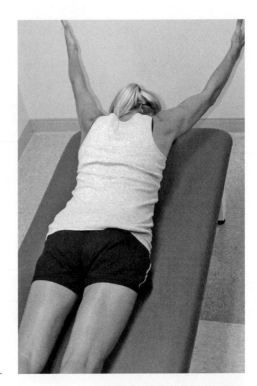

Figure 8-15. Prone lower trapezius.

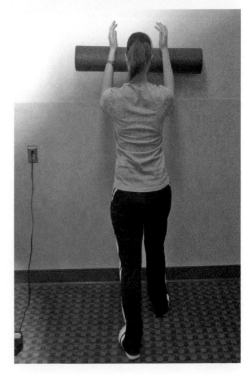

Figure 8-16. Serratus wall slide.

neck pain.[2] Proper seat height allows for comfortable resting positions of the spine and lower extremities by helping maintain a lumbar lordosis. The hips should be slightly elevated above the level of the knees with the feet resting on the floor.[2] The keyboard should be placed at or below the height of the elbows. Forearms should rest on the desk or chair armrests to allow for neutral shoulder, elbow, and wrist postures. This neutral upper extremity posture has consistently demonstrated reduced muscle activity in the upper extremities, thereby decreasing the risk of developing musculoskeletal disorders.[4,15] The computer mouse should be positioned to avoid excessive shoulder abduction and scapular protraction. The monitor should be directly in front of the individual's face (at a distance of ~66 cm) and the top of the monitor should be adjusted to eye level to allow for a neutral head position.[31] It has been shown that less than a 3° upward or downward tilt of the head from a neutral position can have a significant effect on reducing head and neck symptoms.[1]

Postural education and retraining is a necessary component for achieving successful outcomes in patients with PNP. Symptomatic subjects typically demonstrate an increased forward head and shoulder posture[1] and have an increased load in the cervical muscles while performing typing and mousing tasks on the computer.[8] Achieving a neutral spine posture helps equalize load-sharing. This can decrease stress on pain-sensitized structures and improve activation of the deep neck flexors required to maintain cervical lordosis and postural form.[24] To offset the adverse effect of prolonged computer use, the patient should be advised to take 20 to 30 second "microbreaks" every 30 minutes, and not exceed 2 hours while working on the computer. During the microbreaks, the patient should perform basic exercises such as cervical and scapular retraction, thoracic extension, and upper extremity stretching to provide relief to the muscles and joints in the sustained postures.[18]

Falla et al.[16] reported improved activation of spinal stabilizing muscles when subjects sat erect with a neutral posture versus a slumped posture. They also found that instructing an individual to "sit straight up" without cueing was less effective than specific verbal and manual cues to achieve an erect but neutral spine posture. The individuals who received cueing for achieving a neutral spine posture had significantly greater activation of lumbar multifidi and deep neck flexors than those who were simply instructed to "sit straight up."[16,32] To achieve the erect neutral posture, subjects were instructed to achieve the ideal lumbopelvic sitting posture by gently rolling their pelvis forward to rest on the ischial tuberosities, followed by a slight sternal lift, avoiding excessive thoracolumbar extension. Finally, subjects were instructed to lift the occiput minimally to position the head in neutral and to reduce upper cervical extension. The control group was instructed to sit up straight the best they knew how, which resulted in significantly less recruitment of the cervical and lumbar stabilizing muscles. Maintaining a neutral spine posture for prolonged postural activities not only decreases the amount of deleterious stress to the musculoskeletal structures, but also optimally aligns the spine for activation of the deep cervical flexors and lumbar multifidi responsible for maintaining ideal postural form.

In recent years, treatment has focused not only on the biomechanical aspects underlying the development of chronic neck pain, but the psychosocial stressors for long-term management of symptoms. **"Work style"** takes into consideration both the biomechanical and the psychosocial risk factors contributing to the perpetuation of chronic neck pain arising from the imbalance between workload and capacity. A long-term study analyzing the effects of work style interventions showed that a combined intervention of ergonomic and behavioral changes to manage workload resulted in significant long-term reductions in neck and shoulder pain and recovery rate. The behavioral changes included training and education regarding taking adequate rest breaks, strategies to cope with high work demands, and increased body awareness with posture.[14,15] The development of chronic PNP is multifaceted, and involves both intrinsic and extrinsic factors contributing to the perpetuation of symptoms. For long-term success, treatment should involve addressing musculoskeletal impairments with traditional physical therapy interventions, and ergonomic and psychosocial issues that often contribute to perpetuating the condition.

Evidence-Based Clinical Recommendations

SORT: Strength of Recommendation Taxonomy

A: Consistent, good-quality patient-oriented evidence
B: Inconsistent or limited-quality patient-oriented evidence
C: Consensus, disease-oriented evidence, usual practice, expert opinion, or case series

1. Intrinsic factors such as altered muscular control in the cervical and scapular muscles and decreased postural and kinesthetic awareness contribute to the development of postural neck pain. **Grade B**

2. Extrinsic factors such as poor workstation set-up and increased duration of time spent on a video display unit contribute to the development of postural neck pain. **Grade B**

3. Exercises aimed at improving deep neck flexor strength improve the ability to maintain cervical posture and stabilize the cervical spine when performing reaching and upper extremity tasks. **Grade B**

4. Interventions aimed at improving an individual's "work style" may improve the long-term success of treating postural neck pain. **Grade C**

COMPREHENSION QUESTIONS

8.1 Individuals with chronic postural neck pain typically present with which of the following postural positions of the shoulder and neck?

A. Rounded forward shoulders, scapular retraction, mid- and lower-cervical extension and upper-cervical flexion

B. Rounded forward shoulders, scapular protraction, mid- and lower-cervical flexion and upper-cervical flexion

C. Depressed shoulders, scapular retraction, mid- and lower-cervical extension and upper-cervical extension

D. Rounded forward shoulders, scapular protraction, mid- and lower-cervical flexion and upper-cervical extension

8.2 When *initiating* an exercise program for individuals with chronic postural neck pain, early focus should be on *which* of the following?

   A. General cardiovascular exercises

   B. Isometric cervical and shoulder girdle exercises

   C. Strengthening and retraining of the deep cervical flexors

   D. Low-load high repetition neck extension exercises

8.3 Which list represents individual risk factors for chronic postural neck pain?

   A. Female, wearing bifocals, use of a computer mouse for extended periods, psychosocial stressors

   B. Male, psychosocial stressors, use of computer mouse, lower chair

   C. Female, contact lenses, right-hand dominant, infrequent rest breaks

   D. Male, psychosocial stressors, bifocals, infrequent rest breaks

ANSWERS

8.1 **D.** Postural adaptations typically found in the frequent computer user are the forward rounded shoulders and protracted scapulae, mid- and lower-cervical flexion and compensatory upper-cervical extension. Frequently, these postural adaptations are due to inadequate workstation setup and decreased attention to maintaining a neutral spine posture.

8.2 **C.** Research has shown the importance of the training the deep cervical flexors to maintain postural control and alignment for feed-forward stabilization of the cervical spine with upper extremity use.[2,9]

8.3 **A.** Risk factors for developing postural neck pain in office workers include: female sex, frequent computer usage with a computer mouse, eyewear, and psychosocial stressors.[14]

REFERENCES

1. Hoyle JA, Marras WS, Sheedy JE, Hart DE. Effects of postural and visual stressors on myofascial trigger point development and motor unit rotation during computer work. *J Electromyogr Kinesiol.* 2011;21:41-48.

2. Fabrizio P. Ergonomic intervention in the treatment of a patient with upper extremity and neck pain. *Phys Ther.* 2009;89:351-360.

3. Andrews JR, Harrelson GL, Wilk KE. *Physical Rehabilitation of the Injured Athlete.* 3rd ed. Philadelphia, PA: Saunders; 2004.

4. Gerr F, Marcus M, Monteilh C. Epidemiology of musculoskeletal disorders among computer users: lesson learned from the role of posture and keyboard use. *J Electromyogr Kinesiol.* 2004;14:25-31.

5. Johnston V, Souvlis T, Jimmieson NL, Jull G. Associations between individual and workplace risk factors for self-reported neck pain and disability among female office workers. *Appl Ergon.* 2008;39:171-182.

6. Smith L, Louw Q, Crous L, Grimmer-Somers K. Prevalence of neck pain and headaches: impact of computer use and other associative factors. *Cephalgia.* 2009;29:250-257.

7. Magee DJ. *Orthopedic Physical Assessment.* 4th ed. Philadelphia, PA: Saunders; 2002.

8. Szeto GP, Straker LM, O'Sullivan PB. A comparison of symptomatic and asymptomatic office workers performing monotonous keyboard work–1: neck and shoulder muscle recruitment patterns. *Man Ther.* 2005;10:270-280.

9. Szeto GP, Straker LM, O'Sullivan PB. During computing tasks symptomatic female office workers demonstrate a trend towards higher cervical postural muscle load than asymptomatic office workers: an experimental study. *Aust J Physiother.*2009;55:257-262.

10. Falla D, Bilenkij G, Jull G. Patients with chronic neck pain demonstrate altered patterns of muscle activation during performance of a functional upper limb task. *Spine.* 2004;29:1436-1440.

11. Edmondston SJ, Chan HY, Ngai GC, et al. Postural neck pain: an investigation of habitual sitting posture, perception of "good" posture and cervicothoracic kinaesthesia. *Man Ther.* 2007;12:363-371.

12. Falla D, O'Leary S, Fagan A, Jull G. Recruitment of the deep cervical flexor muscles during a postural-correction exercise performed in sitting. *Man Ther.* 2007;12:139-143.

13. Caneiro JP, O'Sullivan P, Burnett A, et al. The influence of different sitting postures on head/neck posture and muscle activity. *Man Ther.* 2010;15:54-60.

14. Bernaards CM, Ariens GA, Hildebrandt VH. The cost-effectiveness of a lifestyle physical activity intervention in addition to a work style intervention on the recovery from neck and upper limb symptoms in computer workers. *BMC Musculoskelet Disord.* 2006;7:80.

15. Bernaards CM, Ariens GA, Knol DL, Hildebrandt VH. The effectiveness of a work style intervention and a lifestyle physical activity intervention on the recovery from neck and upper limb symptoms on computer workers. *Pain.* 2007;132:142-153.

16. Falla D. Unravelling the complexity of muscle impairment in chronic neck pain. *Man Ther.* 2004;9:125-133.

17. Grimmer K. Measuring endurance capacity of the cervical short flexor muscle group. *Aust J Physiother.* 1994;40:251-254.

18. Kisner C, Colby LA. *Therapeutic Exercise: Foundation and Techniques.* 5th ed. Philadelphia: PA: FA Davis Company; 2007.

19. Porterfield JA, DeRosa C. *Mechanical Low Back Pain: Perspectives in Functional Anatomy.* Philadelphia, PA: Saunders; 1991.

20. Wainner RS, Fritz JM, Irrgang JJ, Boninger ML, Delitto A, Allison S. Reliability and diagnostic accuracy of the clinical examination and patient self-report measures for cervical radiculopathy. *Spine.* 2003;28:52-62.

21. Waldrop MA. Diagnosis and treatment of cervical radiculopathy using a clinical prediction rule and a multimodal intervention approach: a case series. *J Orthop Sport Phys Ther.* 2006;36:152-159.

22. Sahrmann S. *Diagnosis and Treatment of Movement Impairment Syndromes.* St. Louis, MO: Mosby; 2002.

23. Edmonston SJ, Wallumrod ME, Macleid F, Kvamme LS, Joebges S, Brabham GC. Reliability of isometric muscle endurance tests in subjects with postural neck pain. *J Manipulative Physiol Ther.* 2008;31:348-354.

24. Jull G, Barrett C, Magee R, Ho P. Further clinical clarification of the muscle dysfunction in cervical headache. *Cephalalgia.* 1999;19:179-185.

25. Fernandez-de-las Penas C, Alonso-Blanco C, Cuadrado ML, Pareja JA. Forward head posture and neck mobility in chronic tension-type headache: a blinded, controlled study. *Cephalalgia.* 2006;26:314-319.

26. Paris SV, Loubert PV. *Foundations of Clinical Orthopaedics.* St. Augustine, FL: Institute Press; 1999.

27. Jull G, Treleaven J, Versace G. Manual examination: is pain provocation a major cue for spinal dysfunction. *Aust J Physiother.* 1994;40:159-165.

28. D'Sylva J, Miller J, Gross A, et al. Cervical Overview Group. Manual therapy with or without physical medicine modalities for neck pain: a systematic review. *Man Ther.* 2010;15:415-433.

29. Miller J, Gross A, D'Sylva J, et al. Manual therapy and exercise for neck pain: a systematic review. *Man Ther.* 2010;15:334-354.

30. Wang WT, Olson SL, Campbell AH, Hanten WP, Gleeson PB. Effectiveness of physical therapy for patients with neck pain: an individualized approach using a clinical decision-making algorithm. *Am J Phys Med Rehabil.* 2003;82:203-218.

31. Wegner S, Jull G, O'Leary S, Johnston V. The effect of a scapular postural correction strategy on trapezius activity in patients with neck pain. *Man Ther.* 2010;15:562-566.

32. Falla D, Jull G, Russell T, Vicenzino B, Hodges P. Effect of neck exercise on sitting posture in patients with chronic neck pain. *Phys. Ther.* 2007;87:408-417.

33. Gross A, Miller J, D'Sylva J, et al. COG. Manipulation or mobilisation for neck pain: a Cochrane Review. *Man Ther.* 2010;15:315-333.

Postsurgical Rehabilitation Status/Post Neck Dissection for Cancer

Douglas Lauchlan

You have been asked by a head and neck surgeon to evaluate a right-hand domi-nant 46-year-old self-employed carpenter. The patient has been complaining of increasing pain in the right shoulder region following a right-sided neck dissection performed 3 months ago. Six months ago, the patient was diagnosed with squa-mous cell carcinoma of the mucosal lining of the head and neck and he has been undergoing intervention for this condition since. Surgical clearance of Levels I to IV of the posterior triangle of the neck was performed and the patient completed 5 weeks of daily radiotherapy to this region. The patient's previous medical history is otherwise unremarkable. Amongst a variety of issues, the patient has been com-plaining of an inability to fully elevate his right upper limb since the surgery. The increasing pain has also caused his sleep to become disturbed. He is aware that he "lacks strength" in his right upper limb in a variety of activities of daily living (ADLs). He reports that his social encounters with other individuals who have undergone head and neck surgery have made him fearful that his physical function will continue to deteriorate and he has concerns for his future quality of life (QOL).

- ► What are the examination priorities?
- ► Based on his health condition, what do you anticipate may be the contributors to activity limitations?
- ► What are possible complications that may limit the effectiveness of physical therapy?
- ► What is his rehabilitation prognosis?
- ► Describe a physical therapy plan of care based on each stage of the health condition.
- ► How might the patient's emotional condition affect rehabilitation?

KEY DEFINITIONS

ACTIVITIES OF DAILY LIVING (ADLs): Typical functional pursuits of the individual based upon his work, hobbies, and general lifestyle both prior to and after surgery

HEAD AND NECK CANCER: Typically relates to cancer of the mucosal lining of the head and neck and most commonly involves the lymph nodes of the neck

NECK DISSECTION: Surgical clearance of all cancerous cells and relevant lymph nodes of the region; commonly called "Levels I to IV clearance" based on the anatomical division of lymph nodes of the neck into distinct groups

QUALITY OF LIFE (QOL): Relates not only to the ability of an individual to perform ADLs, but also to the individual's social interactions with others; commonly takes into consideration both physical and mental health and emotional well-being

SHOULDER: Includes both the glenohumeral and scapulothoracic complex and associated musculature that control position and range of motion (ROM) of the upper limb

Objectives

1. Outline the anticipated physical presentation of the individual at 3 months postsurgical neck dissection and identify the adaptive processes that have likely occurred.
2. Understand the interaction of different neuromusculoskeletal structures causing dysfunction at the shoulder region.
3. Identify appropriate clinical objective measures to monitor change and evaluate the impact of physical therapy interventions.
4. Identify outcome measures for both functional and QOL status for this patient population.
5. Outline the possible emotional and behavioral issues that are likely to impact rehabilitation and recovery.
6. Describe the benefits of a holistic philosophy of care for this patient population.

Physical Therapy Considerations

PT considerations during management of the head and neck cancer survivor with the development of shoulder region pain and disability several months after neck dissection:

▶ **General physical therapy plan of care/goals:** Prevent or minimize loss of ROM of the glenohumeral joint in particular, but also the neck and scapulothoracic regions; restore (as close as possible) local muscle recruitment and static/dynamic postural controls; encourage functional strength gains in associated global muscles of the shoulder region; restore ability to perform ADLs, as able; improve QOL

▶ **Physical therapy interventions:** Patient education regarding regular maintenance of shoulder ROM; passive stretching; joint mobilization; exercises to
promote scapular control; postural and functional re-education resistance training; promotion and reintegration of social and physical activity

▶ **Precautions during physical therapy:** Skin viability and impact of physical
therapy to skin flaps/grafts at neck; potential onset of adhesive capsulitis of the
glenohumeral joint; ongoing medical health status

▶ **Complications interfering with physical therapy:** Social and lifestyle factors
that may impact compliance/engagement of individual to regular physical therapy
sessions; postsurgical activity modifications

Understanding the Health Condition

Despite recent surgical advances, there is still a high mortality rate in individuals requiring surgical clearance of the posterior triangle for head and neck cancer.[1]
Although survival rates are improving, survivors face significant issues relating
to shoulder disability and its impact on QOL. Almost one in every two patients
recovering from head and neck cancer surgery quit working solely due to shoulder
disability; three in every four patients report difficulty returning to everyday tasks
with regards to social and recreational activity.[2] Despite the evolution of surgical
procedures for this condition, shoulder disability is considered an unavoidable byproduct of surgery.[2,3] Although the etiology and pathogenesis of this syndrome are
debated, the existence of postoperative shoulder disability following neck dissection is widely accepted. Patten and Hillel first suggested that postoperative shoulder
disability may be due to adhesive capsulitis of the glenohumeral joint (GHJ) that
is associated with nonuse of the upper limb on the side of surgery during the postoperative period.[4] However, more recently published work in this field has shown
that abnormal scapular motion and control due to temporary or permanent damage to the spinal accessory nerve (CN XI) results in altered GHJ mechanics with
resulting pain and disability.[5,6] The spinal accessory nerve arises from two sources:
the cranial roots from the medulla and the spinal roots from the first five segments of the spinal cord. The nerve makes its passage through the posterior triangle
of the neck to innervate both the sternocleidomastoid and the lower fibers of the
trapezius. Thus, radical surgical clearance of the neck often has an impact on associated neuromusculoskeletal structures of the neck and shoulder region that can result
in symptomatic and asymptomatic developmental movement disorders. Physical
therapy management of shoulder disability following neck dissection is therefore
aimed at creating a holistic and balanced approach to functional return and promotion of normal movement of the shoulder region. Due to the adaptable nature of
the neuromusculoskeletal system, developmental movement disorders may require
time to become established. Shoulder disability commonly presents over the weeks
and months following surgery. Early literature on the development of shoulder problems following neck dissection suggested that partial injury and entrapment of the
spinal accessory nerve, which is the primary motor innervation to the lower fibers
of the trapezius muscle, is the reason for a delayed onset in shoulder disability.[7] This

hypothesis has been supported in recent literature describing that patients commonly do not report symptoms until *weeks* postsurgery.[8] Although the role of the spinal accessory nerve and resulting lower trapezius paresis is recognized, it has been further proposed that this latent onset of pain is more attributable to adhesive capsulitis of the GHJ.[4] The consideration that adhesive capsulitis of the GHJ can result from sustained altered mechanics of the scapulothoracic muscles (regardless of initial etiology) is well recognized in the physical therapy literature.[9-11] Furthermore, the establishment of adhesive capsulitis significantly reduces the effectiveness of physical therapy interventions.[9] The post-neck dissection patient population therefore appears at risk of developing shoulder pain and disability with subsequent resistance to effective physical therapy interventions. Many authors have attempted to throw more light on the nature of this postsurgical shoulder phenomenon termed "Radical Neck Dissection/11th Nerve Syndrome." However, its etiology remains difficult to prove due to the developing nature of the disability. Postoperatively, patients are commonly in pain and demonstrate paresis of the lower trapezius muscle, but there is rarely any capsular shortening or adaptations until 6 to 12 months following surgery.[1,2,4] Recognition that Radical Neck Dissection/11th Nerve Syndrome may be due to the emergence of adhesive capsulitis is significant, but understanding what movement adaptations have led to this clinical state is still unknown.

Panjabi offers a model for physical therapists to understand normal movement and the neuromusculoskeletal factors that may lead to dysfunction.[12] This model suggests that injury to structures belonging to one or more subsystems will result in overall system dysfunction. Figure 9-1 shows how this model can be adapted to the pathodynamics and development of postoperative shoulder disability following neck dissection.

Given that there is a 50% chance of injury to the spinal accessory nerve postsurgery, there are often complex maladaptive movement patterns that arise through these subsystem interactions which relate to eventual shoulder pain and disability.[3,6]

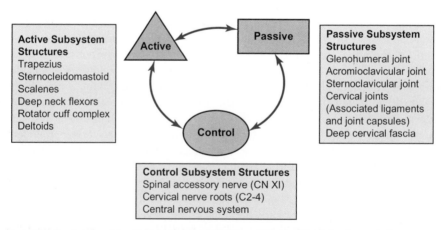

Figure 9-1. A subsystem-based approach to rehabilitation of the shoulder following neck dissection surgery (Reproduced, with permission, from Panjabi MM. The stabilizing system of the spine. Part I. Function, dysfunction, adaptation, and enhancement. *J Spinal Disord.* 1992;5:383-389.)

Despite the development of shoulder pain and disability, it is important to recognize the individual and his immediate healthcare needs. Surviving cancer and the subsequent surgical clearance can have a profound impact on the physical and emotional well-being of this patient population.[13] Therefore, it is of great importance to consider strategies of engagement and participation when establishing a rehabilitation program. The physical therapist should evaluate the person holistically as he improves not only his functional status, but also his social participation in his typical vocational and habitual environment.

Physical Therapy Patient/Client Management

Postoperatively, the physical therapy management of this population can be divided into three domains following the International Classification of Function, Disability and Health: impairments, activity limitations, and participation restrictions.[14] The immediate inpatient management is aimed at the main impairment (injury to neuromusculoskeletal tissues in the aftermath of surgical clearance). Management includes respiratory and airway monitoring, postural advice, and maintenance of active ROM of the shoulder and neck region. After surgery, treatment commonly involves a period of outpatient radiotherapy directed toward the neck/shoulder area. This approach to cancer management is typified by a period of change in the patient's social and daily routines that must incorporate a demanding schedule of treatment. It is important that the physical therapist engages the patient in his shoulder/neck rehabilitation during this period, emphasizing maintenance of GHJ ROM to avoid capsular tightening. During the next phase of rehabilitation, impairments and activity limitations need to be addressed. There is a need to maximize active ROM and return strength and power of the muscles affecting the shoulder and neck region/ upper quadrant. It is important at this stage to recognize the impact of the neural control subsystem and the likely adaptive scapular mechanics due to abnormal neuromuscular control. The typical postsurgical adaptations and potential for postsurgical upper limb disuse has a significant impact on the balance and integration of the other subsystems. The third phase of management focuses on lifestyle participation and reintegration of ADLs including work, hobbies, and typical social interaction.

Examination, Evaluation, and Diagnosis

The physical therapist starts the examination by observing the head, neck, and shoulder structures. Although there are numerous notable observations 3 months following neck dissection surgery (e.g., skin grafting), many of these features are unlikely to impact shoulder function at this stage and will not be discussed. On the side of the neck dissection, decreased muscle mass around the shoulder creates the classic "square-edge" to the deltoid due to the bony prominence of the acromion process being more easily visible. Another common bony point to assess is the spine of the scapula, where significant wasting of the supraspinatus and infraspinatus muscles can be apparent due to disuse atrophy. The patient will most likely adopt the "forward head posture" position with a similarly protracted and elevated scapula.

This leads to two significant postural adaptations: lengthened deep neck flexors (similar adaptation seen post-whiplash[15]) and a reduced subacromial space due to a lack of dynamic stability as the humeral head migrates in a cephalad direction.[11]

Shoulder active range of motion (AROM) should be measured with a goniometer and compared between the affected and unaffected limbs. The affected shoulder often shows reduced glenohumeral elevation with abnormal scapular control due to denervation of the lower trapezius and resulting compensatory *hyperactive* fibers of the upper trapezius.[10] Depending on the stage of adaptive shortening of the GHJ capsule, loss of functional upper limb elevation is likely associated with a combined loss of physiological flexion and abduction of the GHJ. This may also be associated with a tight elastic end feel and pain on testing passive ROM (PROM) of the GHJ. The most limited movements are likely to follow the capsular pattern of restriction at the GHJ (lateral rotation is most restricted, followed by abduction, flexion, and then extension).[16]

Strength testing is unlikely to be painful, but the patient may have selective or global weakness (especially in shoulder abduction) due to the lack of scapular control. The physical therapist should evaluate the postsurgical motor involvement of the spinal accessory nerve. An inability to actively shrug the affected shoulder (upper trapezius fibers) and/or an inability to control the scapulothoracic fixation during active elevation of the upper limb—commonly seen as "winging" of the inferior angle of the scapula (lower trapezius fibers) clearly highlight the presence of an impaired motor output and the likelihood of spinal accessory nerve damage. Thorough neurologic testing should be conducted because the patient may present with decreased or absent sensation, numbness, and/or an associated hypoalgesia or hyperalgesia around the site of the surgery and skin graft. There may be adaptive proprioceptive loss as the subsystems attempt to correct the adaptive imbalances postsurgery.[11]

Significant restrictions in AROM and PROM in the cervical spine are likely to be present due to superficial facial and neck scarring (from the skin graft) and deeper scarring due to the surgical clearance technique. The most affected movements are side bending away from the affected side and rotation toward the affected side. As previously described, a loss of local muscle control (deep neck flexor recruitment) often leads to muscle system imbalances of the head and neck (*e.g.*, hyperactive sternocleidomastoid and upper trapezius). This pattern further contributes to the loss of cervical spine AROM. Often, there is adaptive stiffness and discomfort on palpation and with passive accessory movements of C3 to C5 vertebrae.

Several tests and outcome measures, including goniometry, pain ratings, and passive end feels can be used to identify impairments. Although more commonly used in populations presenting with a traumatic shoulder injury, the Constant shoulder assessment is a widely used and robust tool which could be used to measure the impact of the postsurgical impairment on the individual.[17] QOL can be measured using a variety of instruments. A cancer-specific tool (*e.g.*, University of Washington QOL scale) can be used to measure the impact of rehabilitation on recovery.[18] The **Functional Assessment of Cancer Therapy—Head and Neck (FACTH&N)** has been used to more specifically evaluate the impact of rehabilitation with this population.[5] A more generic QOL measure (SF-36) could be considered for participation.[19] Although there are a number of head and neck cancer outcome measures, the FACTH&N is a multidimensional 39-question self-report QOL outcome measure that allows the therapist to gain specific insight regarding the functional status of the individual and the presence and extent of risk factors which may be associated with an emerging shoulder dysfunction. Choosing the FACTH&N would be preferred since it has been designed specifically for this population and its value and response should hold more validity than the use of non-disease-specific evaluative tools or disease-specific tools that do not focus on functional return. Regardless of the outcome measure selected for monitoring effectiveness of clinical care, measurement of QOL is of great value in determining the meaningfulness of survival to the individual.[20]

Plan of Care and Interventions

The most important aspect of the physical therapy plan of care with respect to the shoulder impairment is to maintain active and passive shoulder ROM as the GHJ capsule becomes tightened due to pain and disuse.[9] Heat, soft tissue massage, and cervical mobilizations can be directed to the neck and upper quadrant in an effort to reduce pain and hyperactivity of the global muscle system.[21] The physical therapist may be limited in being able to achieve normal scapular motion or control due to the likely denervation of the lower trapezius fibers through injury to the spinal accessory nerve (commonly seen as "winging" of the inferior angle of the scapula).[10]

Results from the objective examination should help the therapist rule in or rule out the presence of **adhesive capsulitis** developing at the GHJ. Passive GHJ capsular stretches should be performed to directly manage the adapting soft tissues of the shoulder. Maintenance of the available shoulder ROM is essential through this phase in order to avoid the changes associated with disuse. Although active assisted ROM (AAROM) exercises are commonly used in physical therapy sessions, the ability of the patient to perform these daily at home may be limited due to the nature of the typical equipment used (*i.e.*, over-the-door shoulder pulley system). That said, a creative attempt to promote an active assisted role in maintaining shoulder ROM should be sought, such as holding a cane or stick with both hands and using the unaffected arm to guide the affected arm through all ranges of motion. Progressive active upper extremity exercise can be augmented with graded resistance using (color-coded) therapeutic elastic bands.[5] Progressive resistance can be applied in functional patterns of movement to work on both muscle re-education and neuromuscular recruitment and timing relating to functional patterns of normal movement.[10,11] The physical therapist should address the impact of upper trunk and cervical resting posture on available shoulder ROM. Advice and treatment directed at addressing developmental thoracic kyphosis and increased cervical lordosis should be considered.[22] Simple postural awareness and active stretching should be implemented with the goal of reducing the tendency to adopt these restrictive postures.

Task-specific rehabilitation approaches should be considered for this population. These could be directed toward vocational-related tasks, components of day-to-day duties and general lifestyle requirements, and hobbies or recreational pursuits. Patients should be actively involved in this process of problem solving and goal setting because this enhances ownership and creates shared dialogue between therapist and patient. This shared goal setting approach should be monitored and directed by either party as the patient's needs develop or change. Throughout the patient's episode of care, there should be recognition that shoulder function and strength gains should be developed through an integrative and functionally directed return to activity. This reinforces the patient's understanding of the value and importance of a progressive rehabilitation process approach. In conjunction with developing self-directed rehabilitation habits, the patient must feel that his needs are being met by any prescriptive intervention. In other words, the patient needs to positively value the prescriptive and general advice he has been given. To measure the impact of this rehabilitation approach on the individual, the physical therapist should consider using the Consultation and Relational Empathy (CARE) measure.[23] This measure is designed to evaluate the health practitioner's empathy throughout the consultation and treatment process. Not only is **empathy** strongly linked with understanding the patient's condition, but it is also hugely influential on compliance with directed care.[23] Thus, the likelihood of successful rehabilitation that is dependent on patient compliance with prescribed therapeutic interventions is linked to the degree to which the physical therapist provides empathic care.

Managing the impairment and activity limitations of patients following neck dissection surgery is merely a component of the overall rehabilitation strategy. Patients need to link these traditional physical therapy principles of management to their social inclusion and participation with others. Relationship building and support networks are vital in regaining life focus and a sense of well-being (both from a physical and mental perspective). The physical therapist can measure the patient's self-perceived QOL with the SF-36. If possible, the therapist should observe the patient's natural environment and the many complex influences involved in his sense of well-being and ability to return to performance of ADLs. The therapist should also consider the impact of the patient's reappraisal of the internal criteria that shapes his fundamental values. Many patients may not wish to return to the lifestyle and environments they had prior to diagnosis/surgery.[24] This should be explored on an individual basis and the rehabilitation strategy directed based upon the patient's needs. Simple short-term to long-term goals should be set and re-evaluated as the rehabilitation program progresses. The supportive roles of other healthcare professionals (in particular psychologists and occupational therapists) may be helpful in this process and should be considered as part of the multidisciplinary approach to care.

Evidence-Based Clinical Recommendations

SORT: Strength of Recommendation Taxonomy

A: Consistent, good-quality patient-oriented evidence
B: Inconsistent or limited-quality patient-oriented evidence
C: Consensus, disease-oriented evidence, usual practice, expert opinion, or case series

1. The Functional Assessment of Cancer Therapy—Head and Neck (FACTH&N) is a sensitive multidimensional self-report instrument that measures quality of life and functional status in individuals after neck dissection surgery. **Grade A**

2. Maintenance of glenohumeral joint active ROM and passive capsular stretches prevent the onset of adhesive capsulitis following neck dissection surgery. **Grade C**

3. Increased empathy on the part of the physical therapist throughout the evaluation and treatment process increases patient compliance with prescribed therapeutic interventions and the likelihood of successful rehabilitation that depends on patient compliance. **Grade B**

COMPREHENSION QUESTIONS

9.1 Following surgery for head and neck cancer, a patient visits a physical therapist for the first time due to recent emergence of shoulder pain. She is scared to move the upper limb for fear of injury and damaging her shoulder. List the following treatment goals in order of the *most* likely priority, from highest to lowest.

A. Maintain GHJ ROM

B. Educate on pain values and the beliefs involving pain and damage

C. Improve muscle strength

D. Return to typical ADLs

E. Reduce pain

9.2 A client is referred to a physical therapy clinic by a specialist head and neck surgeon for "rehabilitation of the shoulder" 3 months after undergoing dissection and clearance of the posterior triangle of the neck. After 2 weeks of physical therapy sessions, the patient expresses a desire to stop further treatment. She is not in much pain and is managing most of her ADLs, as long as she does not need to lift her arm above her head. She has a very supportive husband who is "doing everything" for her. What is the *most* appropriate course of action for the physical therapist to pursue?

A. Agree with the client that she has no current deficits or predictable risks for deficits in the future and immediately discharge her from physical therapy.

B. Educate the client about all the risks for decreased ROM and functional decline and suggest a strategy to resolve any conflict and move forward together with agreed goals.

C. Insist that the client continue therapy because she has not met all the goals that the physical therapist has set for her.

D. Educate the client about all the risks for decreased ROM and functional decline, but if she does not agree with your assessment that she needs to continue physical therapy, encourage her husband to continue to perform the overhead activities that she cannot perform.

ANSWERS

9.1 Although every individual must be assessed and managed on a prioritized impairment basis, the likely prioritization here would be **B, E, A, D, C.** A main barrier to rehabilitation is the patient's attitudes and beliefs about pain and damage (option B; *i.e.*, "hurt ≠ harm"). Pain may be modifiable through the use of modalities like transcutaneous electrical nerve stimulation (option E). Maintaining the physiological range of shoulder motion is key to attempting to prevent the onset of adhesive capsulitis of the GHJ joint and the resultant long-term morbidity (option A). Although a return to work may not be possible due to postoperative health concerns and the particular duties and tasks required at work, typical ADLs should be promoted at this stage (option D). Social inclusion and a return to normal recreation and lifestyle may allow a greater sense of physical and emotional well-being, and enhance participation and control, which is commonly reduced in patients who may feel marginalized following their treatment for cancer. An attempt by the therapist to realize the classification of functional domains during the rehabilitation process (impairment, activity limitations and participation restrictions) allows a more holistic, patient-centered approach to the care episode. This should translate to greater patient empowerment and allow more effective management/rehabilitation outcomes. Maintenance of ROM should be considered as ongoing but less essential immediately because capsular shortening and adaptation is unlikely to become established until later in the developmental process. Similarly, traditional progressive resisted global muscle strengthening is likely not an immediate priority until pain and scapular control have been addressed (option C). Establishing an empathetic relationship with the patient is of greater importance in the immediate phase of rehabilitation, in an effort to optimize patient understanding and compliance in a self-directed program of flexibility and strengthening.

9.2 **B.** The key issue to address here is the development of adaptive soft tissue changes through disuse of the upper limb and avoidance of full physiological ROM at the shoulder. With avoidance of full shoulder ROM, there is an increased likelihood of developing adhesive capsulitis of the GHJ with associated pain and disability following a cessation of care at this stage (option A). The client has just begun physical therapy and is unlikely to have developed much adaptive soft tissue shortening at this stage. However, there may be maladaptive scapular motion and poor scapulothoracic control limiting upper limb elevation on the affected side. This may not be holding the client back functionally because she has a supportive husband who may also still be adapting psychologically to the role of caregiver. The client is only 3 to 4 months postsurgery and is likely to have many other commitments to ongoing postoperative care from consultant surgical reviews to oncology, speech and language therapy, dietician and occupational therapy appointments. At this stage following surgery, she may not realize the potential issues associated with her shoulder as the maladaptive cycle of capsular shortening and pain has not become fully established. As much as the physical therapist may wish to persevere with a traditional approach to preventing maladaptive changes at the shoulder region (options C and D), there should be more effort at this juncture to establish the therapeutic relationship—not only with the client but with her husband as well. At this stage, there is often a significant sense of change with regards to her values and belief systems and perhaps also within the relationship she has with her husband. There needs to be acknowledgement that "doing everything" for the client in her "new" postoperative predicament may not be the most appropriate strategy for the couple in the longer term, as there is a need to promote the client's active glenohumeral range and functional involvement in ADLs. Establishing informed and shared objectives for treatment is necessary not only in creating daily routines that can help prevent the onset of adhesive capsulitis of the GHJ but also in enhancing positive behavior toward functional independence and social interactions. There may have to be some negotiation between client and therapist with respect to the level and frequency of contact at this point postoperatively. The physical therapist must recognize the overall impact the surgery and commitment to the postoperative care is having on both the client and her husband. However, regular monitoring of clinical signs should be agreed upon and the client must engage with this on a regular basis. This could be measured through both manual testing of the passive physiological movement available at the GHJ alongside a more holistic functional measure of outcome (*e.g.*, FACTH&N). A shared goal setting and management planning approach should aim to evaluate the effectiveness of any home program which may be undertaken as an alternative to frequent visits to the physical therapy clinic. This gives confidence to the patient that her functional status is being maintained by her *self-directed* approach through promoting a return to typical ADLs where possible.

REFERENCES

1. Hillel AD, Kroll H, Dorman J, Medieros J. Radical neck dissection: a subjective and objective evaluation of postoperative disability. *J Otolaryngol*. 1989;18:53-61.

2. Shone GR, Yardley MP. An audit into the incidence of handicap after unilateral radical neck dissection. *J Laryngol Otol*. 1991;105:760-762.

3. van Wilgen CP, Dijkstra PU, van der Laan BF, Plukker JT, Roodenburg JL. Shoulder complaints after neck dissection; is the spinal accessory nerve involved? *Br J Oral Maxillofac Surg*. 2003;41:7-11.

4. Patten CP, Hillel AD. The 11th nerve syndrome. Accessory nerve palsy or adhesive capsulitis. *Arch Otolaryngol Head Neck Surg*. 1993;119:215-220.

5. McNeely ML, Parliament M, Courneya, KS, et al. A pilot study of a randomized controlled trial to evaluate the effects of progressive resistance exercise training on shoulder dysfunction caused by spinal accessory neurapraxia/neurectomy in head and neck cancer survivors. *Head Neck*. 2004;26: 518-530.

6. Lauchlan DT, McCaul JA, McCarron T. Neck dissection and the clinical appearance of post-operative shoulder disability: the post-operative role of physiotherapy. *Eur J Cancer Care*. 2008;17:542-548.

7. Gordon SL, Graham WP III, Black JT, Black JT, Miller SH. Accessory nerve function and surgical procedures in the posterior triangle. *Arch Surg*. 1977;112:264-268.

8. Hillel AD, Patten C. Neck dissection: morbidity and rehabilitation. In: Jacobs C, ed. *Carcinoma of the Head and Neck: Evaluation and Management*. Boston, MA: Kluwer Academic Publishers; 1990.

9. Stam HW. Frozen shoulder: a review of current concepts. *Physiotherapy*. 1994;80:588-598.

10. Mottram SL. Dynamic stability of the scapula. *Man Ther*. 1997;2:123-131.

11. Hess SA. Functional stability of the glenohumeral joint. *Man Ther*. 2000;5:63-71.

12. Panjabi MM. The stabilizing system of the spine. Part I. Function, dysfunction, adaptation, and enhancement. *J Spinal Disord*. 1992;5:383-389.

13. Lauchlan D, McCaul JA, McCarron T, Patil S, McManners J, McGarva J. An exploratory trial of preventative rehabilitation on shoulder disability and quality of life in patients following neck dissection surgery. *Eur J Cancer Care*. 2011;20:113-122.

14. Ustun TB, Chatterji S, Bickenbach J, Kostanjsek N, Schneider M. The International Classification of Functioning, Disability and Health: a new tool for understanding disability and health. *Disabil Rehabil*. 2003;25:565-571.

15. Jull GA. Deep cervical flexor muscle dysfunction in whiplash. *J Musculoskeletal Pain*. 2000;8: 143-154.

16. Clarkson HM. *Musculoskeletal Assessment: Joint Range of Motion and Manual Muscle Strength*. 2nd ed. Philadelphia, PA: Lippincott Williams & Wilkins; 2000.

17. Constant CR, Murley AH. A clinical method of functional assessment of the shoulder. *Clin Orthop Relat Res*. 1987;214:160-164.

18. Rogers SN, Scott B, Lowe D. An evaluation of the shoulder domain of the University of Washington quality of life scale. *Br J Oral Maxillofac Surg*. 2007;45:5-10.

19. Ware JE Jr, Sherbourne CD. The MOS 36-item short form health survey (SF-36). Conceptual framework and item selection. *Med Care*. 1992;30:473-481.

20. Morton RP, Izzard ME. Quality-of-life outcomes in head and neck cancer patients. *World J Surg*. 2003;27:884-889.

21. Ginn KA, Herbert RD, Khouw W, Lee R. A randomized, controlled clinical trial of a treatment for shoulder pain. *Phys Ther*. 1997;77:802-811.

22. Crawford HJ, Jull GA. The influence of thoracic posture and movement on range of arm elevation. *Physiother Theory Pract*. 1993;9:143-148.

23. Mercer SW, Maxwell M, Heaney D, Watt GC. The consultation and relational empathy (CARE) measure: development and preliminary validation and reliability of an empathy-based consultation process measure. *Fam Pract*. 2004;21:699-705.

24. Schwartz CE, Sprangers MA. Methodological approaches for assessing response shift in longitudinal health-related quality-of-life research. *Soc Sci Med*. 1999;48:1531-1548.

Thoracic Spinal Cord Tumor

Johanna Gabbard

A 47-year-old active female was referred to physical therapy with a 6-week history of right-sided interscapular thoracic back pain and neck stiffness of insidious onset. She felt that the increased intensity of her symptoms might be associated with her recently intensified weight-training program. Her pain was worsening and she was having difficulty getting into a comfortable position at night, although she could eventually get to sleep by adjusting her pillows. Over the past 3 months, she has lost 20 lb, attributing this loss to a planned diet and exercise program she started 6 months ago. Her initial neurologic examination was normal and her signs and symptoms were consistent with a musculoskeletal disorder. The physical therapist provided manual therapy and prescribed therapeutic exercise directed to the cervical and thoracic spine for two sessions over a 7-day period. At the third therapy visit, her back symptoms were unchanged and she noted her legs were feeling "heavy." She also reported having some problems climbing up stairs. The physical therapist repeated the neurologic screen and found that the initial physical therapy diagnosis of mechanical back pain was *not* consistent with new myelopathic signs and symptoms indicative of spinal cord compression. The therapist referred the patient to her primary care provider and an MRI scan was ordered. Subsequently, the patient was diagnosed as having a thoracic meningioma—an intradural extramedullary spinal cord tumor extending from T2 to T5 that was causing thoracic cord compression (Fig. 10-1).

▶ What signs and symptoms are associated with this diagnosis?
▶ What are the most appropriate examination tests?
▶ What are the examination priorities?

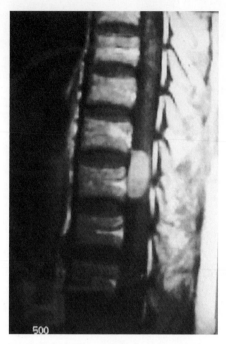

Figure 10-1. T1-weighted sagittal magnetic resonance image showing intradural extramedullary meningioma. (Reproduced from Song KW, Shin SI, Lee JY, Kim GL, Hyun YS, Park DY. Surgical results of intradural extramedullary tumors. *Clin Orthop Surg.* 2009;1:74-80. Figure 1A.)

KEY DEFINITIONS

INTRADURAL EXTRAMEDULLARY TUMOR: Spinal cord tumor that is located within the dura but outside of the spinal cord itself

MENINGIOMA: Slow-growing tumor within the dura; arises from cells of the meningeal covering of the brain and spinal cord

MYELOPATHY: Upper motor neuron disorder caused by compression or ischemia of the spinal cord

SPINAL CORD TUMOR: Abnormal growth of cells in or surrounding the spinal cord

Objectives

1. List the classification of spinal cord tumors.

2. Describe the typical progression of compressive thoracic myelopathy caused by spinal cord tumors.

3. Describe clinical examination findings that are helpful in differentiating musculoskeletal versus non-musculoskeletal pathology.

4. Describe appropriate clinical examination tests that help rule in or rule out musculoskeletal back pain.

Physical Therapy Considerations

PT considerations during examination of the individual with thoracic back pain and progressing neurologic signs and symptoms:

▶ **General physical therapy plan of care/goals:** Medical screening for red flags, neurologic screen at initial and subsequent visits for any patient with clinical presentation of constant midline thoracic pain with insidious onset, failure to improve with conservative medical treatment, weight loss of more than 4.5 kg in 6 months, progressive neurologic changes and positive pathological reflexes

▶ **Physical therapy tests and measures:** Careful patient history, upper and lower quarter neurologic screening tests, dermatome and myotome testing, deep tendon reflexes, assessment for upper motor neuron signs (*e.g.*, Hoffman's sign, clonus, Babinski's sign, inverted supinator reflex, grip and release test)

▶ **Differential diagnoses:** Referred thoracic back pain from visceral structures, spinal cord disease, metastatic disease

▶ **Complications interfering with physical therapy:** Progressive neurologic signs, spinal cord compression

Understanding Health Condition

The thoracic spine is a common site for spinal cord tumors[1] and the most common spinal region for metastatic disease.[2,3] Spinal cord tumors can be either primary or secondary. Primary spinal tumors are formed from cells of the spinal cord or its meningeal coverings. They are much less common than secondary tumors and have an annual incidence in the United States of roughly 0.7 per 100,000 persons.[4] Secondary spinal tumors, or metastatic tumors, comprise the majority of spinal cord lesions. Tumors that most often metastasize to the spine include those from lung, breast, and prostate cancers.[5,6]

Spinal cord tumors are classified according to the anatomical location of the tumor mass in relation to the dura mater and spinal cord. Spinal tumors that arise outside the dura mater are called extradural tumors. These comprise the majority of spinal tumors and include those of metastatic origin. Tumors that arise within the dura are known as intradural tumors and are mostly benign. Intradural tumors are further subdivided into extramedullary tumors (those that originate outside the spinal cord) and intramedullary tumors (those that arise within the substance of the spinal cord itself). Table 10-1 lists common causes of spinal canal lesions based on location.

Spinal meningiomas are classified as intradural, extramedullary primary spinal tumors. These are slow-growing tumors arising from cells of the meningeal covering of the brain and spinal cord. Spinal meningiomas are usually benign and generally do not metastasize. Like most spinal tumors, they typically present with an insidious onset of back pain followed by slow, progressive neurologic disturbances. Spinal meningiomas comprise approximately 25% of all primary spinal tumors in adults and most of these occur in the thoracic spine.[10,11] There is a strong female preponderance and the peak age of occurrence is in the fifth and sixth decade.[10]

Table 10-1 CAUSES OF SPINAL CANAL LESIONS BASED ON SITE OF ORIGIN[7-9]		
Intradural (intramedullary)	Intradural (extramedullary)	Extradural
Syringomyelia Intramedullary tumor (e.g., ependymoma) Inflammation (e.g., abscess, myelitis) Multiple sclerosis	Meningioma Neurofibroma Metastasis (e.g., leptomeningeal seeding or hematogenous)	Herniated disc Spinal stenosis, spondylosis, osteophyte Ligamentum flavum thickening, intraspinal ligament ossification Meningioma Neurogenic tumor (e.g., neurofibroma) Metastasis Vertebral neoplasm with intraspinal extension

Physical Therapy Patient/Client Management

Serious etiologies of back pain such as tumors, fractures, or infections are relatively rare and account for less than 1% of all medical cases seen during spine assessment.[12] Although uncommon, it is incumbent on the physical therapist to be aware of sinister conditions. One of the primary roles of the physical therapist is to demonstrate proficiency in medical screening and clinical reasoning skills throughout the examination to help identify these cases and refer appropriately and expediently.

Back pain arising from underlying serious medical disease can be indistinguishable from benign musculoskeletal pain. However, patients with *thoracic* back pain are proportionately more likely to have serious spinal pathology than patients with cervical or lumbar back pain.[13] This may be secondary to several unique characteristics that render the thoracic region vulnerable to injury or disease. First, the thoracic spine lies in close proximity to many visceral structures; when diseased, viscera can cause local or referred pain.[14] Second, the thoracic spinal cord occupies more space within the spinal canal than its cervical or lumbar counterparts. It is estimated that the spinal cord to spinal canal ratio in the thoracic region is 40% compared to 25% in the cervical region.[15] Thus, the thoracic spine has little tolerance for a space-occupying lesion, such as a herniated disc or spinal tumor. Third, primary spinal cord tumors and metastases are more commonly found in the thoracic region.[2,3] Although the majority of intradural spinal cord tumors are generally benign, marked deterioration of neurologic function can have a profound effect on the patient's health status. Surgical resection is the treatment of choice. Surgical resection has been shown to retard further progression of signs and symptoms, but has been less effective in improving existing neurologic impairments.[16] Therefore, the physical therapist plays a critical role in screening and monitoring for any deterioration of the neurologic status of patients with spinal symptoms and in reducing the risk of late diagnosis of a thoracic spinal lesion.

Examination, Evaluation, and Diagnosis

Signs and symptoms of thoracic spinal cord tumors vary depending on the spinal segments involved and the severity of the lesion. In this patient's case, pain was initially the chief complaint. The patient often presents with midline thoracic pain directly over the spinal lesion, which may or may not be accompanied by pain or discomfort in the shoulder, cervical, upper lumbar, or even anterior chest region. Pain in the latter areas may be more intense than the midline thoracic pain. This pain pattern is a common presentation for many mechanical musculoskeletal conditions, making it very difficult to discern serious pathology from benign musculoskeletal conditions. Despite the mechanical appearance of the complaint, thoracic back pain should always be screened for underlying serious conditions due to the proximity to the visceral systems and the region's vulnerability to metastatic disease and cord compression.[14] General screening for **red flags of possible metastatic or primary spinal tumors** should include questions about: (1) previous personal history of cancer, (2) failure to improve with conservative medical treatment over the past month, (3) age $\geq$ 50 years old, and (4) unexplained weight loss of more than 10 lb in 6 months. In 1988, Deyo and Diehl reported these four positive clinical findings had the highest positive likelihood ratios for detecting the presence of cancer in patients with low back pain.[5] The most sensitive finding in the patient's history when screening for cancer was lack of pain relief from rest (sensitivity > 90%).[5,17] Although the patient in this case has thoracic back pain (not low back pain), positive responses to these questions should lean the physical therapist away from a diagnosis of mechanical back pain. The patient reported weight loss of 20 lb over a 3-month timeframe. She also reported difficulty finding a comfortable position at night due to resting back pain. These positive responses should raise the therapist's index of suspicion and should be explored further to see if there is a reasonable explanation offered for the weight loss and resting night pain. Although the patient provided what appeared to be reasonable explanations for her signs and symptoms, the physical therapist must re-address these issues if the patient fails to respond to expected outcomes.

Particular attention should be paid to the cardiac, pulmonary, gastrointestinal and urogenital systems, which commonly refer pain to the thoracic region.[18] Complaints of cyclical pain, cramping, pressure, symptoms related to food intake or type of food may lead the physical therapist to examine certain visceral structures in more detail. For example, an atypical portrayal of symptoms, such as throbbing, pulsating and pounding are descriptors more common with vascular disorders.

In the absence of red flags that might warrant referral or further diagnostic testing, a comprehensive neuromusculoskeletal examination must be performed to rule out other mechanical structures as the source of the patient's symptoms. Table 10-2 lists differential diagnoses that the physical therapist should consider when a patient presents with thoracic back pain. The differential examination should consider common local etiologies such as muscle or myofascial strain or injury, thoracic facet

Table 10–2   DIFFERENTIAL DIAGNOSES TO CONSIDER FOR PATIENTS PRESENTING WITH THORACIC BACK PAIN

Musculoskeletal Local Sources	Musculoskeletal Referral Sources	Neurological Sources	Non-musculoskeletal Sources
Muscle strain Vertebral or rib fracture Zygapophyseal joint dysfunction Rib dysfunction Ankylosing spondylitis Thoracic disc disease Thoracic disc herniation	Cervical radiculopathy Cervical disc disease Cervical disc herniation	Intercostal neuralgia Cauda equina	Cardiovascular: myocardial infarction, aortic aneurysm, angina Pulmonary: lung cancer, pneumothorax, pulmonary emboli, pleurisy Gastrointestinal: cholecystitis, peptic or gastric ulcer Renal: pyelonephritis, nephrolithiasis Metastatic disease Tuberculosis Inflammatory: multiple sclerosis, acute myelitis

dysfunction, disc herniation, rib joint dysfunction, intercostal neuralgia, or postural syndrome.[19] Local palpation of these areas may reveal excessive muscle guarding or possible localized swelling. Specific palpation and accessory joint testing of the thoracic region often reveals local tenderness and may reveal excessive muscle guarding, local spasm, and/or swelling. There is evidence that spinal manipulative therapy provides some benefit for patients with thoracic and neck pain without neurologic signs.[20,21] However, the therapist should be aware that muscle spasm and relaxation difficulties are common protective signs that may indicate underlying non-musculoskeletal pathology.

The physical therapist should also consider the possibility of regional interdependence and screen for referred etiologies from the cervical spine and shoulder regions.[21-23] These may include cervical facet dysfunction, cervical disc herniation or radiculopathy, primary or referred shoulder dysfunction, local myofascial or referred pain, or postural dysfunction.[19] For this patient with a primary spinal thoracic tumor, manual stress applied to these distant regions would not likely refer pain to the midline.

As the spinal tumor or any space-occupying lesion such as a thoracic disc herniation progresses, the initial complaints of musculoskeletal symptoms progress to signs of neurologic compromise of the spinal cord. Although thoracic radiculopathy caused by intraspinal tumors has been reported, it is unusual; myelopathy from spinal cord compression is the more common clinical presentation.[24] Myelopathy is a pathological condition caused by compression and ischemia of the spinal cord.[25,26] Spinal cord myelopathy typically follows a general progression of signs and symptoms that includes: hyperreflexia, sensory disturbances, clumsiness, ataxia and gait disturbances, balance difficulties, bowel and bladder dysfunction, motor weakness and eventual paraplegia or quadriplegia. Patients with myelopathy in the upper thoracic spine (T1-T4) may complain of weakness and sensory deficits in the hands, arms, shoulders, and legs. Mid-thoracic and lumbar tumors may cause weakness and numbness in the chest, lower trunk, and legs. In the case of thoracic back pain, an upper and lower quarter neurologic screen should be conducted as a component of the physical therapy examination.

Beyond the traditional dermatome, myotome, and deep tendon reflex screening, the physical therapist should select neurologic tests and measures that effectively screen for disease and are highly sensitive. In highly sensitive tests, a negative finding significantly reduces the odds that the disease is present.[27] Clinical tests used to assess for the presence of upper motor neuron signs that may indicate cord compression include: Hoffman's sign, clonus, Babinski's sign, inverted supinator reflex, and the grip and release test. Although commonly used, these tests often show low sensitivity when the results from each test are evaluated individually—that is, a single negative finding cannot rule out the absence of the disease. Cook et al.[26] discussed an examination approach that included a comprehensive patient history, ruling out analogous symptoms of cauda equina syndrome (in which positive findings would prompt an immediate medical referral), and using a **battery of clinical tests to improve the ability to rule out cord compression myelopathy**. These tests, taken as a cluster of findings, can help the physical therapist make a more appropriate physician referral for further diagnostic testing. For detecting space-occupying lesions such as spinal cord tumors, **magnetic resonance imaging (MRI)** is the diagnostic test of choice with relatively high sensitivity (79%-95%) and specificity (82%-88%).[26,28,29] Neither plain film imaging, bone scans, computed tomography (CT) or CT myelography can sufficiently delineate or exclude an intradural tumor and may even delay the diagnosis.[28]

Evidence-Based Clinical Recommendations

SORT: Strength of Recommendation Taxonomy

A: Consistent, good-quality patient-oriented evidence
B: Inconsistent or limited-quality patient-oriented evidence
C: Consensus, disease-oriented evidence, usual practice, expert opinion, or case series

1. Positive answers to screening questions that would lean more toward a cancer etiology of low back pain include: previous personal history of cancer, failure to improve with conservative medical treatment over the past month, age ≥ 50 years old, and unexplained weight loss of ≥ 10 pounds in 6 months. **Grade B**

2. Physical therapists can use careful screening, a comprehensive patient history, and a cluster of screening tests to help rule out a diagnosis of cord compression myelopathy. **Grade B**

3. Magnetic resonance imaging is the preferred diagnostic test for spinal cord tumor. **Grade A**

COMPREHENSION QUESTIONS

10.1 A patient has been referred to physical therapy with a 6-week history of central thoracic back pain that is provoked by cervical spine movements. Which of the following signs or symptoms would cause the physical therapist to pause and seek further clarification or consider referral to a medical provider?

  A. Age over 50 years

  B. Family history of a cardiac disease

  C. Bilateral calf numbness and weakness

  D. Weight loss of 5 lb in past 6 months

10.2 Which of the following signs or symptoms is *not* commonly associated with spinal cord myelopathy?

  A. Spastic gait

  B. Vertigo

  C. Clumsiness

  D. Urinary incontinence

ANSWERS

10.1 **C.** Bilateral signs and symptoms are commonly associated with pathology of the central nervous system and should always be explored further. Bilateral sensory or motor changes can be caused by stenosis of the spinal canal or a space-occupying lesions such as a spinal tumor or herniated disc. A family history of cardiac disease (option B) or age over 50 years (option A) would likely not cause a physical therapist to suspect this clinical presentation. A significant weight loss more suggestive of a cancerous etiology is considered more than 10 lb over a 6-month period (option D).[5]

10.2 **B.** Spinal cord myelopathy, which is caused by compression and ischemia of the spinal cord, results in upper motor neuron symptoms such as hyperreflexia, spasticity, motor disturbances, and poor bladder or bowel control. Although vertigo can be caused by a peripheral or central nervous system disorder, it is not typically associated with upper motor neuron disturbances.

REFERENCES

1. Solero CL, Fornari M, Giombini S, et al. Spinal meningiomas: review of 174 operated cases. *Neurosurgery.* 1989;25:153-160.

2. Kakulas BA, Harper CG, Shibasaki K, Bedbrook GM. Vertebral metastases and spinal cord compression. *Clin Exp Neurol.* 1978;15:127-132.

3. Sioutos PJ, Arbit E, Meshulam CF, Galicich JH. Spinal metastases from solid tumors. Analysis of factors affecting survival. *Cancer.* 1995;1453-1459.

4. Schellinger KA, Propp JM, Villano JL, McCarthy BJ. Descriptive epidemiology of primary spinal cord tumors. *J Neurooncol.* 2008;87:173-179.

5. Deyo RA, Diehl AK. Cancer as a cause of back pain: frequency, clinical presentation, and diagnostic strategies. *J Gen Intern Med.* 1988;3:230-238.

6. Chairners J. Tumours of the musculoskeletal system: clinical presentation. *Curr Orthop*. 1988;2:135-140.

7. Reeder MM, Felson B, Bradley WG. *Reeder and Felson's Gamuts in Radiology: Comprehensive Lists of Roentegen Differential Diagnosis*. 3rd ed. New York: Springler-Verlag Talos; 1993:148-149.

8. Patel SN, Kettner NW, Osbourne CA. Myelopathy: a report of two cases. *J Manipulative Physiol Ther*. 2005;28:539-546.

9. Hudson BR, Cook C, Goode A. Identifying myelopathy caused by thoracic syringomyelia: a case report. *J Man Manip Therapy*. 2008;16:82-88.

10. Sandalcioglu IE, Hunold A, Muller O, Bassiouni H, Stolke D, Asgari S. Spinal meningiomas: critical review of 131 surgically treated patients. *Eur Spine J*. 2008;17:1035-1041.

11. Chamberlain MC, Tredway TL. Adult primary intradural spinal cord tumors: a review. *Curr Neurol Neurosci Rep*. 2011;11:320-328.

12. Sizer PS Jr, Brismee JM, Cook C. Medical screening for red flags in the diagnosis and management of musculoskeletal spine pain. *Pain Pract*. 2007;7:53-71.

13. Boissonnault WG, Bass C. Pathological origins of trunk and neck pain: part I—pelvic and abdominal visceral disorders. *J Orthop Sports Phys Ther*. 1990;12:192-207.

14. Boissonnault WG. *Primary Care for the Physical Therapist: Examination and Triage*. 2nd ed. St. Louis, MO: Saunders; 2011:76-78.

15. Maiman DJ, Pintar FA. Anatomy and clinical biomechanics of the thoracic spine. *Clin Neurosurg*. 1992;38:296-324.

16. Fujiwara K, Yonenobu K, Ebara S, Yamashita K, Ono K. The prognosis of surgery for cervical compression myelopathy. An analysis of the factors involved. *J Bone Joint Surg Br*. 1989;71:393-398.

17. Deyo RA, Rainville J, Kent DL. What can the history and physical examination tell us about low back pain? *JAMA*. 1992;268:760-765.

18. Goodman CC, Snyder TE. *Differential Diagnosis for Physical Therapists: Screening for Referral*. 4th ed. St. Louis, MO: Saunders; 2007.

19. Fruth JS. Differential diagnosis and treatment in a patient with posterior upper thoracic pain. *Phys Ther*. 2006;86:254-268.

20. Campbell BD, Snodgrass SJ. The effects of thoracic manipulation on posterior spinal stiffness. *J Orthop Sports Phys Ther*. 2010;40:685-693.

21. Cleland JA, Childs JD, McRae M, Palmer JA, Stowell T. Immediate effects of thoracic manipulation in patients with neck pain: a randomized clinical trial. *Man Ther*. 2005;10:127-135.

22. Wainner RS. Whitman JM, Cleland JA, Flynn TW. Regional interdependence: a musculoskeletal examination model whose time has come. *J Orthop Sports Phys Ther*. 2007;37:658-660.

23. Bergman GJ, Winters JC, Groenier KH, et al. Manipulative therapy in addition to usual medical care for patients with shoulder dysfunction and pain: a randomized, controlled trial. *Ann Intern Med*. 2004;141:432-439.

24. Renders KJ, Van Wambeke PV, Peers KH, Morlion BJ. A thoracal radiculopathy as the only presenting sign of a meningioma. *J Back Musculoskeletal Rehabil*. 2008;21:63-65.

25. Posner JB. Back pain and epidural spinal cord compression. *Med Clin North Am*. 1987;71:185-205.

26. Cook CE, Hegedus E, Pietrobon R, Goode A. A pragmatic neurological screen for patients with suspected cord compressive myelopathy. *Phys Ther*. 2007;87:1233-1242.

27. Ross MD, Bayer E. Cancer as a cause of low back pain in a patient seen in a direct access physical therapy setting. *J Orthop Sports Phys Ther*. 2005;35:651-658.

28. Abdul-Kasim, K, Thrunher MM, McKeever P, Sundgren PC. Intradural spinal tumors: current classification and MRI features. *Neuroradiology*. 2008;50:301-314.

29. Sze G, Abramson A, Krol G, et al. Gadolinium-DTPA in the evaluation of intradural extramedullary spinal disease. *AJR Am J Roentgenol*. 1988;150:911-921.

Lateral Epicondylalgia

R. Barry Dale

CASE 11

A 44-year-old carpenter has been referred to physical therapy with a diagnosis of right lateral elbow pain. He is right-hand dominant and reports that he has "worked with his hands all his life." His pain has been "off and on" over the last 6 months, but exacerbated while working overtime 2 weeks ago. His past medical history is unremarkable except for prehypertension and recently quitting smoking 8 months ago (0.25 pack per day for ~20 years). He also fell from a ladder 4 years ago and sustained an injury to his neck that was treated with rest, cervical collar, and massage. Recent radiographs of the elbow and shoulder are negative for obvious pathology; however, the cervical spine shows changes consistent with mild degeneration in the right apophyseal joints of C6 and C7. The patient started nonsteroidal anti-inflammatory medication 6 days ago. You are asked to evaluate and treat the patient for 4 weeks before follow-up with his orthopaedic physician. His current complaints are pain in the right elbow and weakness with active gripping, wrist extension, and forearm supination. The pain and weakness limit his ability to work as a carpenter. His goal is to return to work as soon as possible.

► Based on the patient's diagnosis, what are the contributing factors to the condition?
► What are the most appropriate examination tests?
► What are the most appropriate physical therapy interventions?
► What are possible complications that may limit the effectiveness of physical therapy?

KEY DEFINITIONS

CENTRAL SENSITIZATION: Changes within the central nervous system in response to chronic pain resulting in hyperalgesia, a perceptual amplification to noxious stimuli

COUNTERFORCE BRACING: Circumferential orthotic usually comprised an inelastic material worn distal to the lateral humeral epicondyle

LATERAL EPICONDYLALGIA: Pain at the lateral humeral epicondyle, typically at the common extensor tendon; associated with overuse of the wrist extensor muscles

NEOVASCULARIZATION: Growth of new capillaries associated with tissue healing; in tendinopathy, new capillaries may displace collagen and lead to tendon weakening and ultimately failure; free nerve endings accompanying new capillaries likely contribute to pain associated with chronic tendinopathy

TENDINITIS (tendonitis): Relatively *acute* manifestation of a tendon injury associated with hallmark signs and symptoms of inflammation (heat, redness, swelling, pain, and loss of function)

TENDINOPATHY (tendinosis): Painful *chronic* degeneration of a tendon, largely in the absence of classic inflammation; associated with disorganized collagen and neovascularization

Objectives

1. Describe lateral epicondylalgia and identify potential risk factors associated with this diagnosis.
2. Prescribe appropriate manual therapy interventions for a patient with lateral epicondylalgia.
3. Prescribe appropriate joint range of motion and/or muscular flexibility exercises for a patient with lateral epicondylalgia.
4. Prescribe appropriate resistance exercises for a patient with lateral epicondylalgia.
5. Prescribe appropriate adjunctive interventions for a patient with lateral epicondylalgia.

Physical Therapy Considerations

PT considerations during management of the individual with a diagnosis of lateral epicondylalgia:

▶ **General physical therapy plan of care/goals:** Decrease pain; increase muscular flexibility; maintain or prevent loss of range of motion of wrist and elbow joints; increase upper quadrant strength; prevent or minimize loss of aerobic fitness capacity

▶ **Physical therapy interventions:** Patient education regarding functional anatomy and injury pathomechanics; modalities and manual therapy to decrease pain; muscular flexibility exercises; resistance exercises to increase muscular endurance capacity and strength of upper extremity muscles; aerobic exercise program; counterforce bracing

▶ **Precautions during physical therapy:** Monitor vital signs; address precautions or contraindications for exercise, based on patient's pre-existing condition(s)

Understanding the Health Condition

Lateral epicondylalgia is pain experienced at the lateral humeral epicondyle, usually as a result of overuse of the wrist extensor muscles. Other commonly used terms to describe this syndrome are "tennis elbow," lateral epicondylitis, and wrist extensor tendinopathy (tendinitis or tendinosis). Lateral epicondylalgia is becoming the term of choice because the true pathogenesis of this condition is unclear.[1] The predominant complaint for patients with lateral epicondylalgia is pain with active or resisted movements and weakness with wrist extension, supination, and gripping activities. Prevalence in the general population is around 1% to 3% and varies little between males and females.[2,3] Persons in the age range of 45 to 54 years are at the greatest risk for developing the condition and there appears to be an increased risk in individuals who currently smoke or who have smoked tobacco.[2] Individuals are likely to experience the condition in the dominant upper extremity. Persons who participate in forceful and repetitive movements are 5.6 times more likely to develop lateral epicondylalgia than those who do not.[2]

The lateral humeral epicondyle is the origin for the common wrist extensors, and the extensor carpi radialis brevis (ECRB) is most commonly implicated with lateral epicondylalgia.[4,5] Wrist extensors activate during maximal gripping activities to oppose finger and wrist flexion (e.g., when hammering a nail). This partially explains the involvement of the ECRB with gripping activities because the ideal wrist position for maximal grip strength is slight extension of about 15°.[6] Histopathology from individuals presenting with lateral epicondylalgia shows tissue degradation and collagen disorganization within the ECRB.[4,5] Neovascularization and the accompaniment of free nerve endings that give rise to pain are also present.[7] Neurochemicals such as glutamate, substance P, and calcitonin gene-related peptide are abundant and also contribute to tissue sensitivity.[7,8]

While the exact pathogenesis of lateral epicondylalgia is uncertain, the most commonly proposed etiologies are tendinopathies (tendinitis, tendinosis) and radial nerve entrapment.[4] Tendinopathy is distinct from nerve compression, and it is possible that some degree of tendon pathology and nerve entrapment could be present with a patient diagnosed with lateral epicondylalgia. Tendons have lower oxygen consumption and collagen turnover rate than that of other tissues.[7,9] Tissue integrity is a byproduct of the intricate balance between tissue degradation and regeneration. When this balance is disrupted by disproportionate stresses associated with excessive physical activity, it can lead to tendon degradation. Occupational and recreational activities (*e.g.*, carpentry, typing, golf, tennis) may contribute to the development of tendinopathy.[2,10] Distal entrapment of the radial nerve may also contribute to symptoms associated with lateral epicondylalgia.[4] Innervation of the ECRB occurs either via the main branch of the radial nerve, the posterior branch of the radial nerve, or from the superficial branch of the radial nerve.[4] Nayak et al.[4] examined 72 cadaver specimens and found that 29% had a tendinous arch and 11% had a muscular arch in the ECRB musculature. The presence of an arch could compress the nerve during repeated movements, which would result in an entrapment syndrome.

An integrative model of the etiology of lateral epicondylalgia proposed by Coombes, Bisset, and Vicenzo suggests that changes may also occur in local and central pain processing and that motor impairments often accompany local tendon pathology.[8] The affected elbow of individuals with lateral epicondylalgia may experience up to 50% reduced tolerance to pressure-related pain compared to the unaffected elbow. Hypersensitivity over the lateral epicondyle is likely mediated by increased local neurochemicals such as glutamate, substance P, and calcitonin; however, it is also possible that central sensitization associated with altered processing in the spinal cord or brain contributes to abnormal pain sensation.[8,11,12] This may also lead to pain within neurologically related structures such as the cervical spine. For example, there is a high prevalence of neck pain in individuals with lateral epicondylalgia that persists despite adjustments for age and the presence of degenerative joint conditions of the neck.[1,8] Although it is important to recognize the frequent association of neck pain and lateral epicondylalgia, it is equally important to recognize that this association should not be confused with causation.

Motor changes commonly occur with tendinopathies and often lead to performance difficulty with functional and occupational activities. **Grip strength** is detrimentally affected and individuals with lateral epicondylalgia often report significant difficulty carrying grocery bags.[3] It is likely that there is some interaction of the pain system and motor deficits associated with lateral epicondylalgia. Pain-free grip strength is a clinical test that is sensitive to change for patients with lateral epicondylalgia.[13] This test quantifies the interaction between pain and muscle activation during gripping activity with a handgrip dynamometer. As patients recover from lateral epicondylalgia, maximal pain-free grip force should increase.

Physical Therapy Patient/Client Management

Patients with lateral epicondylalgia typically complain of pain at the lateral aspect of the affected elbow. The pain may arise insidiously or suddenly during an activity that uses the common wrist extensors. In early stages, symptoms often resolve as the activity discontinues, but returns upon resumption of activity or exercise. Pain often limits activity participation and symptoms may be present at rest.

Examination, Evaluation, and Diagnosis

The physical therapist must determine if the patient's complaints are localized to the origin of the wrist extensors and whether there is contribution from the cervical spine and/or radial nerve entrapment. The therapist should thoroughly screen and, if necessary, examine the cervical spine to rule out its potential contribution to the patient's clinical presentation. A thorough examination (of any joint) should at least include active range of motion, application of overpressure at end range, passive physiological movements, passive accessory movements, and resistance to movement.[14] The physical therapist notes impairments or limitations and whether the patient's symptoms were reproduced. Provocative physical examination techniques are likely to reproduce the patient's complaint of pain. Most of the examination procedures are either passive stretching or active resistive maneuvers with or without palpation of the wrist extensor muscle group or lateral epicondyle. Physical examination techniques for lateral epicondylalgia are described in Table 11-1 (see page 154). Most of these tests can be performed with the patient sitting on a high plinth.

According to Haker, radial nerve entrapment may be determined by the presence of pain localized approximately two finger breadths inferior to the elbow's flexor crease and medial to the common extensor mass.[5] Other symptoms associated with radial nerve entrapment are night pain, motor dysfunction, and radiating pain into the forearm.[5] The radial nerve tension test determines the presence of neural tension commonly associated with entrapment.[15,16]

Plan of Care and Interventions

There are many interventions from which to choose to treat lateral epicondylalgia. However, the examination should steer the physical therapist toward a selection of potentially beneficial treatments. The potential interventions include manual therapy, exercises, and adjunctive procedures such as modalities.

Manual therapy interventions for lateral epicondylalgia are listed in Table 11-2 (see page 155). **Manual therapy of the cervical and or thoracic spine** could benefit the patient with concomitant neck pathologies, and there is some evidence to show a potential benefit in some individuals with lateral epicondylalgia.[23,24] The decision to address the cervical and or thoracic spine with mobilizations must derive from the results of the initial examination. Cleland, Flynn, and Palmer performed cervical and thoracic intervertebral joint arthrokinematic assessments (described by Maitland[14]) in individuals with lateral epicondylalgia.[24] Hypomobility limitations were treated with mobilization techniques at the involved segments with grade III and IV passive physiological and accessory mobilizations, which were applied in addition to traditional treatments for lateral epicondylalgia.[14,24] Patients receiving manual therapy at the cervical and or thoracic spine improved to a greater extent than individuals that only received treatment at the elbow, but is worthy to note that

Table 11-1 PHYSICAL EXAMINATION TECHNIQUES FOR LATERAL EPICONDYLALGIA

Test	Patient Position	Therapist Action	Findings
Cozen's test or sign[17,18] (active resisted)	Have the patient make a fist, and place patient's elbow in 90° flexion, forearm pronation, and full wrist extension and radial deviation.	Apply maximal resistance to wrist extensors while palpating lateral epicondyle.	Test is positive if patient's symptoms are reproduced.
Thomsen test[5] (active resisted)	Place patient's elbow in full extension with full wrist extension.	Apply maximal resistance to wrist extensors while palpating lateral epicondyle.	Test is positive if patient's symptoms are reproduced.
Handgrip strength test[6] (active resisted)	Patient's shoulder should be in adduction and neutral rotation while seated on a high plinth, elbow flexed at 90° with forearm in neutral pronation/supination, and wrist in ~15° extension. Standardize grip size for consistency (e.g., second position on Jamar dynamometer[6]).	Have patient squeeze dynamometer maximally, which implies that pain is *allowed* during the test (Fig. 11-1).	Record the maximum force produced and compare to the unaffected side.
Pain-free handgrip strength test[5,19-21] (active resisted)	Same position as handgrip strength test.	Have patient squeeze dynamometer with as much force as possible up to the point where pain is encountered. Instruct patient to report when pain occurs (Fig. 11-1).	Record maximum "pain-free" force produced and compare to unaffected side.
Resisted middle finger Maudsley's test[22] (active resisted)	Place patient's shoulder in ~90° flexion, elbow in full extension, forearm in pronation with wrist in neutral with fingers held apart in extension.	Apply resistance into extension at tip of patient's middle finger.	Test is positive if patient's symptoms are reproduced.
Mill's test[17,18] (passive stretch)	Place patient's shoulder at his side, elbow in 90° flexion, forearm in pronation with wrist in full flexion with fingers in full flexion.	While holding the wrist in flexion, move elbow into extension and assess patient's response.	Test is positive if patient's symptoms are reproduced.
Radial nerve tension test[15] (passive stretch)	Place patient's shoulder at his side, elbow in full extension, forearm in pronation with wrist in full flexion with fingers held in full flexion.	Assess for symptom replication.	Test is positive if patient's symptoms are reproduced.
Pain-pressure threshold (passive, digital pressure algometry)[23]	Using a digital pressure algometer, apply force over the origin of the common extensor tendon.	Assess for symptom replication.	Record the maximum force when pain is produced and compare to the unaffected side.

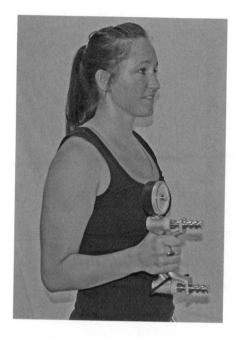

Figure 11-1. Handgrip dynamometer used to measure maximal and pain-free grip strength (Jaymar, Clifton, NJ).

Table 11-2	MANUAL THERAPY INTERVENTIONS FOR LATERAL EPICONDYLALGIA	
Anatomic Region	Technique	Brief Description
Cervical spine	Lateral glides[15,23]	Place patient in supine with affected upper extremity in a position to stretch the radial nerve. Using the webspace of his/her hand, the therapist applies lateral glides at C5/C6 spinal level toward the unaffected side (*e.g.*, for the affected right elbow, the therapist contacts the lateral aspect of the right paraspinal region at level of the C5/C6 segment with his/her right hand, and then produces a straight lateral glide).
Elbow	Mill's manipulation[13]	The patient is sitting with the arm in 90° shoulder abduction and internal rotation (enough to allow olecranon to face upward). Therapist applies small amplitude, high-velocity thrust (grade V) at the end range of elbow extension with forearm in pronation and wrist in full flexion (Fig. 11-2).
	Mulligan mobilizations with movement[25]	Patient identifies an activity that recreates lateral elbow pain and therapist applies a laterally, or posterolaterally directed force (non-thrust) to the radiohumeral joint. Typically, therapist stabilizes the distal humerus with one hand while the other hand contacts the medial forearm and provides a laterally directed mobilization force (Fig. 11-3).
	Transverse friction massage[13,26]	Patient rests comfortably in sitting with affected arm placed on a table at 90° flexion with forearm in supination. Therapist mobilizes soft tissue either across the lateral epicondyle or 1-2 cm distal to the lateral epicondyle with short strokes perpendicular to the common extensor tendon.

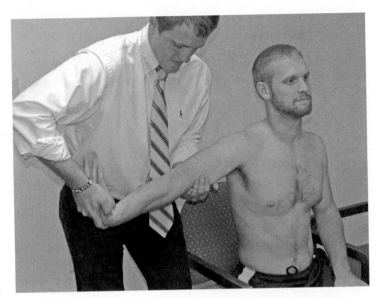

Figure 11-2.
Mill's
manipulation.

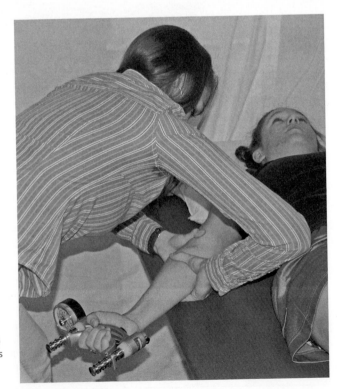

Figure 11-3. Mulligan
mobilizations with
movement (lateral glide)
while the patient performs
a painful movement
(gripping activity).

both groups experienced clinically meaningful improvement over the course of rehabilitation.[24]

Several **mobilization techniques at the elbow** have been described for lateral epicondylalgia: Mill's manipulation, Mulligan mobilization with movement, and soft tissue transverse friction. Typically, a candidate for Mills manipulation has pain emanating from the common extensor tendon at end-range elbow extension with full wrist flexion, pain with palpation over the lateral epicondyle, and pain with gripping and resisted wrist extension.[13] Ideally, radiographs have also demonstrated that the olecranon does not have osteophyte formation. In the absence of imaging, a hard end feel in elbow extension should warn the physical therapist to avoid aggressive maneuvers (author opinion). Vicenzino et al.[21] tested the efficacy of Mulligan mobilization with movement in patients with painful palpation over the lateral epicondyle, painful gripping, and pain with resistance during extension of the second or third finger. Individuals with pain-free grip strength greater than 112 N on the affected side but less than 336 N on the unaffected side, and younger than 49 years of age were more likely to have a favorable response to Mulligan mobilization with movement (clinical prediction rule).

The benefits of joint mobilization and manipulation techniques are most likely mediated by a neurophysiological mechanism, whereas transverse friction massage facilitates tissue remodeling by physical stress.[1]

Exercise interventions for lateral epicondylalgia typically include stretching and strengthening activities (Table 11-3, see page 158).[27-29] The stretching prescription is usually for 30-second holds repeated for 3 to 5 repetitions at least twice per day.[27,28] Strengthening typically includes three sets of 5 to 15 repetitions, and the frequency is typically once per day as part of a daily regimen.[27,29] Exercise provides intrinsic stress to the musculotendinous unit, which stimulates the body to beneficially adapt. Some of the adaptations include increased tissue resiliency and reduced neovascularization.[30,31] A comprehensive program should include both stretching and strengthening activities for the major muscle groups of the upper extremity.

Many **adjunctive and physical modalities** have been proposed to benefit lateral epicondylalgia (Table 11-4, see page 159). Historically, modalities have been used to decrease local inflammation. Physical therapy modalities include various physical forms of energy such as cryotherapy, low intensity ultrasound, phototherapy, and low-level laser. The effectiveness of these modalities has been mixed in the literature.[20,32,33] More recent interventions (e.g., phototherapy, low intensity ultrasound, and low-level laser) attempt to stimulate changes in the tissue histology and do not target inflammation, especially if the condition is chronic.[7,20,32,34-36]

Orthotic management typically includes various forms of **counterforce bracing**.[37,38] These braces are thought to redistribute force along the common extensor tendon and away from the origin at the lateral epicondyle. There has been some evidence to show improvement with functional grip strength and pain with counterforce bracing.[38] However, a comprehensive review by Struijs et al.[37] did not draw definitive conclusions on the effectiveness of counterforce bracing.

Table 11-3	EXERCISE INTERVENTIONS FOR LATERAL EPICONDYLALGIA	
Technique	**Muscle Group**	**Brief Description**
Stretching	Wrist extensors	Begin with elbow in 90° flexion, full forearm pronation, and flex the wrist. Progress by holding the wrist in full flexion while extending the elbow (Fig. 11-4).
	Wrist flexors	Begin with elbow in 90° flexion, full forearm supination, and then extend the wrist. Progress by holding the wrist in full extension while extending the elbow.
	Forearm supinators	Begin with elbow in 90° flexion, and then pronate the forearm.
	Forearm pronators	Begin with elbow in 90° flexion, and then supinate the forearm.
	Radial nerve tension (stretch)	Have patient depress the scapula, internally rotate the shoulder, fully extend the elbow (the forearm pronates automatically when the elbow extends with the glenohumeral joint internally rotated), and flex wrist and fingers.
Strengthening	Grip strength	Begin with gentle gripping activities (below pain threshold) with the elbow in flexion and neutral pronation/supination. Progress with increasing squeeze intensity, and by placing the elbow extension and forearm in pronation.
	Wrist extension (isotonic)	Begin with elbow in 90° flexion, the forearm in full pronation, and then extend wrist with the weight of the hand only. Initially progress by increasing resistance and later by extending elbow.
	Wrist extension (eccentric emphasis)[28,29]	Option 1: Begin with elbow in 90° flexion, the forearm in full pronation, and then extend wrist passively (use the other hand). Once wrist is extended, lower into flexion under eccentric control of wrist extensors. Initially progress by increasing resistance and later by extending elbow. Option 2: FlexBar regimen (Fig. 11-5).
	Wrist flexion	Begin with elbow in 90° flexion, the forearm fully supinated, and then flex wrist with the weight of the hand only. Initially progress by increasing resistance and later by extending elbow.
	Forearm supination	Begin with elbow in 90° flexion and full forearm pronation. Supinate forearm with the weight of the hand only. Progress by increasing resistance.
	Forearm supination (eccentric emphasis)	Begin with elbow in 90° flexion and full forearm pronation. Supinate forearm passively (use the other hand, or gravity). Once forearm is supinated, lower into pronation under eccentric control of supinators. Progress by increasing resistance.
	Forearm pronation	Begin with elbow in 90° flexion and full forearm supination. Pronate forearm with the weight of the hand only. Progress by increasing resistance.

Table 11-4   SELECTED ADJUNCTIVE INTERVENTIONS FOR LATERAL EPICONDYLALGIA

Intervention Category	Specific Intervention	Brief Description
Counterforce bracing	Proprietary orthotic	Orthotic strap placed around the affected forearm just distal to the lateral epicondyle.
Modalities	Ultrasound[39] (low intensity)	Low intensity ultrasound with a frequency of 1.5 MHz, duty cycle of 20%, and spatial average intensity of 30 mW/cm². Note that this is a special ultrasound application (Exogen, Smith and Nephew Inc., Memphis, TN).
	Phototherapy[20]	Polarized (waves move on parallel planes) polychromy (wide range of wavelengths, 480-3400 nm) incoherent (nonsynchronized) and low-energy (40 mW/cm²) light applied at an operating distance of 5-10 cm 3 times per week for 4 weeks may reduce symptoms.
	Low-level laser[35]	Wavelength of 904 nm with low output (5-50 mW) directed at the tendon insertion on the lateral epicondyle over an area of 5 cm² with a dose of 0.25-1.2 J per treatment area appear to be most effective form of low-level laser application.
	Electrical therapy[40]	The patient sits comfortably and holds a ground electrode in the affected hand while resting the arm on a table. The therapist applies the probe electrode to local tender points around the lateral epicondyle. Noxious interrupted, low-frequency (4 Hz) direct current is applied for 30 s, and each tender point is stimulated 3 times for 6 treatment sessions.

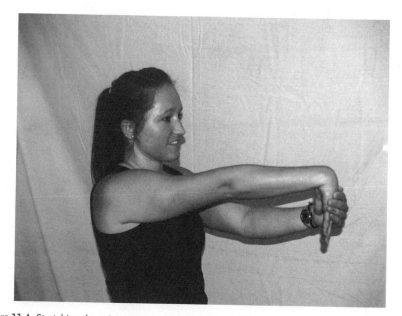

Figure 11-4. Stretching the wrist extensors with the elbow in full extension.

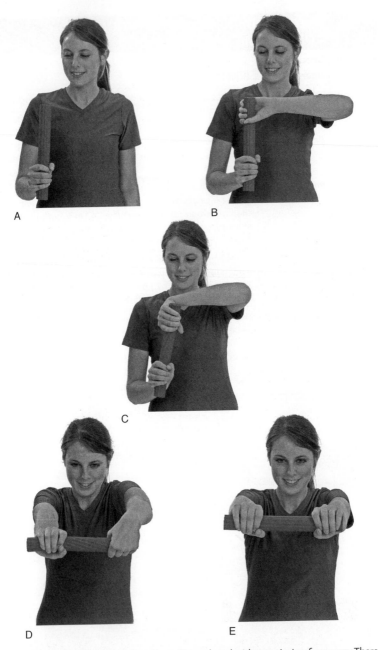

Figure 11-5. The FlexBar "Tyler Twist" regimen (Reproduced with permission from www.Thera-BandAcademy.com and permission from The Hygenic Corporation). **A.** The FlexBar is held at the bottom end by the (right) affected hand with the wrist placed in full extension. **B.** The top end of the FlexBar is held by the unaffected hand, while the affected side is maintained in extension. **C.** The unaffected hand twists the FlexBar by actively flexing the wrist. **D.** The patient then moves the FlexBar to a parallel position to the floor, which places the affected elbow into extension while maintaining the wrist in extension. **E.** The affected wrist slowly allows the FlexBar to "untwist" (eccentric wrist extension) while the unaffected wrist maintains a flexed position.

Evidence-Based Clinical Recommendations

SORT: Strength of Recommendation Taxonomy
A: Consistent, good-quality patient-oriented evidence
B: Inconsistent or limited-quality patient-oriented evidence
C: Consensus, disease-oriented evidence, usual practice, expert opinion, or case series

1. Pain-free grip strength is a sensitive examination sign for documenting impairment associated with lateral epicondylalgia. **Grade A**

2. Manual therapy of the cervical spine is effective for management of lateral epicondylalgia for those individuals who have a cervical spinal pathology contributing to their symptoms. **Grade B**

3. Mobilization techniques at the elbow and stretching and strengthening exercises are effective interventions for treating lateral epicondylalgia. **Grade B**

4. Adjunctive interventions such as low-intensity ultrasound, phototherapy, and low-level laser may be effective treatment for lateral epicondylalgia. **Grade C**

5. Counterforce bracing may be effective for management of lateral epicondylalgia. **Grade C**

COMPREHENSION QUESTIONS

11.1 Patients with lateral epicondylalgia are *most* likely to have impairments with which of the following activities of daily living?
   A. Reaching overhead
   B. Holding a briefcase
   C. Typing on a keyboard
   D. Opening a drawer

11.2 Which of the following manual therapy interventions directly targets the contractile tissue of the lateral elbow?
   A. Lateral glides of the cervical spine
   B. Transverse friction massage of the origin of the wrist extensors
   C. Wrist flexor stretch (by movement into wrist extension)
   D. Mobilization with movement (lateral glide) to radiohumeral joint

11.3 Which of the following muscles is *most* commonly implicated in the tendinopathy associated with lateral epicondylalgia?
   A. Extensor carpi radialis brevis
   B. Flexor carpi ulnaris
   C. Supinator
   D. Pronator teres

ANSWERS

11.1 **B.** Holding or carrying objects requires static grip strength. In patients with lateral epicondylalgia, grip strength impairment is well documented and pain-free grip strength is considered a very useful clinical assessment measure.

11.2 **B.** All of these interventions have some evidence to support their use in the treatment of lateral epicondylalgia; however, transverse friction massage is the only intervention that directly targets the contractile tissue of the common extensor tendon.

11.3 **A.** Extensor carpi radialis brevis is the most commonly affected muscle of the lateral elbow musculature with respect to tendinopathy.

REFERENCES

1. Vicenzino B, Cleland JA, Bisset L. Joint manipulation in the management of lateral epicondylalgia: a clinical commentary. *J Man Manip Ther.* 2007;15:50-56.

2. Shiri R, Viikari-Juntura E, Varonen H, Heliovaara M. Prevalence and determinants of lateral and medial epicondylitis: a population study. *Am J Epidemiol.* 2006;164:1065-1074.

3. Walker-Bone K, Palmer KT, Reading I, Coggon D, Cooper C. Prevalence and impact of musculoskeletal disorders of the upper limb in the general population. *Arthritis Rheum.* 2004;51:642-651.

4. Nayak S, Ramanatha L, Krishnamurthy A, et al. Extensor carpi radialis brevis origin, nerve supply and its role in lateral epicondylitis. *Surg Radiol Anat.* 2010;32:207-211.

5. Haker E. Lateral epicondylalgia: diagnosis, treatment, and evaluation. *Crit Rev Phys Rehabil Med.* 1993;5:129-154.

6. Bhargava AS, Eapen C, Kumar SP. Grip strength measurements at two different wrist extension positions in chronic lateral epicondylitis-comparison of involved vs. uninvolved side in athletes and non athletes: a case-control study. *Sports Med Arthrosc Rehabil Ther Technol.* 2010;2:22.

7. Abate M, Silbernagel KG, Siljeholm C, et al. Pathogenesis of tendinopathies: inflammation or degeneration? *Arthritis Res Ther.* 2009;11:235.

8. Coombes BK, Bisset L, Vicenzino B. A new integrative model of lateral epicondylalgia. *Br J Sports Med.* 2009;43:252-258.

9. Vailas AC, Tipton CM, Laughlin HL, Tcheng TK, Matthes RD. Physical activity and hypophysectomy on the aerobic capacity of ligaments and tendons. *J Appl Physiol.* 1978;44:542-546.

10. Smidt N, Lewis M, VAN DER Windt DA, Hay EM, Bouter LM, Croft P. Lateral epicondylitis in general practice: course and prognostic indicators of outcome. *J Rheumatol.* 2006;33:2053-2059.

11. Sran M, Souvlis T, Vicenzino B, Wright A. Characterisation of chronic lateral epicondylalgia using the McGill pain questionnaire, visual analog scales, and quantitative sensory tests. *Pain Clinic.* 2002;13:251-259.

12. Wright A, Thurnwald P, Smith J. An evaluation of mechanical and thermal hyperalgesia in patients with lateral epicondylalgia. *Pain Clinic.* 1992;5:221-227.

13. Nagrale AV, Herd CR, Ganvir S, Ramteke G. Cyriax physiotherapy versus phonophoresis with supervised exercise in subjects with lateral epicondylalgia: a randomized clinical trial. *J Man Manip Ther.* 2009;17:171-178.

14. Maitland GD, Hengeveld E, Banks K, English K. *Maitland's Vertebral Manipulation.* 7th ed. Edinburgh: Elsevier Butterworth-Heinemann; 2005.

15. Elvey RL. Treatment of arm pain associated with abnormal brachial plexus tension. *Aust J Physiother.* 1986;32:225-230.

16. Vicenzino B, Neal R, Collins D, Wright A. The displacement, velocity and frequency profile of the frontal plane motion produced by the cervical lateral glide treatment technique. *Clin Biomech.* 1999;14:515-521.

17. Evans RC. *Illustrated Orthopedic Physical Assessment.* 3rd ed. St. Louis, MO: Mosby; 2009.

18. Cook C, Hegedus EJ. *Orthopedic Physical Examination Tests: An Evidence-Based Approach.* Upper Saddle River, NJ: Pearson Prentice Hall; 2008.

19. Stratford PW, Levy DR. Assessing valid change over time in patients with lateral epicondylitis at the elbow. *Clin J Sport Med.* 1994;4:88-91.

20. Stasinopoulos D. The use of polarized polychromatic non-coherent light as therapy for acute tennis elbow/lateral epicondylalgia: a pilot study. *Photomed Laser Surg.* 2005;23:66-69.

21. Vicenzino B, Smith D, Cleland J, Bisset L. Development of a clinical prediction rule to identify initial responders to mobilisation with movement and exercise for lateral epicondylalgia. *Man Ther.* 2009;14:550-554.

22. Roles NC, Maudsley RH. Radial tunnel syndrome: resistant tennis elbow as a nerve entrapment. *J Bone Joint Surg Br.* 1972;54:499-508.

23. Vicenzino B, Collins D, Wright A. The initial effects of a cervical spine manipulative physiotherapy treatment on the pain and dysfunction of lateral epicondylalgia. *Pain.* 1996;68:69-74.

24. Cleland J, Flynn T, Palmer J. Incorporation of manual therapy directed at the cervicothoracic spine in patients with lateral epicondylalgia: a pilot clinical trial. *J Man Manip Ther.* 2005;13:143-151.

25. Mulligan B. *Manual Therapy: "NAGS," "SNAGS," "MWMS," etc.* 4th ed. Wellington, NZ: Plane View Services Ltd; 1999.

26. Brosseau L, Casimiro L, Milne S, et al. Deep transverse friction massage for treating tendinitis. *Cochrane Database Syst Rev.* 2002;(4):CD003528.

27. Martinez-Silvestrini JA, Newcomer KL, Gay RE, Schaefer MP, Kortebein P, Arendt KW. Chronic lateral epicondylitis: comparative effectiveness of a home exercise program including stretching alone versus stretching supplemented with eccentric or concentric strengthening. *J Hand Ther.* 2005;18:411-420.

28. Svernlov B, Adolfsson L. Non-operative treatment regime including eccentric training for lateral humeral epicondylalgia. *Scand J Med Sci Sports.* 2001;11:328-334.

29. Tyler TF, Thomas GC, Nicholas SJ, McHugh MP. Addition of isolated wrist extensor eccentric exercise to standard treatment for chronic lateral epicondylosis: a prospective randomized trial. *J Shoulder Elbow Surg.* 2010;19:917-922.

30. Ohberg L, Alfredson H. Effects on neovascularisation behind the good results with eccentric training in chronic mid-portion Achilles tendinosis? *Knee Surg Sports Traumatol Arthrosc.* 2004;12:465-470.

31. Ohberg L, Lorentzon R, Alfredson H. Eccentric training in patients with chronic Achilles tendinosis: normalised tendon structure and decreased thickness at follow up. *Br J Sports Med.* 2004;38:8-11.

32. Manias P, Stasinopoulos D. A controlled clinical pilot trial to study the effectiveness of ice as a supplement to the exercise programme for the management of lateral elbow tendinopathy. *Br J Sports Med.* 2006;40:81-85.

33. Oken O, Kahraman Y, Ayhan F, Canpolat S, Yorgancioglu ZR, Oken OF. The short-term efficacy of laser, brace, and ultrasound treatment in lateral epicondylitis: a prospective, randomized, controlled trial. *J Hand Ther.* 2008;21:63-67.

34. Kohia M, Brackle J, Byrd K, Jennings A, Murray W, Wilfong E. Effectiveness of physical therapy treatments on lateral epicondylitis. *J Sport Rehabil.* 2008;17:119-136.

35. Bjordal JM, Lopes-Martins RA, Joensen J, et al. A systematic review with procedural assessments and meta-analysis of low level laser therapy in lateral elbow tendinopathy (tennis elbow). *BMC Musculoskelet Disord.* 2008;9:75.

36. Buchbinder R, Green SE, Youd JM, Assendelft WJ, Barnsley L, Smidt N. Shock wave therapy for lateral elbow pain. *Cochrane Database Syst Rev.* 2005;(4):CD003524.

37. Struijs PA, Smidt N, Arola H, Dijk CN, Buchbinder R, Assendelft WJ. Orthotic devices for the treatment of tennis elbow. *Cochrane Database Syst Rev.* 2002;(1):CD001821.

38. Jafarian FS, Demneh ES, Tyson SF. The immediate effect of orthotic management on grip strength of patients with lateral epicondylosis. *J Orthop Sports Phys Ther.* 2009;39:484-489.

39. Fu SC, Hung LK, Shum WT, et al. In vivo low-intensity pulsed ultrasound (LIPUS) following tendon injury promotes repair during granulation but suppresses decorin and biglycan expression during remodeling. *J Orthop Sports Phys Ther.* 2010;40:422-429.

40. Reza Nourbakhsh M, Fearon FJ. An alternative approach to treating lateral epicondylitis. A randomized, placebo-controlled, double-blinded study. *Clin Rehabil.* 2008;22:601-609.

Degenerative Spondylolisthesis

Ted Weber

A 60-year-old semi-retired female with a diagnosis of degenerative spondylolisthesis (DS) was referred to physical therapy by an orthopaedic spine surgeon. She first experienced pain about 4 weeks ago after walking a golf course and using a pull cart during a tournament. She indicates that she generally rides in a golf cart; however, use of golf carts was prohibited during tournament play. She notices that her pain is localized to her central low back, buttocks, and posterior thighs. Her symptoms worsen as the day progresses. She denies bowel or bladder signs/symptoms, sensation changes, weakness, or episodes of her legs "giving way." She is moderately overweight (BMI = 28 kg/m^2) and does not participate in a regular exercise program aside from her biweekly golf game. Her previous medical history includes a history of episodic low back pain and a cesarean section associated with the birth of her second child 35 years ago. She has a history of hyperlipidemia and type 2 diabetes mellitus. Her goals are to reduce her pain to allow her to cook meals for her family and to resume 18 holes of golf twice weekly without use of a golf cart.

► Based on the patient's diagnosis, what do you anticipate may be the contributing factors to her condition?
► What are the most appropriate examination tests?
► What are the most appropriate physical therapy interventions?
► What are possible complications that may limit the effectiveness of physical therapy?
► What is her rehabilitation prognosis?

KEY DEFINITIONS

DEGENERATIVE SPONDYLOLISTHESIS (DS): Acquired anterior displacement of one vertebra over the subjacent vertebra, associated with degenerative changes and without a disruption or defect in the vertebral ring

NEUROGENIC CLAUDICATION: Pain, paresthesias, and cramping of one or both legs due to neurologic compromise; typically brought on by standing or walking and relieved with sitting

SEGMENTAL INSTABILITY: Decreased capacity of the spine's stabilizing system to maintain the spinal neutral zones within physiological limits so that there are no neurologic deficits, major deformities, or incapacitating pain

SPINAL STENOSIS: Narrowing of the central spinal canal or intervertebral foramen at a single or multiple levels that can compress nerves and adjacent structures

SPONDYLOLYSIS: Defect in the pars interarticularis portion of the vertebrae; typically occurs in the lower lumbar vertebrae

SPONDYLOSIS: Degenerative changes in the intervertebral discs and osteophytic changes in the associated vertebral bodies

Objectives

1. Describe degenerative spondylolisthesis (DS) and potential risk factors associated with this condition.

2. Provide appropriate educational interventions for the individual with DS.

3. Design and implement manual therapy interventions to address the impairments common to individuals with DS.

4. Prescribe appropriate strength, endurance, flexibility, and motor control exercises for individuals with DS.

Physical Therapy Considerations

PT considerations during management of the individual with a diagnosis of degenerative spondylolisthesis:

▶ **General physical therapy plan of care/goals:** Decrease pain; educate patient regarding self-care and monitoring of condition; educate patient regarding pain mechanisms and psychosocial effects; improve strength, endurance, flexibility, and stability of lower extremities and spine; improve motor control of spinal stabilizers in recreational and functional activities; establish regular aerobic exercise regimen; return patient to recreational golf and activities of daily living (ADLs) with minimal symptoms

▶ **Physical therapy interventions:** Patient education regarding pathoanatomy and natural history of condition, red flags necessitating return to physician, pain mechanisms, and psychosocial effects; manual therapy interventions to address impairments identified in initial evaluation; flexibility, strength, endurance, and motor control exercises for spine and lower extremities; segmental activation of deep spinal stabilizers and incorporation into functional activities; general aerobic conditioning

▶ **Precautions during physical therapy:** Monitor baseline and exercise vital signs (especially given cardiovascular disease risk factors); monitor exacerbation of symptoms associated with therapy; monitor for yellow flags

▶ **Complications interfering with physical therapy:** Monitor for red flags such as progression of neurologic signs and symptoms

Understanding the Health Condition

Degenerative spondylolisthesis (DS) is an acquired disorder of the spine that results in the anterior displacement of one vertebra over the subjacent vertebra (Fig. 12-1).[1] Unlike spondylolytic spondylolisthesis, DS occurs in the absence of a pars interarticularis defect.[1] DS usually affects older individuals (> 40 years of age),[1] is 5 to 6 times more common in females[2] and 3 times more common in persons of African American descent.[3] The increased incidence in females

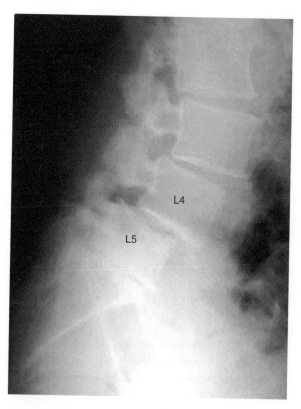

Figure 12-1. Lateral lumbar spine x-ray demonstrates a 25% anterior slippage of L4 on L5 due to a defect in the L4 pars interarticularis. This is called *spondylolisthesis.* (Reproduced with permission from Brunicardi FC, Andersen DK, Billiar TR, Dunn DL, Hunter JG, Matthews JB, Pollock RE, eds. *Schwartz's Principles of Surgery.* 9th ed. New York: McGraw-Hill; 2010. Figure 42-26.)

is surmised to be due to generalized ligamentous laxity due to hormonal influences. Other potential risk factors include pregnancies, generalized joint laxity, and hyperlordosis.[1]

The disease process typically begins in the second decade of life as primary degeneration of the intervertebral disc leads to loss of disc height, segmental laxity, annulus encroachment on the neural foramen, and buckling and hypertrophy of the ligamentum flavum.[4-6] The initial microinstability contributes to increased loading of the facet joints, facet hypertrophy, cartilage degradation, and stretching of the facet joint capsules, which allow forward displacement of the segment.[5] Anterior displacement combined with degenerative changes such as facet joint hypertrophy and malalignment and osteophyte formation narrow the spinal canal, which results in stenosis.[6] The tensile strength of the spinal ligaments diminishes with age, allowing further forward displacement of the affected vertebra.[7] Aging may also result in diminished muscle mass of the lumbar stabilizers[6] (e.g., multifidi, erector spinae, quadratus lumborum) and inadequate muscular stabilization.[1]

DS typically occurs at the L4-L5 segment.[1] The coronal orientation and strong iliolumbar ligaments of the L5-S1 segment prevent forward displacement at that motion segment and transmit forces superiorly.[1,5] The L4-L5 segment, however, typically has facets that are sagittally oriented and has less ligamentous support.[1,5] Patients with DS have been shown to have more pronounced sagittal plane facet joint alignment compared with those without DS.[8] Similarly, the incidence of DS is four times greater in the presence of a sacralized L5.[2] Patients with DS at the L4-L5 segment typically demonstrate L5 nerve root signs; however, patients with severe stenosis also demonstrate involvement of the L4 nerve root.[5]

The anterior displacement of the superior vertebra is generally mild (mean displacement of 14%). However, since the neural arch is intact, small amplitudes of movement can result in stenosis and compression of the cauda equina.[2] Progression of the slippage occurs in 30% to 34% of patients, but rarely does this slip exceed 25% to 30% of the width of the inferior vertebra.[5,9] Most patients with DS and without neurologic deficits respond well to conservative care.[10] Progression of the anterior displacement is associated with participation in occupations or activities that require repetitive flexion of the spine.[10]

Physical Therapy Patient/Client Management

Conservative care (education, exercise, manual therapy, lifestyle management, oral medication) is the treatment of choice for most patients, although surgery is often recommended for patients with lower extremity symptoms.[1,5] The rehabilitation prognosis for patients with DS is generally good, with only 10% to 15% of patients seeking surgical treatment.[1] Matsunaga and colleagues[9] found that progression of vertebral slippage occurred in only 34% of patients and found no correlation between the progression of slippage and clinical symptoms. Seventy-six percent of patients without neurologic symptoms remained so at the 10-year follow-up.[9] In contrast, of those that exhibited neurologic symptoms at the initial evaluation (*e.g.*, neurogenic claudication, bowel and bladder signs), 83% demonstrated worsening of these symptoms without surgery.

Medications such as nonsteroidal anti-inflammatories, acetaminophen, opioids, glucocorticoids, muscle relaxants, and antidepressants may be prescribed by the patient's physician.[1,4] Epidural injection of a glucocorticoid may also be used to alleviate edema resulting from chemical irritation and mechanical compression of neural tissue. The efficacy of epidural injections has not been well established in patients with DS and spinal stenosis.[1,4,10,11] Physical therapists should monitor patients for adverse drug reactions (ADRs) such as gastric upset/ulcer or allergic reactions. Opioids commonly result in constipation and can reduce blood pressure to dangerous levels in hypotensive patients; dependence is also a concern. Opioids and muscle relaxants interfere with a patient's ability to work, perform ADLs, and/or safely drive or operate machinery. Glucocorticoids commonly affect mood, elevate blood pressure and blood glucose, and may interfere with sleep. Moreover, they may accelerate bone mineral loss.

The primary goals of physical therapy are to educate the patient about symptom management and to enable her to return to her prior level of ADLs and recreational activities with minimal symptoms. Physical therapy interventions are specific to patient impairments and include education regarding joint protection and body mechanics, spine and lower extremity strengthening, motor control exercises, manual therapy, and aerobic conditioning.

Examination, Evaluation, and Diagnosis

Patients with DS most commonly present with low back pain, but may also present with any combination of neurogenic claudication, bowel/bladder signs and symptoms and radiculopathy.[1,11] Pain usually worsens over the course of the day and with changes in position (*e.g.*, sitting to standing).[1] Leg pain that frequently shifts from side to side is common and independent of neurologic signs.[1] In addition, cold feet, altered gait, leg(s) "giving way" and restless legs syndrome are sometimes seen.[1] Patients with DS and associated stenosis may have leg and buttock pain that is exacerbated by walking and relieved by forward flexion and/or activities that create more space in the central canal, such as forward flexion or walking while pushing a shopping cart.[5] As the central canal narrows, neurogenic claudication can result from mechanical irritation of the cauda equina or from local exercise-induced ischemia.[4]

Patients with DS generally show restrictions in lumbar motion—especially active extension—as a result of narrowing of the spinal canal with this movement direction.[5] Weakness is observed in 15% to 20% of patients, typically affects the L5 myotome, and usually does not result in functionally significant losses of strength.[5] Loss of reflexes is generally not diagnostic as most healthy older patients demonstrate an age-related reduction in reflexes.[5] Straight leg raises are generally negative.[1]

Diagnostic imaging is typically used to confirm the clinical diagnosis of DS.[1] Standing lateral and flexion-extension lateral radiographs are used to quantify instability and diagnose DS, defined as greater than 4 mm of slippage.[5,10] This criterion has a high false positive rate, as demonstrated by positive imaging in 42% of *asymptomatic* individuals.[12] MRI is the most appropriate technique for assessing the effects of spinal stenosis associated with DS on neural structures.[1,5,10] Occult DS, which cannot be seen on supine radiographs, can sometimes be detected with axially loaded MRI.[1] Computed tomography can provide imaging of facet orientation and pathology and can be used in patients with a contraindication to MRI.[5] Myelograms can further enhance imaging of nerve root entrapment and central canal stenosis.[1] Electromyography (EMG) is used to differentiate neuropathy from neurogenic claudication in patients with diabetes mellitus and/or peripheral neuropathy.[5]

There are two commonly used classification systems that grade the *degree* of anterior displacement of the vertebra in spondylolisthesis. The Meyerding classification divides a spondylolisthesis into four grades with increasing severity of translation (25%, 50%, 75%, 100%).[3] The other method, attributed to Taillard, describes the slip as a percentage of the anteroposterior displacement of the top vertebra on the subjacent vertebra.[3] The Marchetti-Bartolozzi classification system describes the *etiology* of the spondylolisthesis, differentiating between acquired (traumatic, postsurgical, pathologic, and degenerative) and developmental forms of spondylolisthesis.[3]

A comprehensive physical therapy examination should be conducted to rule out red flags such as cauda equina syndrome, spinal fracture, and neoplasm. Table 12-1 provides a summary of examination techniques suggested for the patient with DS. Adjacent structures, especially the thoracic spine, sacroiliac joint (SI) joints, and hips, should be screened as potential sources and/or contributors to low back pain and dysfunction. Neurologic screening should be conducted to assess the involvement of myotomes, dermatomes, and reflexes and to establish baseline criteria for monitoring progression of the condition.

Spinal range of motion (ROM) should be measured with an inclinometer and any aberrant movements (*e.g.*, instability catch, painful arc of motion, Gowers' sign,

Table 12-1	EXAMINATION TECHNIQUES FOR THE PATIENT WITH DEGENERATIVE SPONDYLOLISTHESIS	
Test Name	**Procedure**	**Findings**
Active spinal flexion and extension	The patient is in the standing position. The physical therapist stands behind the patient with the inclinometer held at the T12/L1 vertebral level. The patient is asked to bend down (flex forward) as far as possible while keeping the knees straight. After returning to the starting position, the patient is instructed to extend backward as far as possible.[13]	Active spinal ROM Identification of pain at specific range(s) of motion Movement restrictions Identification of aberrant movements during active spinal motion, including: instability catch, painful arc of motion, Gowers' sign, reversal of lumbopelvic rhythm
Hip AROM/PROM, and special tests	All cardinal planes of motion Thomas, Ely's, and Ober's tests	Restrictions in hip AROM/PROM that may result in adverse or painful movement of the spine

(Continued)

Table 12-1   EXAMINATION TECHNIQUES FOR THE PATIENT WITH DEGENERATIVE SPONDYLOLISTHESIS (CONTINUED)

Test Name	Procedure	Findings
Passive hip joint mobility	The patient lies supine with the pelvis fixated with a belt. The therapist grasps the distal femur with both hands and applies a distraction force. A traction strap can also be utilized to increase the force applied. Additional assessment techniques are described by Maitland[14]	Hyper/hypomobility
Posterior-anterior (PA) lumbar/thoracic mobility testing	The patient lies prone on the table. A posterior to anterior directed force is applied to the target spinal levels in the lumbar and thoracic regions[15]	Mobility of the segment is judged as hypomobile or hypermobile
Direct interventions applied to increase mobility or stability, respectively
Prone instability test	Test Position #1: Patient lies prone on the table with her trunk supported by table and her legs over the edge; her feet are resting on the floor. Therapist provides a PA pressure to the lumbar spine in area(s) of suspected instability. Test Position #2: Patient then lifts her legs and therapist again applies PA pressure.[13]	Pain in the first position that is eliminated in the second position with therapist-applied PA pressure implies lumbar instability.
Lateral musculature test (side support test)	The patient is sidelying with the top foot in front of the bottom foot. Using the lower elbow for support, the patient lifts the hips off the table with only the feet and elbow in contact with the table. Maximal hold time is recorded in seconds.[13]	Time that patient is able to maintain position indicates trunk muscle endurance
Lumbar extension endurance test	The patient is positioned in prone with a pillow under the abdomen. While maintaining pelvic stabilization via gluteal contraction, the patient is asked to hold the sternum off the floor as long as possible.[13]	Time that patient is able to maintain position indicates trunk extensor muscle endurance.
If hold time is < 5 s, the test is positive for poor lumbar extensor endurance.
Straight leg raise	The patient is supine and the inclinometer is placed just below the tibial tubercle. The therapist raises the leg to the maximal pain-free range while maintaining the knee in full extension.[13]	If radicular symptoms occur at a ROM < 70°, suggests less favorable prognosis.
Active straight leg raise	The patient is supine and asked to lift both legs off the table and hold that position for 5 s.[13]	Time that patient is able to maintain position indicates trunk flexor muscle endurance.
If hold time is < 5 s, the test is positive for poor trunk flexor muscle endurance.

or reversal of lumbopelvic rhythm) should be noted. These signs may indicate an inability to control lumbar motion and suggest a need for stabilization exercises.[13] Lower extremity active and passive ROM should be measured since restrictions in these structures may influence spinal motion. A positive straight leg raise may be indicative of radicular symptoms and may suggest a less favorable prognosis.[13] Endurance capacity of the spinal muscles can be assessed by using the extensor endurance test and lateral muscular endurance test (*i.e.*, the side support test).[16] The active straight leg test can be used to establish trunk flexion strength.[17]

Posterior-anterior passive accessory intervertebral movements should be tested at each thoracolumbar level. Findings of hypermobility or hypomobility at these articulations can be used to direct interventions[18] and/or determine prognosis.[13] The prone instability test should also be conducted for both assessment and prognostic capabilities.[13] Sacroiliac, thoracic, and hip joint mobilities should also be assessed because restrictions in these joints can affect lumbar motion.[18]

Outcome measures such as the Patient Specific Functional Scale,[19] the Modified Oswestry Disability Questionnaire[20] and the Fear Avoidance Beliefs Questionnaire[21] should be used to identify patient-centered goals, measure disability, and identify yellow flags/suggest prognosis, respectively.

Plan of Care and Interventions

Conservative care should be the initial choice of treatment for most patients with spondylolisthesis, regardless of the presence of neurologic symptoms.[11] Unfortunately, there is insufficient evidence to determine optimal conservative treatment protocols for patients with DS.[1,4,13,22,23] Most studies that have examined conservative care for low back pain have broad inclusion criteria and failed to recognize its heterogeneous nature.[13] Moreover, these studies suffer from methodological flaws, including: lack of a control group and/or randomization of subjects, small sample size, inadequate follow-up, and outcome assessments that lack validation.[4] Clinicians therefore must rely on sparse clinical evidence, biological principles, an understanding of biomechanics, and sound clinical reasoning in the development of conservative approaches. Comorbidities and the wide range of functional capabilities typical in this population also need to be considered in treatment planning. An individualized treatment approach should be created for each patient, focusing on education, manual therapy, and therapeutic exercise.[4,24]

The basic concepts of pathoanatomy and biomechanics in DS should form the foundation of patient education. These principles help the patient understand the rationale for physical therapy, how to decrease symptom exacerbation, and how to minimize stresses that might lead to further degeneration. Specifically, the patient should be taught to avoid end range spinal movements, especially flexion, that place further stress on the passive stabilizing structures.[24] Lifting in spinal flexion and/or rotation can greatly magnify these stresses, regardless of the load; therefore, proper lifting techniques should be taught.[24] Conversely, maintenance of a slightly flexed lumbar spine/posterior pelvic tilt can increase the cross-sectional area of the spinal canal and neural foramen and improve stenotic symptoms. Fatigue may diminish the ability of active stabilizing structures to maintain an ideal posture.[13] Therefore, it is important that the patient gains sufficient strength of the lower extremity and spinal musculature to support correct lifting postures as well as adequate endurance to allow maintenance of correct posture throughout the day. Pacing strategies should also be taught to prevent excessive fatigue that might lead to compromise of correct posture.

A mechanical description of the patient's pathoanatomy should include a discussion of the patient's likely favorable prognosis and how physical therapy interventions can contribute to a successful outcome. Unhelpful beliefs (*e.g.*, movement worsens symptoms or causes harm, catastrophizing, poor expectation for recovery, fear avoidance behaviors) have been shown to influence outcomes in patients with back pain.[25] Such beliefs should be screened for and specifically addressed in the educational component of physical therapy. Interventions that specifically address these factors have demonstrated improved outcomes.[26]

Some studies suggest that treatments that focus solely on anatomical sources of pain should be replaced by or enhanced with an activity-based approach that facilitates the resumption of normal activities *despite* the presence of pain.[25,26] The physical therapist can assist the patient in the identification of activities or situations that cause discomfort, such as prolonged overhead activities, axial loading (*e.g.*, lifting, carrying a backpack), or postural faults and suggest more appropriate movement and postural strategies. Additional information regarding the identification and management of psychological factors is beyond the scope of this case study and can be found elsewhere.[27,28]

Manual therapy interventions such as mobilization of spinal segments and the lower extremity should be included for hypomobile joints. A recent systematic review, including one high-quality randomized control trial, concluded that manual therapy combined with exercise may be beneficial for patients with spinal stenosis.[29] Since many patients with DS frequently present with stenotic symptoms and deficits in flexibility and mobility similar to those with spinal stenosis, it is reasonable to surmise that similar manual techniques may be beneficial for this population. Manual techniques should be directed at articulations that were identified as hypomobile in the examination and may contribute to adverse biomechanical stress at that spondylolisthetic segment.

Whitman and colleagues[18] found that a flexion-based exercise regimen combined with body weight-supported treadmill walking and manual therapy was superior to a program that utilized treadmill walking, flexion exercises, and subtherapeutic ultrasound in patients with stenosis. By reducing the compressive loading of the spine, body weight-supported walking increases the cross-sectional area of the neural canal relative to weightbearing positions.[30] Subjects were provided sufficient unloading to allow them to walk without symptoms with a goal of reducing body weight support as tolerated. Given the difficulty of obtaining body weight-support training apparatuses in most clinical settings, similar therapeutic effects may be obtained via the unloading effects of aquatic exercise therapy.[4] Progression of weightbearing tolerance could be achieved by varying the depth of water. Manual therapy techniques in the study by Whitman et al.[18] included both thrust and non-thrust mobilizations, manual stretching of musculotendinous structures of the spine and lower extremity, and trunk and lower extremity strengthening exercises. The authors emphasized that manual techniques were applied to multiple regions of the body (thoracic/lumbar spine, pelvis, hip, and ankle) depending on impairments identified in the initial examination. Normalizing hip ROM is of particular importance in patients with DS because restrictions, especially in hip extension, can result in excessive spinal extension. Manual techniques such as distraction or anterior mobilization of the hip joint, soft tissue mobilization and stretching of the iliopsoas, tensor fascia lata and rectus femoris are often well suited for patients with DS.

Therapeutic exercises should be prescribed not only to address deficits in strength and ROM, but also to address the increased motor control demands required by an unstable spine (Table 12-2). By definition, patients with DS have at least one motion segment with attenuation of the structural support typically provided by the discs, ligaments, joint capsules, and bony architecture. Panjabi collectively referred to these structures as the "passive subsystem."[31] Development of tension in the passive subsystem is particularly important for spinal stability in movements occurring at end range. In the middle ranges of motion—termed the "neutral zone"—the passive subsystem provides minimal resistance but may instead serve to sense movement, providing feedback to the neural control subsystem.[31] The active subsystem, consisting of the spinal muscles and tendons, is predominantly responsible for providing stability in ranges where tension from the passive subsystem is minimal. Fritz and colleagues[24] hypothesized that an increase in the size of the neutral zone relative to total ROM places greater demands on the active subsystem and the neural control subsystem that supports it. Evidence for increased reliance on the active subsystem to provide stability is seen in patients with spinal instability who experience pain in mid-ranges of movement rather than at end range, present with an instability catch, painful arc of motion, the Gowers' sign, or reversal of lumbopelvic rhythm.[13] In addition, increased postural sway,[32,33] slower reaction times,[34] and impaired activation of deep stabilizers in anticipation of limb movements and loads[35,36] may suggest altered

Table 12-2 THERAPEUTIC EXERCISES FOR THE PATIENT WITH DS		
Exercise Name	Starting Position	Exercise Technique
Single/double knee-to-chest	Supine	Patient brings one or both legs to the chest, inducing lumbar flexion. In the single knee exercise, the contralateral leg is kept straight and flush with the table.
Lumbar rotation stretch	Sidelying	The patient lies on left side. The left leg is straight and the right hip and knee are flexed. The right foot is placed in the left leg's popliteal space and the right knee is allowed to descend toward the floor as the torso rotates to the right.
Foam roller extension (Fig. 12-2)	Supine	The patient lies with a foam roller under the stiff/hyperkyphotic thoracic segments and, while maintaining a neutral or flexed cervical and lumbar spine, the patient extends the thoracic spine over the roller.

(Continued)

Table 12-2 THERAPEUTIC EXERCISES FOR THE PATIENT WITH DS (*CONTINUED*)

Exercise Name	Starting Position	Exercise Technique
Transversus abdominis/Internal Oblique activation (Fig. 12-3)	Initially in supine or sidelying Progression to seated, standing, and functional activities that previously caused pain	The therapist palpates the abdomen ~1 inch medial and slightly inferior to the anterior superior iliac spine. The patient is directed to draw the abdomen away from the therapist's fingers as he/she exhales. Alternatively, the patient can be directed to lift the pelvic floor (females can be directed to lift the vagina, males can perform a lift of the testes). The therapist should feel gentle flattening of the abdomen. Movement of the spine, bulging of the abdomen, and compression of the rib cage should not occur. (For review of this treatment approach and progression, see Richardson and Jull[37] and Richardson et al.[38])
Segmental multifidus activation (Fig. 12-4)	Sidelying	With the patient sidelying, the therapist palpates the spine adjacent to the spinous processes at the level of the DS. The patient is directed to cause the muscles underlying the therapist's fingers to gently bulge. Alternatively, the patient can be directed to try to draw the posterior superior iliac spines together. The therapist should feel a gentle development of muscle tension. Rapid contraction of superficial musculature, indicating activation of lumbar erector spinae musculature, should not be felt. (For review of this treatment approach and progression, see Richardson and Jull[37] and Richardson et al.[38])
Posterior pelvic tilt (Fig. 12-5)	Initially supine, followed by standing against wall, and then standing unsupported	Deep stabilizer activation (transversus abdominis, internal obliques, multifidi) is initiated as described above and followed by tilting the pelvis posteriorly and flattening lumbar spine against the supporting surface. The thoracic and cervical regions of the spine are maintained in a neutral posture.
Side plank (Fig. 12-6)	Sidelying	Deep stabilizer activation is initiated as described above. The patient places the right elbow directly beneath the shoulders, then lifts the body off the ground, supporting its weight on the right knee and elbow. The spine and hips are maintained in neutral position (Fig. 12-6A). The exercise may be progressed by using the feet (rather than the knees) as a base of support (Fig. 12-6B).
Quadruped with UE/LE movement (Fig. 12-7)	Quadruped	Deep stabilizer activation is initiated as described above. Maintaining a neutral spinal posture, the patient flexes one upper extremity (Fig. 12-7A), or extends one lower extremity (Fig. 12-7B), or flexes and extends the contralateral upper extremity and lower extremity, respectively (Fig. 12-7C).

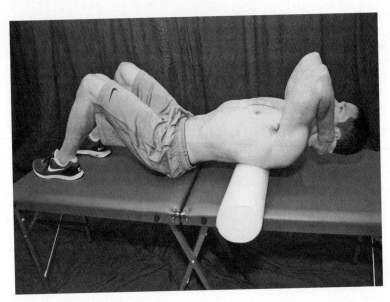

Figure 12-2. Foam roller extension exercise.

neural control in patients with low back pain due to spinal instability. These findings emphasize the importance of assessing quantity *and* quality of movement and training the neural control subsystem to restore muscular control throughout the middle ranges of motion (*e.g.*, progressively introducing unstable surfaces, therapy balls, and functional activities in exercise regimens).[24,37] Poor movement quality becomes

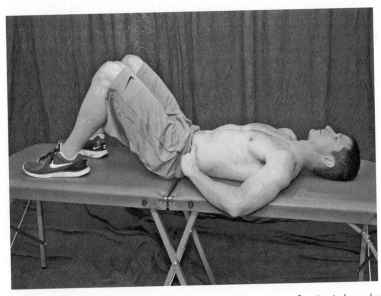

Figure 12-3. Transversus abdominis/internal oblique activation. Patient performing independent palpation—drawing his abdomen away from his fingers as he exhales.

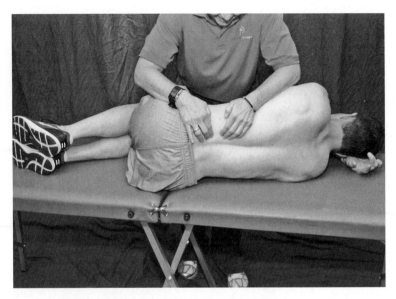

Figure 12-4. Segmental multifidus activation.

evident when the patient has lost activation of her active subsystem structures (*e.g.*, deep abdominals, multifidi) and experiences pain in mid-range movements and/or returns to her previous compensatory stabilization strategies (*e.g.*, the Gowers' sign).

Although few high quality studies have specifically evaluated stabilization exercises for patients with spondylolisthesis, a recent systematic review by McNeely

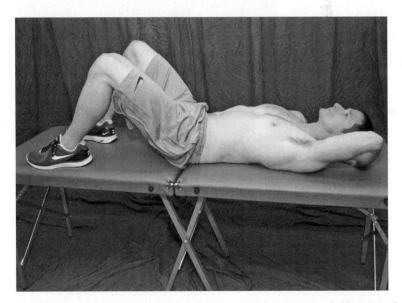

Figure 12-5. Posterior pelvic tilt. Patient contracts transversus abdominis/internal oblique muscles and then tilts the pelvis posteriorly and flattens the lumbar spine against the supporting surface.

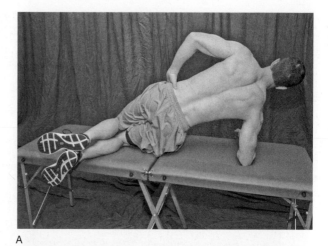

A

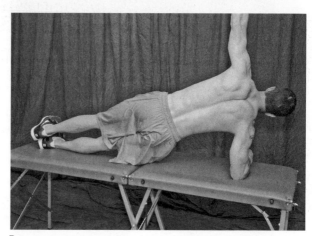

Figure 12-6. Side plank.   B

and colleagues[22] identified one study that met criteria for inclusion and was rated as strong. In this study, O'Sullivan and colleagues[39] had patients with symptoms associated with isthmic spondylolysis (pars interarticularis fracture) or spondylolisthesis perform either a 10-week **spinal stabilization exercise regimen** as originally described by Richardson and Jull[37] or general exercise activities (control group). The authors hypothesized that low back pain and dysfunction in this population sample was attributable to the inability of the motor control system (i.e., neural control subsystem) to appropriately coordinate trunk muscle contraction to stabilize the unstable segment. Subjects in the spinal stabilization group initially learned to perform an isolated contraction of the deep abdominal muscles (transversus abdominis and internal obliques) with coactivation of the lumbar multifidus at the level of the defect. Training progressively added limb movements and was later followed by incorporation of specific muscle activation into activities that had previously aggravated the subjects' symptoms. Because dysfunction in this population was hypothesized to result from a motor control deficit, the authors emphasized the necessity

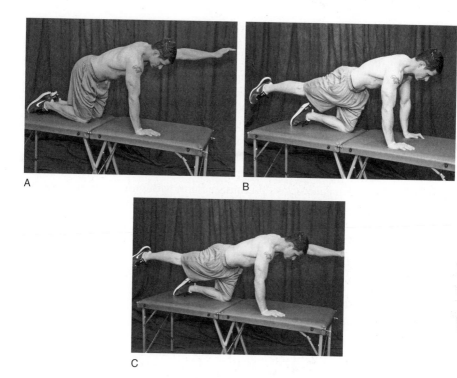

Figure 12-7. Spinal stabilization exercises. Quadruped progression with upper extremity and lower extremity movement.

of progressing a patient only when an isolated contraction of the deep musculature could be reliably performed. When compared to the control group, the spinal stabilization group demonstrated improvements in pain and function as measured by the Oswestry Disability Index that were maintained at 30 months.[39]

Most patients with DS report that lumbar flexion eases their symptoms and a recent clinical practice guideline[40] recommends a **flexion-based approach** for patients with that directional preference. A flexion-based approach emphasizes the strengthening of lumbar flexors (abdominals) and stretching of tight structures that inhibit lumbar flexion (*e.g.*, lumbar extensors, hip flexors and associated capsular and ligamentous structures). Fritz et al.[24] suggested strengthening the abdominal muscles, especially the rectus abdominis, in patients with spinal instability. McGill,[41] however, found high levels of compressive and shear forces are imparted on the spine during curl-up exercises and suggested side planks (Fig. 12-6) as a suitable alternative for strengthening the abdominal musculature. Regardless of exercise(s) chosen, the patient should be taught how to posteriorly rotate the pelvis to promote lumbar flexion, initially in the supine position, and then progressed to a standing posture. As the patient becomes more adept at controlling the pelvic orientation, she can be taught to find symptom-easing positions while walking and performing other functional or recreational activities.

Distally, tight anterior hip structures can result in anterior pelvic tilt and lumbar extension when the patient is standing or in the mid-stance through terminal stance phases of gait.[42] Stretching the iliopsoas, rectus femoris, tensor fascia lata, anterior hip adductors, and ankle plantar flexors and strengthening the hip extensors and posterior hip abductors facilitates the maintenance of a flexed lumbar posture. Stretching the lumbar extensors and improving thoracic extension through self-mobilization with a foam roller can assist the patient in assuming a more comfortable posture. Improved hamstring ROM allows greater forward flexion without demanding end range lumbar flexion that may lead to further stress on the posterior lumbar structures and exacerbation of the forward slip. Despite the general acceptance of a flexion-based approach in patients with stenotic symptoms, a recent review asserts that exercise regimens that utilize this approach have not been shown to be definitively better than other approaches.[4] Because patients with spinal stenosis have also demonstrated paraspinal muscle denervation[43] and impaired trunk extensor muscle function,[44] strengthening the spinal extensors may be beneficial for this population. Sinaki and colleagues[45] concluded that, although a flexion-based strength regimen was superior to an extension-based approach in patients with spondylolisthesis, exercises that target the spinal extensors may be beneficial. They suggested avoiding exercises that move the patient into spinal extension (e.g., isometric contractions or those that move the patient from a flexed lumbar position to a neutral position). Rather, spinal stabilization exercises should be performed in a **quadruped position** using single arm or leg extension or contralateral arm/leg extension (Fig. 12-7) because this position has been shown to activate the spinal extensors without excessively loading the spine compared to trunk extension in prone which imparted much greater loading forces.[46]

Aerobic exercise is beneficial for treating nonspecific low back pain[4], but has not been specifically validated for the treatment of DS. Regardless, aerobic exercise is suggested with the therapeutic goals of improving cardiovascular fitness, decreasing fear avoidance behavior, modulating pain, managing body weight, improving hemodynamic factors at the affected neural and musculoskeletal structures, and managing other comorbidities such as peripheral artery disease, diabetes mellitus, and coronary artery disease.[42] Stationary cycling is an excellent choice for aerobic activity since it promotes spinal flexion and helps reduce the potential for neurogenic claudication.[1] Swimming, aquatic therapy, and body weight-supported walking have also been suggested as appropriate forms of conditioning for patients with DS.[1,18]

Recent efforts have been directed at identifying patients who would most benefit from therapeutic exercise programs. Hicks and colleagues[13] developed a **clinical prediction rule to predict the success** of a stabilization program in patients with spinal instability. The authors utilized an 8-week stabilization program that incorporated exercise principles similar to the study conducted by O'Sullivan et al.[39] and found that age <40 years was the strongest predictor of success as defined by a 50% or greater improvement in the Oswestry Disability Index (+LR = 3.7, 95% CI = 1.6-8.3). The authors suggested that younger patients may have responded better to spinal stabilization exercises because increased age is associated with reduced muscle mass. As such, more than 8 weeks may be required to elicit gains in muscular strength sufficient to create clinically meaningful stability in older patients. Even in the presence of widespread frailty and comorbidities, significant strength gains have been demonstrated even in nonagenarian patients when sufficient intensity is utilized.[47] Given the wide range of impairments, comorbidities, and functional goals in patients with DS, the therapist must utilize creativity in exercise selection, modification, and progression to address each patient's deficits so that she can achieve her functional goals.

Surgery may be considered in patients who have not responded to conservative care and who have persistent leg pain, progressive neurologic deficits, and a significant reduction in quality of life.[4,5] Some studies have shown that **patients with DS and neurologic symptoms** are more likely to exhibit deterioration of their condition without surgery[10] and show greater improvement in pain, function, and overall satisfaction with surgery relative to conservative care at four-year follow-up.[47-49] Spinal fusion has been shown to be more effective at relieving lower extremity symptoms than low back pain.[4,50] However, these studies did not evaluate long-term outcomes and poorly described or controlled for conservative care. It is also important to note that surgical interventions carry significant morbidity and mortality rates, especially in older patients.[51-54] Surgical interventions, especially complex fusions, have risen dramatically in the recent past and have resulted in a concomitant rise in life-threatening adverse events, length of hospital stays, rehospitalizations, mortality, and costs.[54] Major medical complications, including cardiopulmonary events or cerebrovascular accidents, have been shown to occur in 4.7% of patients over 66 years of age who received a single-level fusion and 5.2% of those undergoing complex fusions.[54] These data should not be used to frighten patients, but rather to fully inform them of the potential risks and benefits involved and desirability of aggressively pursuing conservative approaches to care.

Evidence-Based Clinical Recommendations

SORT: Strength of Recommendation Taxonomy

A: Consistent, good-quality patient-oriented evidence
B: Inconsistent or limited-quality patient-oriented evidence
C: Consensus, disease-oriented evidence, usual practice, expert opinion, or case series

1. Most individuals with degenerative spondylolisthesis do not require surgery and experience decreased pain and improved function with conservative care. **Grade A**

2. Manual therapy interventions for hypomobile spinal segments and lower extremity joints improves perceived recovery, pain, function, and walking tolerance in patients with stenotic symptoms. **Grade B**

3. A specific exercise regimen aimed at strengthening the deep spinal stabilizers improves function and decreases pain in patients with spondylolisthesis. **Grade B**

4. Spinal flexion-based treatment protocols may improve low back pain and function in individuals with degenerative spondylolisthesis. **Grade B**

5. Exercises for strengthening spinal extensors may improve patient outcomes but should be performed in a range that avoids lumbar extension (*e.g.*, quadruped position). **Grade C**

6. Younger age (<40 years) predicts success with spinal stabilization treatment protocols in patients with spinal instability. **Grade B**

7. Patients with degenerative spondylolisthesis and neurologic signs and symptoms are more likely to demonstrate deterioration in symptoms and signs without surgery. **Grade A**

COMPREHENSION QUESTIONS

12.1 Which statement is true regarding degenerative spondylolisthesis?

A. Instability typically occurs at the L5/S1 segment as a result of the sagittal orientation of the facets at this segment.

B. Most patients with this condition eventually require surgery as the disc continues to degenerate with continued aging.

C. Conservative care is the treatment of choice for most patients, regardless of the presence of neurologic signs.

D. Radiological signs closely correlate with clinical signs and progression of the condition.

12.2 A patient with DS that presents with low back pain but without associated neurologic symptoms should be told that her prognosis is:

A. Poor. Symptoms seldom resolve and the patient eventually requires surgery.

B. Unknown. Symptoms improve or worsen without identifiable prognostic factors.

C. Good in the short term, but the prognosis worsens over time with most patients eventually requiring surgery.

D. Good. Most patients do well with conservative care and without surgery.

ANSWERS

12.1 **C.** Even though studies have shown that most patients with leg symptoms will continue to deteriorate without surgery,[10] conservative care is initially recommended for most patients. It is important to note that these studies poorly define or control for conservative care.

12.2 **D.** Most patients with DS and without neurologic deficits respond well to conservative care[10] and only 10% to 15% of patients with DS eventually seek surgery.[1] Progression of vertebral slippage was shown to occur in only 34% of patients and no correlation was found between the progression of slippage and clinical symptoms.[9] Seventy-six percent of patients without neurologic symptoms remained so at the 10-year follow-up. Progression of the slip is associated with participation in occupations or activities that require repetitive flexion of the spine.[10]

REFERENCES

1. Kalichman L, Hunter DJ. Diagnosis and conservative management of degenerative lumbar spondylolisthesis. *Eur Spine J.* 2008;17:327-335.

2. Rosenburg NJ. Degenerative spondylolisthesis. *J Bone Joint Surg.* 1975;57:467-474.

3. Butt S, Saifuddin A. The imaging of lumbar spondylolisthesis. *Clin Radiol.* 2005;60:533-546

4. Atlas SJ, Delitto A. Spinal stenosis: surgical versus nonsurgical treatment. *Clin Orthop Relat Res.* 2006;443:198-207.

5. Herkowitz HN. Spine update. Degenerative lumbar spondylolisthesis. *Spine.* 1995;20:1084-1090.

6. Benoist M. Natural history of the aging spine. *Eur Spine J.* 2003;12:S86-S89.

7. Panjabi MM, Goel VK, Takata K. Physiologic strains in the lumbar spine ligaments. An in vitro biomechanical study 1981 Volvo Award in Biomechanics. *Spine.* 1982;7:192-203.

8. Grobler LJ, Robertson PA, Novotny JE, Pope MH. Etiology of spondylolisthesis. Assessment of the role played by facet joint morphology. *Spine.* 1993;18:80-91.

9. Matsunaga S, Ijiri K, Hayashi K. Nonsurgically managed patients with degenerative spondylolisthesis: a 10- to 18-year follow-up study. *J Neurosurg.* 2000;93:194-198.

10. Watters WC III, Bono CM, Gilbert TJ, et al. North American Spine Society. An evidence-based clinical guideline for the diagnosis and treatment of degenerative lumbar spondylolisthesis. *Spine J.* 2009;9:609-614.

11. Vibert BT, Sliva CD, Herkowitz HN. Treatment of instability and spondylolisthesis: surgical versus nonsurgical treatment. *Clin Orthop Relat Res.* 2006;443:222-227.

12. Hayes MA, Howard TC, Gruel CR, Kopta JA. Roentgenographic evaluation of the lumbar spine flexion-extension in asymptomatic individuals. *Spine.* 1989;14:327-331.

13. Hicks GE, Fritz JM, Delitto A, McGill SM. Preliminary development of a clinical prediction rule for determining which patients with low back pain will respond to a stabilization exercises program. *Arch Phys Med Rehabil.* 2005;86:1753-1762.

14. Maitland GD. *Peripheral Manipulation.* 3rd ed. Boston, MA: Butterworth-Heinemann; 1991.

15. Maitland GD, Hengeveld, E, Banks K, English K. *Maitland's Vertebral Manipulation.* 7th ed. Edinburgh: Elsevier Butterworth-Heinemann; 2005.

16. McGill SM, Childs A, Liebenson C. Endurance times for low back stabilization exercises: clinical targets for testing and training from a normal database. *Arch Phys Med Rehabil.* 1999;80:941-944.

17. Waddell G, Somerville D, Henderson I, Newton M. Objective clinical evaluation of physical impairment in chronic low back pain. *Spine.* 1992;17:617-628.

18. Whitman JM, Flynn TW, Childs JD, et al. A comparison between two physical therapy treatment programs for subjects with lumbar spinal stenosis: a randomized clinical trial. *Spine.* 2006;31:2541-2549.

19. Young IA, Cleland JA, Michener LA, Brown C. Reliability, construct validity, and responsiveness of the neck disability index, patient-specific functional scale, and numeric pain rating scale in patients with cervical radiculopathy. *Am J Phys Med Rehabil.* 2010;89:831-839.

20. Fritz JM, Irrgang JJ. A comparison of the modified Oswestry low back pain disability questionnaire and the Quebec back pain disability scale. *Phys Ther.* 2001;81:776-788. Erratum in: *Phys Ther.* 2008;88:138-139.

21. Waddell G, Newton M, Henderson I, Somerville D, Main CJ. A fear-avoidance beliefs questionnaire (FABQ) and the role of fear-avoidance beliefs in chronic low back pain and disability. *Pain.* 1993;52:157-168.

22. McNeely ML, Torrance G, Magee DJ. A systematic review of physiotherapy for spondylolysis and spondylolisthesis. *Man Ther.* 2003;8:80-91.

23. Spratt KF, Weinstein JN, Lehmann TR, Woody J, Sayre H. Efficacy of flexion and extension treatments incorporating braces for low-back pain patients with retrodisplacement, spondylolisthesis, or normal sagittal translation. *Spine.* 1993;18:1839-1849.

24. Fritz JM, Erhard RE, Hagen BF. Segmental instability of the lumbar spine. *Phys Ther.* 1998;78:889-896.

25. Linton SJ, Shaw WS. Impact of psychological factors in the experience of pain. *Phys Ther.* 2011;91:700-711.

26. Nicholas MK, Linton SJ, Watson PJ, Main CJ. "Decade of the Flags" Working Group. Early identification and management of psychological risk factors ("yellow flags") in patients with low back pain: a reappraisal. *Phys Ther.* 2011;91:737-753.

27. Nicholas MK, George SZ. Psychologically informed interventions for low back pain: an update for physical therapists. *Phys Ther.* 2011;91:765-776.

28. Butler DS, Moseley GL. *Explain Pain.* Adelaide: Noigroup Publications; 2003.

29. Reiman MP, Harris JY, Cleland JA. Manual therapy interventions for patients with lumbar spinal stenosis: a systematic review. *NZ J Physiother.* 2009;37:17-28.

30. Willen J, Danielson B, Gaulitz A, Niklason T, Schonstrom N, Hansson T. Dynamic effects on the lumbar spinal canal: axially loaded CT-myelography and MRI in patients with sciatica and/or neurogenic claudication. *Spine.* 1997;22:2968-2976.

31. Panjabi MM. The stabilizing system of the spine. Part I. Function, dysfunction, adaptation, and enhancement. *J Spinal Disord.* 1992;5:383-389.

32. Luoto S, Taimela S, Hurri H, Pyykko I, Alaranta H. Psychomotor speed and postural control in low back pain patients. A controlled follow up study. *Spine.* 1996;21:2621-2627.

33. Nies N, Sinnott PL. Variations in balance and body sway in middle-aged adults. Subjects with healthy backs compared with subjects with low back dysfunction. *Spine.* 1991;16:325-330.

34. Luoto S, Hurri H, Alaranta H. Reaction times in patients with chronic low back pain. *Eur J Phys Med Rehabil.* 1995;5:47-50.

35. Hodges PW, Richardson CA. Inefficient muscular stabilization of the lumbar spine associated with low back pain. A motor control evaluation of transversus abdominis. *Spine.* 1996;21:2640-2650.

36. Hodges PW, Richardson CA. Contraction of the abdominal muscles associated with movement of the lower limb. *Phys Ther.* 1997;77:132-142.

37. Richardson CA, Jull GA. Muscle control-pain control. What exercises would you prescribe? *Man Ther.* 1995;1:2-10.

38. Richardson C, Hodges PW, Hides J; Manipulation Association of Chartered Physiotherapists. *Therapeutic Exercise for Lumbopelvic Stabilization: A Motor Control Approach for the Treatment and Prevention of Low Back Pain.* 2nd ed. Elsevier; 2004.

39. O'Sullivan PB, Phyty GD, Twomey LT, Allison GT. Evaluation of specific stabilizing exercise in the treatment of chronic low back pain with radiologic diagnosis of spondylolysis or spondylolisthesis. *Spine.* 1997;22:2959-2967.

40. Fritz JM, Cleland JA, Childs JD. Subgrouping patients with low back pain: evolution of a classification approach to physical therapy. *J Orthop Sports Phys Ther.* 2007;37:290-302.

41. McGill SM. Distribution of tissue loads in the low back during a variety of daily and rehabilitation tasks. *J Rehabil Res Dev.* 1997;34:448-458.

42. Backstrom KM, Whitman JM, Flynn TW. Lumbar spinal stenosis-diagnosis and management of the aging spine. *Man Ther.* 2011;16:308-317.

43. Leinonen V, Määttä S, Taimela S, et al. Paraspinal muscle denervation paradoxically good lumbar endurance, and an abnormal flexion-extension cycle in lumbar spinal stenosis. *Spine.* 2003;28: 324-331.

44. Keller TS, Szpalski M, Gunzburg R, Spratt KF. Assessment of trunk function in single and multi-level spinal stenosis: a prospective clinical trial. *Clin Biomech.* 2003;18:173-181.

45. Sinaki M, Lutness MP, Ilstrup DM, Chy CP, Gramse RR. Lumbar spondylolisthesis: retrospective comparison and three-year follow-up of two conservative treatment programs. *Arch Phys Med Rehabil.* 1989;70:594-598.

46. Callaghan JP, Gunning JL, McGill SM. The relationship between lumbar spine load and muscle activity during extensor exercises. *Phys Ther.* 1998;78:8-18.

47. Weinstein JN, Tosteson TD, Lurie JD, et al. SPORT Investigators. Surgical versus nonsurgical therapy for lumbar spinal stenosis. *N Engl J Med.* 2008;358:794-810.

48. Pearson AM, Lurie JD, Blood EA, et al. Spine patient outcomes research trial: radiographic predictors of clinical outcomes after operative or nonoperative treatment of degenerative spondylolisthesis. *Spine.* 2008;33:2759-2766.

49. Weinstein JN, Lurie JD, Tosteson TD, et al. Surgical compared with nonoperative treatment for lumbar degenerative spondylolisthesis. Four-year results in the Spine Patient Outcomes Research Trial (SPORT) randomized and observational cohorts. *J Bone Joint Surg Am.* 2009;91:1295-1304.

50. Deyo RA. Back surgery: who needs it? *N Engl J Med.* 2007;356:2239-2243.

51. Reindl R, Steffen T, Cohen L, Aebi M. Elective lumbar spinal decompression in the elderly: is it a high risk operation? *Can J Surg.* 2003;46:43-46.

52. Ragab AA, Fye MA, Bohlman HH. Surgery of the lumbar spine for spinal stenosis in 118 patients 70 years of age or older. *Spine.* 2003;28:348-353.

53. Carreon LY, Puno RM, Dimar JR II, Glassman SD, Johnson JR. Perioperative complications of posterior lumbar decompression and arthrodesis in older adults. *J Bone Joint Surg Am.* 2003; 85-A:2089-2092.

54. Deyo RA, Mirza SK, Martin BI, Kreuter W, Goodman DC, Jarvik JG. Trends, major medical complications, and charges associated with surgery for lumbar spinal stenosis in older adults. *JAMA.* 2010;303:1259-1265.

Spondylolisthesis in Young Athlete

Danny J. McMillian

An 18-year-old high school football player is referred to an outpatient physical therapy clinic after an evaluation for persistent central low back pain. The orthopaedist established a diagnosis of type IIB, grade II spondylolisthesis at L5/S1. He reports no history of specific trauma. His pain is aggravated by prolonged standing or walking, lifting weights (especially overhead), and bending backward or twisting. Sitting or lying down with his hips and knees bent relieves the pain. His medical history is otherwise unremarkable. The patient's goal is to return to football as soon as possible.

▶ What are the examination priorities?
▶ What examination signs may be associated with this diagnosis?
▶ Based on the patient's diagnosis, what do you anticipate may be the contributing factors to his condition?
▶ What are the most appropriate physical therapy interventions?
▶ What are possible complications that may limit the effectiveness of physical therapy?
▶ Identify the psychological or psychosocial factors apparent in this case.

KEY DEFINITIONS

CORE STABILITY: Ability of muscles within the "core" region (abdomen, lumbar spine, pelvis, and hips) to protect (*i.e.*, stabilize) the lumbar spine from potentially injurious forces and to create and/or transfer forces between anatomic segments during functional movements

DYSPLASTIC SPONDYLOLISTHESIS: Translational displacement of one vertebral segment on another caused by congenital deficiency of the posterior elements of the spine

SPONDYLOLISTHESIS: Translational displacement or nonanatomic alignment of one vertebral segment on another

SPONDYLOLYSIS: Defect or abnormality of the pars interarticularis of the vertebral arch

Objectives

1. Describe spondylolisthesis and identify potential risk factors associated with this diagnosis.

2. Prescribe joint range of motion and/or muscular flexibility exercises for a patient with spondylolisthesis.

3. Prescribe motor control exercises for a young athlete with spondylolisthesis.

Physical Therapy Considerations

PT considerations during management of the individual with a diagnosis of spondylolisthesis:

▶ **General physical therapy plan of care/goals:** Decrease pain; increase pain-free range of motion and muscular flexibility; increase spine and lower quadrant strength, endurance and motor control; maintain or improve aerobic fitness capacity

▶ **Physical therapy interventions:** Patient education regarding functional anatomy and injury pathomechanics; modalities and manual therapy to decrease pain and improve joint motion; muscular flexibility exercises; resistance exercises to increase muscular strength and endurance of the core and lower extremities; aerobic exercise program

▶ **Precautions during physical therapy:** Address precautions or contraindications for exercise, based on the patient's pre-existing condition(s); identify and avoid postures and loading conditions that are likely to exacerbate the condition

▶ **Complications interfering with physical therapy:** Potential for further anterior translation of the L5 vertebra with neurologic impairment of the lower extremities

Understanding the Health Condition

Spondylolisthesis is defined as translational displacement or nonanatomic alignment of one vertebral segment on another.[1] It is most common in the lumbar spine at the L5-S1 segment and it is usually associated with bilateral spondylolytic defects at the pars interarticularis (Fig. 13-1). In most cases, the pathology is caused by repeated mechanical stress and the condition occurs incrementally, with the spectrum ranging from a stress reaction that is undetectable with plain radiographs to a frank fracture.[2]

Mechanical stress to the pars interarticularis is greatest with spinal extension and rotational forces.[3] For this reason, it is most commonly seen among young athletes involved in football blocking, overhead lifting, tennis serving, baseball pitching, gymnastics, and the butterfly swim stroke.[4] In fact, spondylolysis and spondylolisthesis are the **most common spinal injuries in young athletes**. The incidence of spondylolysis for young athletes seeking care for low back pain has been reported at 47% compared to 5% for the general population.[5] In contrast, the same researchers also reported an 11% incidence of disc-related back pain in adolescent athletes compared to a 48% incidence of discogenic back pain in the nonathletic adult population. The prevalence of spondylolisthesis stabilizes in adulthood, and the etiology of new occurrences after this time are usually considered to be degenerative in nature.[1] Degenerative spondylolisthesis is nearly six times more likely to occur in women than men.[6] The classifications of spondylolisthesis by type[7] and severity[8] are described in Tables 13-1 and 13-2, respectively.

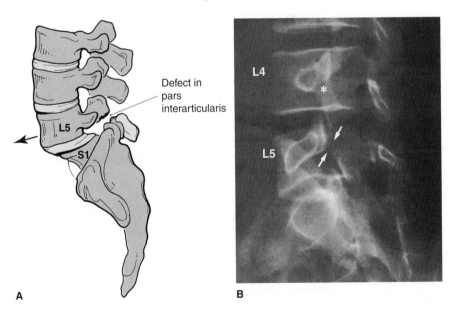

Defect in pars interarticularis

L4

*

L5

S1

A   **B**

Figure 13-1. A. Diagram of spondylolisthesis of L5 over S1 caused by spondylolysis of L5. **B.** Oblique plain film of lumbar spine demonstrates a spondylolysis or pars defect on the right side at L5 (arrows). Note the intact pars at L4 (*). (Reproduced with permission from Chen MY, Pope TL, Ott DJ, eds. *Basic Radiology*. 2nd ed. New York: McGraw-Hill; 2011. Figure 13-12 A and B.)

Table 13-1 WILTSE CLASSIFICATION OF TYPES OF SPONDYLOLISTHESIS	
Type I Dysplastic/congenital	Congenital abnormalities of the upper sacrum or the arch of L5 permit the olisthesis (slip) to occur: • Type IA: dysplastic posterior elements and facets; usually associated with spina bifida • Type IB: dysplastic articular process with sagittal-oriented facet joints • Type IC: other congenital abnormalities, such as failure of formation or segmentations producing spondylolisthesis
Type II Isthmic	Lesion within the pars interarticularis: • Type IIA: lytic fatigue fracture • Type IIB: elongation (microfracture healed with elongation) • Type IIC: acute fracture secondary to trauma
Type III Degenerative	Long-standing intersegmental instability, such as within the apophyseal joints, permitting slippage
Type IV Traumatic	Due to fractures in areas of the bony hook other than the pars interarticularis
Type V Pathological	Results from generalized or localized bone disease (*e.g.,* osteogenesis imperfecta, Paget's disease)

The pain associated with symptomatic spondylolisthesis can degrade motor control of the spine, leading to unbalanced loading of spinal structures.[9] Therefore, ensuring optimal motor control of the lumbopelvic region and entire kinetic chain is a priority. Optimizing functional core stability is one strategy to improve and maintain control of the spinal region. Core stability has been defined by Hodges as the restoration or augmentation of the ability of the neuromuscular system to control and protect the spine from injury or reinjury.[10] Core stability can be conceptualized as a product of trunk muscle capacity for control (strength and endurance) and the coordination and control of those same muscles to improve control of the lumbar spine and pelvis.[10] Deficits in motor control of the trunk have been associated with not only back pain, but also increased risk of lower extremity injury.[11]

Table 13-2 MEYERDING CLASSIFICATION OF SPONDYLOLISTHESIS SEVERITY[1]	
Grade	Percentage of Vertebral Translation*
1	0%-25%
2	26%-50%
3	51%-75%
4	76%-100%
5	100%

*Calculated as the distance of translation divided by the A-P diameter of the inferior vertebral body X 100%.

Physical Therapy Patient/Client Management

There are several potentially effective interventions for the patient with spondylolisthesis. Therapeutic exercises should be prescribed to optimize neuromuscular responsiveness and to alleviate soft tissue restrictions that would promote excessive lordosis.[12-14] Manual therapy is indicated to address identified mobility impairments above and below the area of the spondylolisthesis. Because this patient is experiencing only intermittent pain related to provocative activities, the routine use of modalities and medications is not an essential component of management. Other patients with this condition might present with a greater need for pain management and may benefit from selected modalities and analgesic medications. It is important to note that patients with spondylolisthesis appear to have no greater disability from their back pain than the general public.[15] The implication of this finding is that clinicians should be wary of attributing *all* back pain in this population to the spondylolisthesis.

The primary goal for this patient and others of a similar age and activity level is to return to pain-free, unrestricted activity with minimal risk for further tissue trauma. This patient expressed interest in returning to football "as soon as possible." The therapist must ensure that the patient has realistic expectations about the prognosis and expected rehabilitation timeline. Education of the patient should also ensure he has a thorough understanding of the requirements for returning to his sport. Because the patient's diagnostic category, type IIB, suggests tissue healing is complete, the primary determinant of readiness for return to play will be the patient's ability to demonstrate dynamic stability of the spine during loading conditions that simulate football.

Examination, Evaluation, and Diagnosis

Although the patient has received a full diagnostic examination by the orthopaedist, the physical therapist should perform a thorough neuromusculoskeletal examination to confirm the patient's current status and guide the rehabilitation plan of care. While many individuals with this condition are asymptomatic, individuals presenting with type II spondylolisthesis usually report central low back pain of varying intensity. The pain is often described as dull and aching. Symptoms radiating to the buttocks and posterior thigh are not uncommon, although true radicular symptoms are more likely with degenerative spondylolisthesis (type III), because disc and facet degeneration often combine to narrow the neural foramina. Most often, patients report that their pain is aggravated by prolonged standing or walking and bending backward or twisting. The pain is often relieved by sitting or lying down with the hips and knees bent.

Physical examination should start with observation of posture. Although patients commonly present with an anterior tilt of the pelvis and increased lumbar lordosis, the patient in pain might present with decreased lordosis related to muscle guarding.[2] Gait stride might be shortened in order to decrease rotational stress to the spine or to accommodate tight hamstrings.[2] While any active movement of the spine might be limited in this patient, spinal extension is most likely to recreate his pain. Similarly, passive extension and passive accessory movements of the spondylolytic

L5/S1 segment (*e.g.*, posterior to anterior glides) are likely to provoke the patient's pain. The physical therapy examination must include muscle length testing with particular concern for tightness that might promote excessive lumbar lordosis (*e.g.*, iliopsoas, rectus femoris, tensor fascia lata). The therapist should evaluate whether the patient is able to activate deep trunk muscles (transversus abdominis and multifidi), and have the patient perform functional movement tests to identify patterns that suggest inadequate control of the kinetic chain.

The diagnosis of spondylolisthesis can be established with plain radiographs.[1] Oblique views aid in the identification of spondylolysis and flexion-extension films are used to measure instability. When radicular and other neurologic signs are present, MRI and CT myelogram assist in determining the site and degree of stenosis or impingement.[1]

Plan of Care and Interventions

Physical therapy interventions should address findings from the musculoskeletal examination. Interventions often include manual therapy and therapeutic exercise to address impaired joint kinematics, muscular tightness, muscular weakness, and motor control. Most patients with spondylolisthesis benefit from therapeutic interventions to improve both mobility and dynamic stability.

Patients with spondylolisthesis often present with *decreased* mobility in the thoracic spine, hip, lumbar extensor muscles, and muscles that anteriorly tilt the pelvis. Since one objective for the patient with symptomatic spondylolisthesis is to achieve dynamic stabilization of the lumbar spine, impaired mobility of the regions above (thoracic spine) and below (hip) has the potential to greatly limit functional mobility.[16] Optimizing thoracic and hip mobility might allow the patient to dynamically stabilize the lumbar spine. Manipulation, mobilization, stretching, and range of motion exercises are all potentially appropriate intervention options in the thoracic spine and hip regions. Because the spondylolisthesis increases the spinal extension moment, interventions are also aimed at reducing the tension on posterior lumbar structures. Spinal flexion exercises are normally indicated to decrease the load on posterior vertebral tissues.[17] Such exercises might reduce tension in lumbar extensor muscles and stretch passive and active structures of the posterior lumbar spine.[18] Examples of flexion exercises include: supine-knees-to-chest, trunk curl-ups, and seated or quadruped lumbar flexion. Last, the physical therapist must optimize length of the **muscles that anteriorly tilt the pelvis**. Through their attachments to the pelvis, several muscles have the potential to exacerbate a spondylolisthesis by promoting an anterior tilt of the pelvis when shortened. Thus, static and/or dynamic stretching of tight iliopsoas, rectus femoris, and tensor fascia lata muscles should be included in the exercise program.[19]

Deficits in **dynamic trunk stability** have been associated with back pain,[11] and strategies to improve spinal stabilization have been used to decrease pain and functional disability in patients with spondylolisthesis.[12] Table 13-3 presents a three-phased approach, based on a training strategy by Smith et al.[20] that could be used to decrease pain and functional disability in patients with spondylolisthesis. The purpose of the first phase (phase I) is to develop kinesthetic awareness, provide foundational motor control, and to improve endurance during slow-velocity, limited-excursion

Table 13-3 PHASED EXERCISE APPROACH TO IMPROVING DYNAMIC STABILITY FOR ATHLETES WITH SPONDYLOLISTHESIS

Phase and Primary Focus	Exercise/Activity	Technique
Phase I Focus on developing kinesthetic awareness, foundational motor control, and endurance during slow-velocity, limited-excursion movements	Establish the neutral position of the pelvis ("neutral spine")	Perform this activity in various functional positions (*e.g.*, supine, quadruped, seated and standing). Exercise consists of isolated, rhythmic anterior and posterior tilting of the pelvis, with each set of repetitions stopping at a midpoint between anterior and posterior extremes of motion. Manual facilitation techniques from the therapist might be necessary to initiate isolated pelvic movement.
	Activation of the transversus abdominis (TrA) and multifidi muscles. Activation of the TrA and multifidi should be confirmed with each new exercise added in phase I. Once confirmed, the abdominal bracing strategy can be used to activate the core musculature.	This activity should be performed in various functional positions. The transversus abdominis (TrA) may be activated by drawing the naval toward the spine and slightly upward. The patient or therapist may confirm its activation by palpating for tension just medial and inferior to the anterior superior iliac spine. Multifidus activation is monitored by palpation (either by the patient or therapist) immediately lateral to the relevant lumbar spinous process as the patient attempts to "swell" the muscle into the palpating digit(s). The contractions of both TrA and multifidi should be gentle and not disturb a rhythmic breathing pattern. Observe for loss of the pelvic neutral position, as this likely indicates that global trunk muscles are attempting to compensate for poor activation of deep stabilizers. Activation of the pelvic floor muscles may facilitate coactivation of the TrA and multifidi. (The patient can be advised to contract as if stopping the flow of urine.)
	Quadruped limb elevation progression	From the quadruped position, establish the neutral position of the pelvis. Provide progressive challenges to this stable position by lifting and extending the limbs away from the trunk. Begin with single arm and leg lifts, then progress to reciprocal arm/leg lifts (Fig. 13-2). Do not elevate the limbs beyond parallel with the spine. Stop the progression if the neutral position is not maintained.

(Continued)

Table 13-3 PHASED EXERCISE APPROACH TO IMPROVING DYNAMIC STABILITY FOR ATHLETES WITH SPONDYLOLISTHESIS (CONTINUED)

Phase and Primary Focus	Exercise/Activity	Technique
	Abdominal curl-ups	Begin in the supine position with one leg straight, the other flexed at the hip and knee, and the pelvis and lumbar spine in a neutral position. The curl-up is performed by raising the head and the upper shoulders off the floor. The motion takes place in the thoracic spine—*not* the lumbar or cervical region. To begin, the hands are placed under the lumbar region to monitor movement of the lumbar spine (Fig. 13-3A). Hold the curl-up for several seconds, then return smoothly to starting position and repeat as indicated. Progress exercise by using one or all of the following techniques: raising the elbows, placing the hands on the head (Fig. 13-3B), lifting the straight leg. Stop progression if the neutral position is not maintained.
	Supine bridge	From supine, hooklying position (knees bent about 90°), gently squeeze gluteus maximus bilaterally. Slowly increase activation of this muscle until the hips rise a few inches from the floor. Ensure neutral position of the pelvis is maintained. Hold several seconds, then return smoothly to starting position and repeat as indicated. To reduce tendency to extend the lumbar spine rather than the hip, consider fully flexing one hip and performing a single-leg support bridge.
	Side bridge	Begin in modified sidelying with the hips and knees flexed and the upper body supported through forearm contact with the ground. Press through the forearm to establish protective stabilization of the shoulder girdle, and then gradually lift the pelvis from the ground. The pelvis should translate forward as it lifts so that sagittal plane alignment of the knees, hips, and shoulders is achieved. Stop elevation of the hips when frontal plane alignment of the spine and thighs is achieved. Hold several seconds, and then return smoothly to the starting position and repeat as indicated. Progress this exercise by starting with the knees extended, with the foot of the top leg on the ground directly in front of the foot of the bottom leg (Fig. 13-4).
	Standing rotational resistance	Begin in standing with the pelvis and lumbar spine in neutral and trunk muscles engaged with a gentle, bracing contraction. To train for control of rotational forces, begin with a cable or elastic cord positioned at chest level in the transverse plane. The handle attached to the resistance is initially held close to the chest (Fig. 13-5A). Perform the exercise by slowly extending the elbows to increase transverse plane loading (Fig. 13-5B). Hold several seconds, and then return smoothly to the starting position and repeat as indicated. Ensure stability is maintained in all planes of motion.

Phase II		
Progress to higher velocity, more dynamic multiplanar endurance, strength, power, and coordination challenges incorporating upper and lower extremity movements	Lunge progression	Begin by performing body-weight lunges in the cardinal planes. Ensure both lower extremity alignment and pelvis/lumbar spine stability throughout the movement. Progress the activity by adding a balanced load (e.g., weight vest, medicine ball) held at the center of the chest. Reduce the load and then position it away from the midline.
	Medicine ball throws	A medicine ball that bounces and a solid wall can be used to train reactive stability by progressively rapid, short-range throws and catches. Progress the load, speed, and volume of exercise as indicated. For the chest pass, begin about 6 ft from the wall in an athletic stance with the ball held close to the chest (Fig. 13-6A). Maintain the stance, neutral pelvis, and spine position as throws become progressively faster. For rotational passes, turn 90° away from the wall and assume the athletic stance with the ball just lateral to the outermost thigh, which bears most of the weight initially (Fig. 13-6B). Ensure sufficient hip/knee flexion, hip internal rotation, and vertical alignment of the ankle/knee/hip of the outer leg. The thoracic spine is also rotated away from the wall. Push off the outer leg and "unwind" the outside leg, hip, and thoracic spine in order to create the rotational force for the throw. The arms should act primarily as tethers to transfer the force created in the legs and thoracic spine.
	Multiplanar challenges using an exercise ball	An exercise ball can be used to create an unstable surface that challenges trunk motor control. From the plank position with the legs supported on the ball (Fig. 13-7A), flex the hips to draw the knees toward the chest (Fig. 13-7B). Do not allow the lumbar spine to drop into extension. From the plank position with the forearms supported on the ball, shift forearm pressure in all directions to include circular motions. With the upper back supported on the ball, slowly roll side to side (Fig. 13-7C) to engage rotational stabilizers.
	Lifting an asymmetrical load	Place an appropriate weight beside the patient at a height that permits optimal trunk and lower extremity alignment (Fig. 13-8A). Lift the weight while maintaining trunk stability (Fig. 13-8B). Observe for aberrant movement, primarily in the frontal plane.
	Asymmetrical push-press into split-squat	Start with an appropriate weight in one hand at shoulder level (Fig. 13-9A). Perform a push-press by flexing slightly at the hips and knees, then quickly extend the hips and knees while guiding the weight overhead (Fig. 13-9B). Maintaining arm and trunk alignment, perform split squats or lunges (Fig. 13-9C). Key points of execution include: arm alignment perpendicular to the ground, maintenance of neutral lumbopelvic position, and frontal plane alignment of forward hip and knee.

(Continued)

Table 13-3   PHASED EXERCISE APPROACH TO IMPROVING DYNAMIC STABILITY FOR ATHLETES WITH SPONDYLOLISTHESIS (CONTINUED)

Phase and Primary Focus	Exercise/Activity	Technique
Phase III Activity-specific skill simulations, with emphasis on mastery of component motions that present the greatest challenge to neutral spine alignment. Listed here are suggestions appropriate for a football lineman.	Sled push	First, match the height of the handle to the requirements of the patient. After selecting an appropriate load, have the patient demonstrate an athletic stance (flexed at the hips and knees) with a neutral pelvis and core activation. Maintain the neutral pelvis because force production for the sled push is achieved through powerful extension of the hips, knees and ankles (Fig. 13-10).
	Isometric, axial loading	Use a barbell and weight rack hooks to create an isometric, axial load (Fig. 13-11). The barbell is placed under the hooks that are normally used to support the barbell on the rack. This simulates a common force as football lineman struggle for position. Ensure the athlete maintains the lumbopelvic neutral position throughout the application of force, generally in 3-4 s increments. As the athlete demonstrates proficiency, adjust the rate of force application and the degree of loading to simulate realistic conditions.
	Standing trunk rotation with unilateral "punch"	Cable or elastic resistance may be used to create resistance to combined leg/trunk/arm rotation, simulating a common movement in many sports. Most of the rotation for this exercise is produced at the hips and thoracic spine. Ensure that the pelvis and lumbar spine remain in the neutral position (Fig. 13-12A). Observe for compensatory trunk movement in the sagittal and frontal planes as the athlete "punches" his arm forward (Fig. 13-12B).

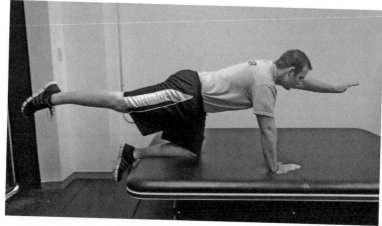

Figure 13-2. Quadruped limb elevation progression.

movements. Most activities are directed at the pelvis and lumbar spine. However, integration of activities involving the extremities should begin as soon as basic core stabilization is demonstrated. In the only randomized, controlled trial to study the effect of specific core training on patients with spondylolysis or spondylolisthesis, O'Sullivan et al.[12] provided evidence to support the use of specific training for the

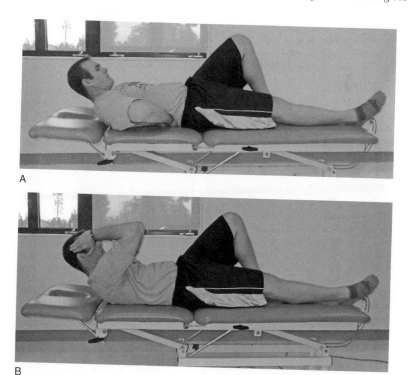

Figure 13-3. Abdominal curl-up. **A.** Elbow lift progression. **B.** Hands-on-head progression.

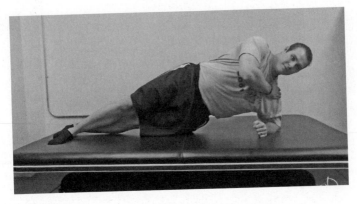

Figure 13-4. Side bridge.

deep abdominal muscles combined with coactivation of the lumbar multifidi. This study, along with support for the role of deep abdominal and lumbar multifidi activation training in the treatment of chronic low back pain[10] has influenced many physical therapists to consider such training as the foundation of their approach to motor control for the patient with lumbar impairments. However, there remains controversy as to the *best* strategy for promoting foundational motor control of the trunk.

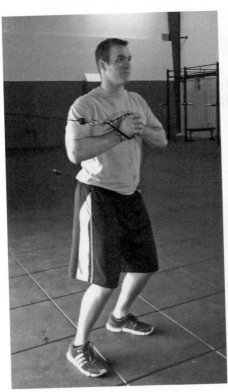 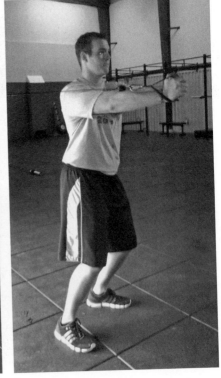

A

B

Figure 13-5. Standing rotational resistance. **A.** Starting position. **B.** Ending position.

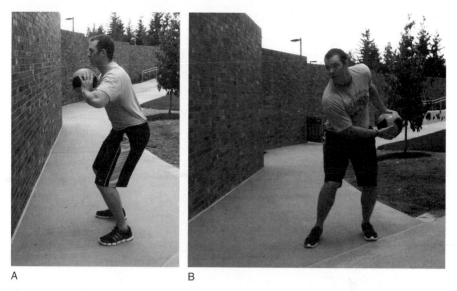

A   B

Figure 13-6. Medicine ball throws. **A.** Medicine ball chest pass. **B.** Medicine ball rotational pass.

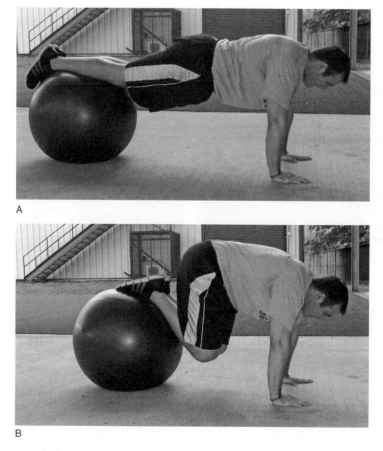

A

B

Figure 13-7. Multiplanar challenges with exercise ball. **A.** Exercise ball plank. **B.** Plank with leg tucks. **C.** Exercise ball twist.

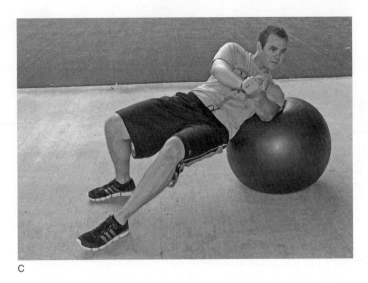

C

Figure 13-7. (*Continued*)

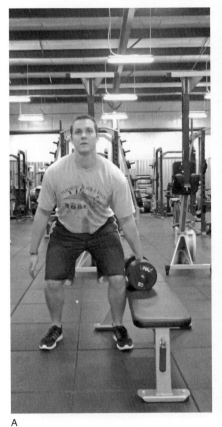

A

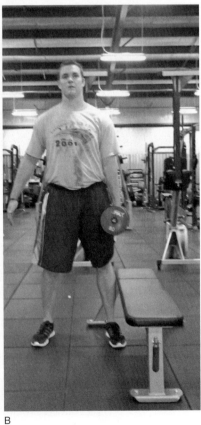

B

Figure 13-8. Asymmetrical lift. **A.** Starting position. **B.** Ending position.

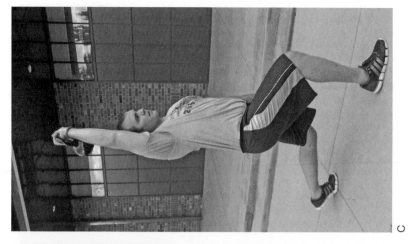

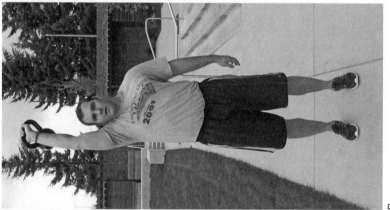

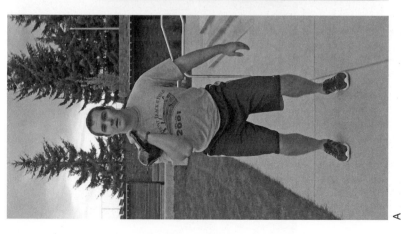

Figure 13-9. Asymmetrical push-press. **A.** Starting position. **B.** Ending position. **C.** Asymmetrical overhead split squat.

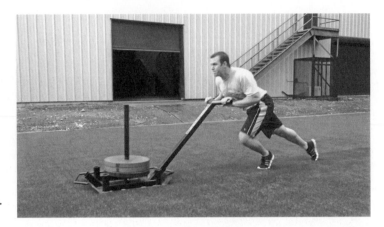

Figure 13-10. Sled push.

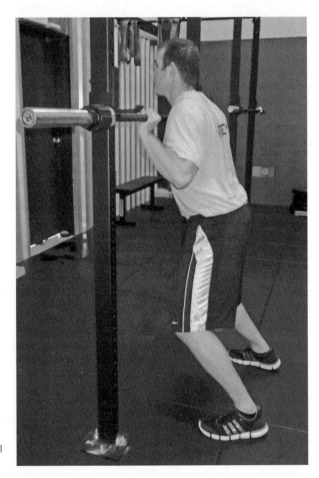

Figure 13-11. Isometric axial trunk loading.

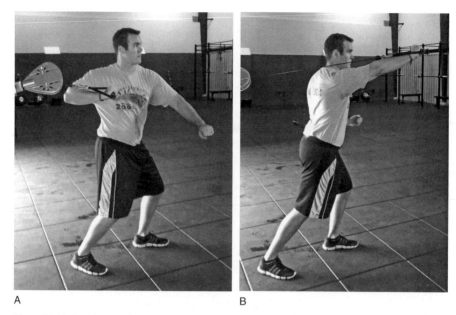

Figure 13-12. Standing trunk rotation. **A.** Starting position. **B.** Ending position with unilateral "punch."

The common practice of first achieving bilateral activation of the transversus abdominis (*e.g.*, using the abdominal drawing-in maneuver in which the patient is instructed to draw the umbilicus toward the spine and upward, while palpating for transversus abdominis contractions medial and inferior to the anterior superior iliac spines) before all stabilization training has been called into question.[22-24] Evidence from Grenier and McGill suggests that abdominal bracing (co-contraction of all abdominal and low back muscles) provides greater trunk stability than isolated activation of the transversus abdominis.[23] Given uncertainty in the literature about the optimal means for dynamically stabilizing the trunk, a reasonable middle ground might be as follows: early in the rehabilitation of a patient with low back impairments, establish the patient's ability to activate deep stabilizers such as the transversus abdominis and multifidi in static positions; then, as exercise and activities are progressed, place primary emphasis on alignment, coordination, and energy efficiency of movement rather than pre-activation of muscles that might or might not be a part of the optimal motor program for a given task. During phase II of training to improve dynamic stability of the lumbar spine, progressive loads, speed, and excursion are introduced to challenge the newly gained lumbar stability. More complex, integrated movements are introduced as indicated based on the patient's proficiency with simple movements and his activity and sport requirements. The last phase of dynamic stability training includes activity-specific skill simulations, with emphasis on mastery of component motions that present the greatest challenge to neutral spine alignment. Factors to consider are occupational and sport-specific loads, acceleration, velocity, coordination, and endurance. Traditional training modes for a particular sport should be re-evaluated in light of the patient's unique impairments and risks. In the present case, the traditional practice of heavy-resistance squatting for football lineman should be reconsidered in light of evidence that such activity is associated with hyperextension of the lumbar spine, thus potentially exacerbating conditions such as spondylolysis and spondylolisthesis.[25]

Evidence-Based Clinical Recommendations

SORT: Strength of Recommendation Taxonomy

A: Consistent, good-quality patient-oriented evidence
B: Inconsistent or limited-quality patient-oriented evidence
C: Consensus, disease-oriented evidence, usual practice, expert opinion, or case series

1. Spondylolisthesis and spondylolysis are the most common spinal injuries in young athletes, especially in those sports that require spinal extension and rotational forces. **Grade A**

2. Stretching tight muscles that anteriorly tilt the pelvis is an effective component of conservative care for spondylolisthesis. **Grade C**

3. Specific exercises aimed to improve dynamic trunk stability are associated with less pain and better function for patients with spondylolisthesis. **Grade B**

COMPREHENSION QUESTIONS

13.1 Which pain-provoking activity is *least* likely to raise suspicion of spondylolisthesis as an etiology of low back pain?

    A. A gymnastic floor routine

    B. Triathlon training

    C. Intensive practice of the tennis serve

    D. Intensive practice of the golf swing (driving)

13.2 Select the *most* appropriate exercise strategy for the rehabilitation of patients with spondylolisthesis.

    A. Flexion range of motion exercises; stretching tight muscles that promote anterior pelvic tilt; foundational motor control exercises for deep core stabilizers

    B. Extension range of motion exercises; stretching tight muscles that promote anterior pelvic tilt; activity-specific skill simulations with emphasis on mastery of component motions that present the greatest challenge to neutral spine alignment

    C. Flexion range of motion exercises; stretching tight muscles that promote anterior pelvic tilt; foundational motor control exercises for deep core stabilizers; progression to activity-specific skill simulations with emphasis on mastery of component motions that present the greatest challenge to neutral spine alignment

    D. Flexion range of motion exercises; stretching tight muscles that promote anterior pelvic tilt; progressive resistance exercise for all core muscles

ANSWERS

13.1 **B.** Activities involving extension of the lumbar spine are most likely to provoke symptoms in the presence of spondylolisthesis.[2-4] When axial loads and rotation are added to extension, the forces on posterior vertebral structures are increased.[3] The components of triathlon training (crawl-stroke swim, bicycling, and running) have only modest extension moments and range of motion requirements. The other three activities listed have significant spinal extension and rotational components.

13.2 **C.** Range of motion exercises that promote flexion are better tolerated than extension.[17] Stretching is most effective when applied to muscles whose shortened length promotes anterior tilt of the pelvis. Activation of the deep stabilizers is often impaired in patients with low back pain.[9] Therefore, specific exercises to promote activation are indicated.[12] When consistent activation of the deep stabilizers has been achieved, progressing to activity-specific challenges allows the therapist to determine whether skills learned in previous simple exercises will transfer to goal-directed activities.[20,21]

REFERENCES

1. Metz LN, Deviren V. Low-grade spondylolisthesis. *Neurosurg Clin N Am.* 2007;18:237-248.

2. Herman MJ, Pizzutillo PD, Cavalier R. Spondylolysis and spondylolisthesis in the child and adolescent athlete. *Orthop Clin N Am.* 2003;34:461-467.

3. Chosa E, Totoribe K, Tajima N. A biomechanical study of lumbar spondylolysis based on a three-dimensional finite element method. *J Orthop Res.* 2004;22:158-163.

4. O'Connor FG, d'Hemecourt PA, Nebzydoski M. Spondylolysis: a practical approach to an adolescent enigma. In: Seidenberg PH, Beutler AI, eds. *The Sports Medicine Resource Manual.* Philadelphia, PA: Saunders; 2008:418-421.

5. Micheli LJ, Wood R. Back pain in young athletes. Significant differences from adults in causes and patterns. *Arch Pediatr Adolesc Med.* 1995;149:15-18.

6. Vibert BT, Sliva CD, Herkowitz HN. Treatment of instability and spondylolisthesis: surgical versus nonsurgical treatment. *Clin Orthop Relat Res.* 2006;443:222-227.

7. Wiltse LL, Newman PH, Macnab I. Classification of spondylolysis and spondylolisthesis. *Clin Orthop Relat Res.*1976;117:23-29.

8. Meyerding HW. Spondylolisthesis: surgical treatment and results. *Surg Gynecol Obstet.* 1932;54:371-377.

9. Hodges PW, Richardson CA. Relationship between limb movement speed and associated contraction of the trunk muscles. *Ergonomics.*1997;40:1220-1230.

10. Hodges PW. Core stability exercise in chronic low back pain. *Orthop Clin N Am.* 2003;34:245-254.

11. Zazulak BT, Hewett TE, Reeves NP, Goldberg B, Cholewicki J. Deficits in neuromuscular control of the trunk predict knee injury risk: a prospective biomechanical-epidemiologic study. *Am J Sports Med.* 2007;35:1123-1130.

12. O'Sullivan PB, Phyty GD, Twomey LT, Allison GT. Evaluation of specific stabilizing exercise in the treatment of chronic low back pain with radiologic diagnosis of spondylolysis or spondylolisthesis. *Spine.* 1997;22:2959-2967.

13. O'Sullivan PB. Lumbar segmental "instability": clinical presentation and specific stabilizing exercise management. *Man Ther.* 2000;5:2-12.

14. Macedo LG, Maher CG, Latimer J, McAuley JH. Motor control exercise for persistent, nonspecific low back pain: a systematic review. *Phys Ther.* 2009;89:9-25.

15. Frennered AK, Danielson BI, Nachemson AL. Natural history of symptomatic isthmic low-grade spondylolisthesis in children and adolescents: a seven-year follow-up study. *J Pediatr Orthop.* 1991;11:209-213.

16. Van Dillen LR, Bloom NJ, Gombatto SP, Susco TM. Hip rotation range of motion in people with and without low back pain who participate in rotation-related sports. *Phys Ther Sport.* 2008;9:72-81.

17. Sinaki M, Lutness MP, Ilstrup DM, Chu CP, Gramse RR. Lumbar spondylolisthesis: retrospective comparison and three-year follow-up of two conservative treatment programs. *Arch Phys Med Rehabil.* 1989;70:594-598.

18. Brotzman SB. Low back injuries. In: Brotzman SB, Wilk KE, eds. *Clinical Orthopaedic Rehabilitation.* Philadelphia, PA: Mosby; 2003:557-558.

19. Sampsell E. Rehabilitation of the spine following sports injury. *Clin Sports Med.* 2010;29:127-156.

20. Smith CE, Nyland J, Caudill P, Brosky J, Caborn DN. Dynamic trunk stabilization: a conceptual back injury prevention program for volleyball athletes. *J Orthop Sports Phys Ther.* 2008;38:703-720.

21. Kibler WB, Press J, Sciascia A. The role of core stability in athletic function. *Sports Med* 2006;36:189-198.

22. Allison GT, Morris SL, Lay B. Feedforward responses of transversus abdominis are directionally specific and act asymmetrically: implications for core stability theories. *J Orthop Sports Phys Ther.* 2008;38:228-237.

23. Grenier SG, McGill SM. Quantification of lumbar stability by using 2 different abdominal activation strategies. *Arch Phys Med Rehabil.* 2007;88:54-62.

24. Brown SH, Vera-Garcia FJ, McGill SM. Effects of abdominal muscle coactivation on the externally preloaded trunk: variations in motor control and its effect on spine stability. *Spine.* 2006;31:E387-E393.

25. Walsh JC, Quinlan JF, Stapleton R, FitzPatrick DP, McCormack D. Three-dimensional motion analysis of the lumbar spine during "free squat" weight lift training. *Am J Sports Med.* 2007;35:927-932.

Low Back Pain: Manipulation

Carl DeRosa

CASE 14

A 52-year-old male self-refers to physical therapy for evaluation and treatment of low back pain. He states that he has had recurrent bouts of low back pain over the past 12 years and for most of those episodes, the back pain tends to resolve to his satisfaction. On occasion, he has had to see his family doctor for episodes that did not resolve. In most instances, he was given nonsteroidal anti-inflammatory medication and a small booklet describing low back exercises. He feels that these exacerbations of pain now last longer and the bouts seem more frequent. This most recent back pain episode began 7 days ago. He is a university professor and does not want this episode to cause him to miss work as several of his past episodes have done.

▶ What are key questions to ask in order to further clarify the patient's complaints and provide direction for the examination?
▶ What are the most appropriate physical therapy interventions?
▶ What is his rehabilitation prognosis?

KEY DEFINITIONS

ACUTE, SUBACUTE, AND CHRONIC LOW BACK PAIN (LBP): Classic description of the course of LBP using a temporal guideline; acute is typically considered to last 0 to 4 weeks, subacute from 1 to 3 months, and chronic more than 3 months; most common back complaints are exacerbations of a recurrent back condition, which compounds these classic descriptors

CHRONIC PAIN SYNDROME: Syndrome in which the psychosocial and behavioral aspects of pain far exceed the mechanical or chemical nociceptive influences present; chronic pain syndrome is distinct from chronic LBP

CLINICAL PREDICTION RULE: Use of a specific combination of signs, symptoms, and aspects of history and physical examination to predict the probability of success with a particular intervention strategy

MANIPULATION: Physical intervention intended to direct a specific force into a targeted region of the body (often a joint) identified by rate of force application and location within the range of motion (beginning, middle, or end of available range); distinction between mobilization and manipulation is typically related to *rate* of force application (*i.e.*, manipulation is a *high* velocity thrust)

RADICULAR PAIN: Pain most often due to an inflammatory state of the nerve root, which lowers the nerve root's threshold to mechanical stimulus (either tension or compression)

REFERRED PAIN: Pain felt at a distance from the actual anatomical source of involvement or injury; due to extensive innervation of spinal tissues, pain can be felt in the lower quarter due to involvement of low back tissues (or in the upper quarter due to involvement of cervical tissues), irrespective of involvement of the nerve roots in the region

SEGMENTAL INSTABILITY: Displacement or aberrant motion between two bony segments that results when a force is applied; it is a biomechanical entity distinct from hypermobility; most typical types are translational motions due to applied shear loads

Objectives

1. List key aspects of the history and physical examination that would provide evidence that the low back pain a patient is experiencing is *not* radicular in nature.

2. Describe how the clinical prediction rule for manipulation can be utilized in the management strategy for a patient presenting with LBP.

3. Provide a rationale for the use of therapeutic exercise in conjunction with manipulation to optimize the prognosis for a patient presenting with exacerbation of a recurrent low back condition.

4. Describe how to triage the patient presenting with LBP and pain into the lower extremity into either a radicular pain category or a nonradicular pain category.

Physical Therapy Considerations

PT considerations during management of the individual with a diagnosis of mechanical low back pain:

▶ **General physical therapy plan of care/goals:** Decrease pain in rapid and cost-effective manner; begin graded, active, spinal activity program progressing to therapeutic exercise focused on enhancing neuromuscular performance

▶ **Physical therapy interventions:** Spinal mobilization or manipulation to specific regions with primary intent of modulating pain; resistance exercises to increase muscular strength and endurance (especially of spinal extensors, abdominals, and hip musculature); exercises to improve motor control and overall aerobic fitness; education regarding position, loads, and activities that have the potential to exacerbate this specific clinical problem as determined by the pathomechanics gleaned via the physical examination

▶ **Precautions during physical therapy:** No contraindications present for pain modulation techniques chosen; monitor that leg pain symptoms do not extend distal to the knee; exercise overload must remain within the physiologic limits of patient's spinal condition

▶ **Complications interfering with physical therapy:** Psychosocial factors affecting prognosis including fear of movement and low expectation of recovery; exacerbation of pain following manipulation intervention; distal referral of symptoms as a result of manipulation or exercise regimen

Understanding the Health Condition

Low back pain is the most prevalent form of musculoskeletal discomfort reported by adults.[1] The prevalence of LBP is not as dependent on the degenerative processes associated with aging as might be expected. Low back pain continues through young and middle adulthood, but at the sixth decade, it appears to plateau and then decline in the later decades of life.[2] Socioeconomic factors are also important to consider because they are recognized as potential risk factors for lumbar pain and disability, ultimately contributing to its direct and indirect costs. A higher prevalence of LBP has been linked to such factors as lower educational levels,[1] unskilled laborers,[3] and workers with physically demanding job responsibilities.[4] The total costs of LBP in the United States exceed $100 billion per year with two-thirds being indirect costs due to lost wages and reduced productivity.[5]

The great majority of the costs of LBP are associated with management of the *chronic* disorder. This has significant influence on the goals of treatment and the physical therapist's approach toward management of the condition. Comprehensive care for the patient presenting with LBP includes attempts to manage the disorder as it immediately presents in the clinic. However, perhaps more importantly, management involves utilizing interventions and appropriate patient education strategies to minimize the potential for the acute, simple LBP episode to evolve into a chronic pain syndrome. In addition, the physical therapist must recognize that the majority of nonsurgical LBP episodes presenting in the physical therapy clinic are recurrent phenomena (*i.e.*, the patient often presents with an exacerbation of his chronic back condition). Thus, the focus of intervention strategies is to help prevent recurrences, or at a minimum, provide information or strategies in order to help the patient self-manage his recurrent back problem.

There are numerous reasons why recurrent back problems are so prevalent. The tissues of the spine undergo physiological changes due to aging and due to injury. As a result of such changes, the ability of the tissues to tolerate forces, especially those forces that traverse the lumbopelvic region due to weightbearing and movement, are not easily attenuated by the low back tissues. When those forces exceed the physiological capacity of the tissues, pain occurs due to mechanical or chemical activation of the tissue nociceptive system.

In the low back (as in other areas of the musculoskeletal system), the mechanical loading capacity of tissues lowers as we age.[6] Because the low back is a hub of weightbearing, injuries can occur even with the simplest routine activities of daily living. This lifetime accumulation of such injuries, coupled with normal aging and degenerative processes, renders the back susceptible to re-injury. For example, the spinal segment can be viewed similar to a three-legged stool, with the front leg of the stool representing the intervertebral disc, and the back two legs of the stool represented by the right and left apophyseal joints. Apophyseal joint arthritis alone, or in combination with degeneration of the annulus fibrosus, results in an intervertebral segment that has less ability to tolerate forces such as tension, compression, and shear. Such degenerative changes result in the loss of inherent spinal stability. The breakdown of these tissues can result in aberrant motion between vertebral segments, resulting in segmental instability. Partial thickness degeneration of the facets of the apophyseal joints results in a segment that can no longer tolerate compressive loading when compared to normal, healthy tissue.[7] When compression exceeds the physiological capacity of this compromised tissue, discomfort or pain results.

Any structure within the spine that is innervated and provides afferent input to the central nervous system has the capacity to elicit symptoms of LBP. Tissues and structures including the dura mater and nerve roots, apophyseal joints, annulus fibrosus, bone, ligaments, fascia, and muscle all exhibit the capacity to generate pain when damaged. Despite a reasonable understanding of tissue injury and tissue innervation, identification of the *precise* anatomical structure causing a patient's episode of pain is not always possible. In fact, in many low back conditions, the presence of abnormal imaging findings (radiographs, computerized tomography, magnetic resonance imaging) has no correlation to the presence or absence of clinical symptoms.[8-10] Thus, treatment of LBP using a pathoanatomical model of care is often futile and costly.

One of the few tissues in the spine that can be implicated with some degree of confidence as the patient's source of pain is the nerve root. When the nerve root is involved in the pain syndrome, a very distinct set of symptoms and/or signs is present. There are two nerve root conditions: nerve root compression and nerve root irritation. Nerve root compression can result in true neurologic findings such as muscle weakness, reflex changes, and/or sensory disturbances. Nerve root irritation, which is often due to the abnormal chemical milieu that results from intervertebral disc lesions, presents with a distinct set of symptoms (as opposed to signs). Symptoms of nerve root irritation include: leg pain greater than back pain, clearly demarcated region of lower extremity pain, pain often below the knee, a highly disturbing and distressing type of pain, reproduction of lower extremity pain with neural tension tests (especially positive straight leg raise), and sharp peripheralizing pain with gentle spinal motions. Common examples of the latter include sharp and rapidly peripheralizing pain into the legs with slight degrees of active or passive lumbar flexion, or lumbar rotation of the lumbar spine. Any direction of motion can result in peripheralization of true nerve root irritation. The hallmark is the remarkably small amount of motion necessary to elicit such a dramatic pain response.

Low back conditions that are nonradicular in nature (*i.e.*, not due to nerve root irritation or nerve root compression), present differently especially in regards to referral into the lower extremity. Any innervated tissue in the low back can refer pain into the lower extremity. These nonradicular pain patterns typically present as conditions in which the pain in the low back is more aggravating and more of a concern to the patient than the discomfort in the lower extremity. The lower extremity discomfort with nonradicular syndromes is not as clearly demarcated and the quality of pain is not as disconcerting as true radicular pain. This is in contrast to the individual with nerve root (radicular) pain in which the lower extremity pain is often the more problematic complaint than the pain in the low back. Therefore, an important goal of the examination (history and physical) is for the physical therapist to discern whether the LBP and leg pain that the patient presents with is radicular pain (*i.e.*, true nerve root problem) or nonradicular pain (*i.e.*, pain felt in the back and referred to the lower extremity due to injury to any low back structure such as apophyseal or sacroiliac joints, muscle, ligament, fascia, etc.)

Physical Therapy Patient/Client Management

The **management strategy for the patient presenting with an exacerbation of a recurrent LBP problem** should be focused on rapid relief of pain followed by progressing the patient toward an active exercise program to improve the strength of the trunk and extremity musculature. Improving the health of the neuromuscular system after achieving pain relief is an essential component of management because the priority of treatment should be to minimize recurrences and minimize the potential for the mechanical back pain problem to evolve into a chronic pain syndrome.[11-14]

Examination, Evaluation, and Diagnosis

The examination of a patient self-referred for LBP requires two initial triages. The first is to determine if the presenting pain is nonmechanical or mechanical in origin. Nonmechanical pain is pain referred from pelvic or abdominal viscera or a neoplasm, pain of vascular origin, or pain associated with other medical conditions. Nonmechanical pain refers to pain not typically made worse with mechanical loading. A systems review and questions regarding recent weight loss, fevers, past medical history, night pain, bowel or bladder disturbances, and recent surgeries are essential elements of the history and physical examination for the patient with LBP. Mechanical disorders typically have some pain resolution with rest or relief from weightbearing and a pain pattern that can be correlated with activity, motion, or applied loads. Familiar pain can often be provoked with specific lumbopelvic motions, positions, or in response to specifically applied loads to the joints or soft tissues. In the absence of these phenomena, further medical evaluation is indicated.

The second triage is to ascertain whether the patient's pain complaint is radicular or nonradicular. Careful questioning regarding the pain pattern should be addressed early in the examination: "Is the back pain worse than the leg pain?" Or conversely, "Is the leg pain more disconcerting than the back pain?" Affirmative answers to these questions help the therapist determine if the condition is more likely nonradicular or radicular, respectively. In addition, a sickening quality to the pain, pain that is below the knee, and pain that is clearly demarcated in a dermatomal distribution are all strong indicators of radicular pain. A complaint of weakness in the lower extremity can also indicate a radicular disorder. If the history reveals suspicion of a radicular condition, confirmatory tests must be done in the physical examination such as straight leg raising, Slump testing, myotome and reflex assessments, and dermatome screening.

An acute episode of pain also presents an opportunity to determine if the clinical prediction rule for manipulation can be used. Key aspects of the history and the physical examination help determine whether the patient meets some or all of the criteria for regional lumbopelvic manipulation. Research has suggested that patients meeting such criteria can experience significant changes in pain pattern and perception of pain with the application of manipulation, advice to remain active, and a prescribed course of exercise.[15,16] **Patients most likely to benefit from a regional lumbopelvic manipulation** exhibit the following: duration of symptoms less than 16 days, no symptoms distal to the knee, lumbar hypomobility, at least one hip with more than 35° range of passive internal rotation, and Fear Avoidance Belief Questionnaire (FABQ) score less than 19. The probability of a successful outcome with lumbar manipulation increased from 45% to 95% with the presence of four or more of these examination findings.[15] The criteria presented in this clinical prediction rule are most suggestive of nonradicular etiologies of pain that would benefit from the use of manipulation as an intervention. This illustrates why the second triage of determining whether the syndrome is radicular or nonradicular in nature is important.

Subsequent to the publication of this clinical prediction rule, a pragmatic rule was suggested that helps to simplify the prediction of which patients with LBP are likely to experience dramatic improvement in pain and perception of disability with regional lumbopelvic manipulation.[17] Two factors in this pragmatic rule helped predict improvement: duration of symptoms less than 16 days and no symptoms distal to the knee. Subjects in this study had a moderate to large shift in probability of a successful outcome following application of low back manipulation. The clinical application of this rule may be illustrated by an example. A family practice physician examining a patient for LBP may want to determine whether referral to a physical therapist for spinal manipulation may be indicated. The physical therapist simply needs to ask the patient about the duration of his symptoms and whether they extend distal to the knee. This decreases the need for the family practice physician to have the patient complete the Fear Avoidance Beliefs Questionnaire and perform an examination of hip range of motion and spinal mobility.

This clinical prediction rule has been further validated with two different manipulation techniques: the regional lumbopelvic manipulation and the rotary lumbopelvic manipulation.[18] Combining manipulation and stabilization exercises for patients meeting this clinical prediction rule may be of even greater benefit, especially since one of our goals is to minimize recurrences.[19] Reductions of pain and disability are reasonable goals if the history and physical examination reveal predictors meeting the clinical prediction rule for LBP.

For the current patient, his subjective history contained three of the five predictors (duration of symptoms 7 days, no pain below the knee, and administered FABQ score >19) as to whether he would benefit from application of manipulation, advice to remain active, and a prescribed course of exercise. The physical examination will reveal whether the remaining two predictors are present (lumbar hypomobility and hip internal rotation range of motion). The physical examination should start with the patient in the standing position. Assessment includes: frontal plane and sagittal plane posture; active motion of the lumbar spine in forward bending, forward bending and sidebending combined, backward bending, backward bending and sidebending combined, overpressure in each of these directions, and the effect of the pain pattern with these repeated motions, and gait analysis.

In the supine position, hip active and passive ROM can be assessed and various sacroiliac provocative stresses applied through the lever of the femur. Full flexion of the hips begins to flex the pelvis on the lumbar spine, which then can be compared to the results found with standing active flexion. Straight leg raise testing can be performed and lower extremity myotomes and reflexes effectively screened in this position.

In the prone position, hip ROM can be further assessed, in particular the internal and external ROM.[20] Additional sacroiliac stresses can be applied, followed by posterior to anterior (PA) spring tests over the lumbar spine, which place a compressive force through the apophyseal joints and a shear stress between adjacent lumbar spinal segments. The response to compression and shear stresses over the lumbar spine should be compared to the results of the extension, and extension-sidebending tests that were performed during the standing portion of the examination. Posterior to anterior forces over individual lumbar spinous processes, or bilaterally over the region of the lumbar transverse processes can be used to determine hypomobility, as well as to determine if such a compression and shear force applied to the lumbar spine reproduces the patient's familiar pain.

The intent of the physical examination is not to precisely identify the anatomical structure considered to be at fault (a pathoanatomical model), but rather to determine those loads or positions that reproduce a patient's familiar pain (a pathomechanical model). Figure 14-1 shows several parts of the physical examination that uniquely

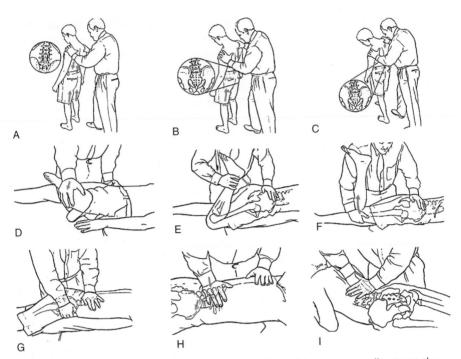

Figure 14-1. A. Overpressure in backward bending. The physical therapist manually retracts the scapulae to focus the extension force in the upper part of the lumbar spine. A gradual vertical force from above causes extension. **B.** Backward bending, sidebending to the left, and slight rotation to the right, with a superior-to-inferior overpressure applied to the right shoulder. **C.** Modification of standing examination to increase the extension, compression, and shear stresses in the left lumbosacral triangle by positioning the left lower extremity in extension, then having the patient backward bend and sidebend to the left. The examiner applies overpressure with the right hand. The patient's response to this end-range extension and compression is evaluated. **D.** The patient's left lower extremity is put into the FABER position (passive flexion, abduction, external rotation). As the examiner directs the femur toward the table, this stresses the left sacroiliac joint and produces a small rotary force to the lumbosacral junction. **E.** Passive knee flexion in prone is tested to assess the length of the rectus femoris. If this muscle is decreased in length, passive knee flexion can cause anterior torsional stress to the ilium that is transferred up to the lumbar spine as lumbosacral extension, which increases facet compression and shear stress. Anterior rotary movement of the pelvis before the knee reaches 90° of flexion is a positive sign. **F.** Prone passive femoral extension. The examiner lifts the femur beyond the point where the anterior thigh musculature and joint capsule become taut. This results in extension up through the remaining lumbar spine segments. **G.** Prone application of passive compressive and shear force to the pelvis and spine. The examiner pushes down with the top hand and up with the bottom hand until the two forces meet. A positive finding is reproduction of the familiar symptoms. **H.** Prone posterior-to-anterior rotary force imparted to the posterior superior iliac spine and right ilium. Intent is to determine is movement provokes familiar pain. **I.** Application of end-range stress to the lumbar spine in extension. The patient is asked to come up on his elbows. The examiner's index and middle fingers of one hand are placed on either side of the spinous process. The examiner's other hand is placed over the index and middle fingers to direct a force to the inferior articulating processes. (Reproduced with permission from Carl DeRosa, PT, PhD, FAPTA.)

place compressive and shear loads over the lumbar spine. Information gained from determining the nociceptive mechanics (*i.e.*, which positions and stresses reproduce the patient's symptoms) can then be utilized to prescribe the activity and exercise portions of the intervention.

Plan of Care and Interventions

This patient was carefully examined and the physical therapist determined that his LBP was of mechanical origin and that it was back pain with a nonradicular component. The patient's primary complaint is pain and his secondary complaints are related to loss of function (concern about recurrences, fear of not being able to continue his work, unable to perform normal activities of daily living without fear of pain exacerbation). Therefore, the history and physical exam suggest that the focus of intervention should be to relieve his pain rapidly and to provide strategies to maximize his physical health (especially his overall strength) to minimize the likelihood of recurrences. With the age-related breakdown of the specialized connective tissues of the spine (*e.g.*, intervertebral discs, apophyseal joints), the neuromuscular system becomes the primary means by which loads must be attenuated. Thus, attention to improving neuromuscular efficiency, especially of his trunk and hips must be an important aspect of care.

The patient met criteria for the clinical prediction rule for LBP and the regional lumbopelvic manipulation was used with success. This manipulation was performed by applying the intervention with the patient in the supine position because this followed the original clinical prediction rule, but success might also have been predicted utilizing a lumbar rotary type manipulation.[18] In order to document the manipulation of choice in a manner that is understandable and reproducible, the manipulation was documented in the manner suggested by Mintken et al.[21,22] Documentation in this manner allows the intervention to be clearly understood and potentially replicated, and avoids using biomechanical descriptions of manipulation techniques that have little scientific evidence. This model suggested a documentation standard for manipulation techniques utilizing the following six descriptors: rate of force application, location in range of available movement, direction of force, target of force, relative structural movement, and patient position. Thus, the technique applied to this patient was documented as a high velocity, end range, left rotational force to the left ilium on the lumbar spine in supine (Fig. 14-2).

After the patient's pain resolves to a satisfactory level with the manipulation intervention, the results of the physical examination can be utilized to develop a series of **stabilization exercises** intended to improve trunk motor control and strength. The initial exercise prescription incorporates the results of the physical examination by determining pain-free positions and movements. Initial training should focus on strengthening the abdominal muscles and low back extensors. Such exercises have the ability to improve perceived disability in both the short- and long-term in patients with recurrent LBP.[23] The patient should be instructed to report any peripheralization of pain during exercises or activities of daily living.

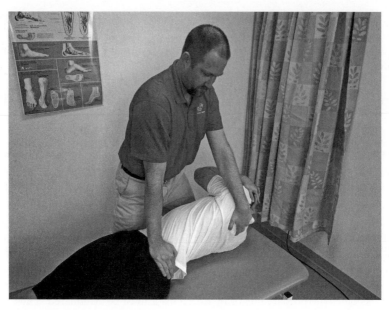

Figure 14-2. Manipulation technique: high velocity, end range, left rotational force to the left ilium on the lumbar spine in the supine position.

The physical therapist must emphasize to the patient that the goal is *centralization* of pain (*i.e.*, pain is felt in a more proximal location in response to repeated movements or sustained positions). The concept of centralizing pain should be utilized as a means to determine when to increase the frequency and intensity of his exercise program.[24] Carefully administered exercises emphasizing motor control are effective for nonspecific, nonradicular LBP. Motor control exercises for the spine are more than teaching a patient the "neutral" position of the spine. Instead, the physical therapist must incorporate the results of the physical examination to determine the motions and positions of the lumbar spine that have the least potential to exacerbate the pain pattern. With some patients, that may mean more of a flexion bias, and in others an extension bias. The results ascertained in the physical examination dictate the control of the spine necessary for pain-free activity. A systematic review of 14 randomized controlled trials concluded that motor control when used in isolation or in conjunction with additional interventions decreased LBP and disability.[25,26]

In addition to stabilization exercises, the patient should be prescribed **progressive endurance exercises and dynamic exercises** at a higher intensity. For this patient, the following exercises serve as excellent strengthening stimuli for the trunk and hip musculature: air squats (proper squat exercises without weight with close attention to form), squat thrusts (squats with an overhead press maneuver at the end), kettlebell swings emphasizing hip motion, dynamic plank exercises (plank position with alternating hip flexion), and standing pulley exercises emphasizing pulling motions, rowing motions, and hip rotary motions, being careful to avoid lumbar rotary motions. Lumbar rotation is especially important to monitor because it places excessive compressive loads to the lumbar apophyseal joints, and tensile stresses to the annulus fibrosus. Programs including the exercises above have also been shown to have a positive effect on patients who have recurrent exacerbations of a chronic back problem.[27,28]

Evidence-Based Clinical Recommendations

SORT: Strength of Recommendation Taxonomy

A: Consistent, good-quality patient-oriented evidence

B: Inconsistent or limited-quality patient-oriented evidence

C: Consensus, disease-oriented evidence, usual practice, expert opinion, or case series

1. To minimize back pain recurrences and the potential for a mechanical back pain problem to evolve into a chronic pain syndrome, the management strategy for patients presenting with an exacerbation of recurrent LBP should focus on rapid pain relief followed by progression toward strengthening exercises of the trunk and extremity musculature. **Grade A**

2. Lumbopelvic manipulation is effective for treating low back pain in individuals demonstrating specific history and physical exam criteria. **Grade A**

3. Spinal stabilization and progressive endurance exercises for the trunk and hip musculature are effective interventions to manage acute, subacute, or recurrent low back pain. **Grade B**

COMPREHENSION QUESTIONS

14.1 Which of the following pain characteristics is *least* likely to be caused by nerve root irritation?

    A. Leg pain greater than back pain

    B. Pain in the lower extremity that is clearly demarcated as opposed to general aching

    C. Back pain that is made worse with lifting

    D. Pain below the knee

14.2 Manipulation can be considered an intervention of choice for a patient presenting with low back pain when:

    A. Pain is below the knee and made worse with spinal extension.

    B. Onset of symptoms is within a 2-week time period and generalized hypomobility can be determined with posterior to anterior spring testing of lumbar spine.

    C. More muscle spasm and guarding is detected on one side compared to the opposite side.

    D. Slump test and straight leg raise test are positive.

ANSWERS

14.1 **C.** Increased intradiscal pressure, which occurs during lifting when the spine is flexed, is associated with disc pathology. Leg pain greater than back pain (option A) and pain below the knee (option D) are typical indicators of nerve root pain. Pain in the lower extremity that is clearly demarcated suggests a specific referral pattern (*e.g.*, dermatomal pattern) that could be due to irritation of a nerve root (option B).

14.2 **B.** Options A and C have no evidence-based correlation with the utilization of spinal manipulation. Positive Slump test and straight leg raise tests (option D) are more indicative of nerve root pathology, which can be a contraindication for manipulation.

REFERENCES

1. Picavet HS, Schouten JS. Musculoskeletal pain in the Netherlands: prevalences, consequences and risk groups, the DMC(3)-study. *Pain.* 2003;102:167-178.

2. Goetzel RZ, Hawkins K, Ozminkowski RJ, Wang S. The health and productivity cost burden of the "top 10" physical and mental health conditions affecting six large U.S. employers in 1999. *J Occup Environ Med.* 2003;45:5-14.

3. Papageorgiou AC, Macfarlane GJ, Thomas E, Croft PR, Jayson MI, Silman AJ. Psychosocial factors in the workplace—do they predict new episodes of low back pain? Evidence from the South Manchester Back Pain Study. *Spine.* 1997;22:1137-1142.

4. Lee P, Helewa A, Goldsmith CH, Smythe HA, Stitt LW. Low back pain: prevalence and risk factors in an industrial setting. *J Rheumatol.* 2001;28:346-351.

5. Katz JN. Lumbar disc disorders and low-back pain: socioeconomic factors and consequences. *J Bone Joint Surg Am.* 2006;88 Suppl 2:21-24.

6. Leveille SG. Musculoskeletal aging. *Curr Opin Rheumatol.* 2004;16:114-118.

7. Dunlop RB, Adams MA, Hutton WC. Disc space narrowing and facet joints. *J Bone Joint Surg Br.* 1984;66:706-710.

8. Wiesel SW, Tsourmas N, Feffer HL, Citrin CM, Patronas N. A study of computer-assisted tomography. I. The incidence of positive CAT scans in an asymptomatic group of patients. *Spine.* 1984;9: 549-551.

9. Boden SD, Davis DO, Din TS, Patronas NJ, Wiesel SW. Abnormal magnetic-resonance scans of the lumbar spine in asymptomatic subjects. A prospective investigation. *J Bone Joint Surg Am.*1990;72:403-408.

10. Savage RA, Whitehouse GH, Roberts N. The relationship between the magnetic resonance imaging appearance of the lumbar spine and low back pain, age, and occupation in males. *Eur Spine J.* 1997;6:106-114.

11. Airaksinen O, Brox JI, Cedraschi C, et al. COST B13 Working Group on Guidelines for Chronic Low Back Pain. Chapter 4. European guidelines for the management of chronic nonspecific low back pain. *Eur Spine J.* 2006;15 Suppl 2:S192-300.

12. Chou R, Qaseem A, Snow V, et al. Clinical Efficacy Assessment Subcommittee of the American College of Physicians; American Pain Society Low Back Pain Guidelines Panel. Diagnosis and treatment of low back pain: a joint clinical practice guideline from the American College of Physicians and the American Pain Society. *Ann Intern Med.* 2007;147:478-491.

13. Savigny P, Watson P, Underwood M. Guideline Development Group. Early management of persistent non-specific low back pain: summary of NICE guidance. *BMJ.* 2009;338:b1805.

14. Rainville J, Hartigan C, Martinez E, Limke J, Jouve C, Finno M. Exercise as a treatment for chronic low back pain. *Spine J*. 2004;4:106-115.

15. Flynn T, Fritz J, Whitman J, et al. A clinical prediction rule for classifying patients with low back pain who demonstrate short-term improvement with spinal manipulation. *Spine*. 2002;27: 2835-2843.

16. Childs JD, Fritz JM, Flynn TW, et al. A clinical prediction rule to identify patients with low back pain most likely to benefit from spinal manipulation: a validation study. *Ann Int Med*. 2004;141: 920-928.

17. Fritz JM, Childs JD, Flynn TW. Pragmatic application of a clinical prediction rule in primary care to identify patients with low back pain with a good prognosis following a brief spinal manipulation intervention. *BMC Fam Prac*. 2005;6:29.

18. Cleland JA, Fritz JM, Kulig K, et al. Comparison of the effectiveness of three manual therapy techniques in a subgroup of patients with low back pain who satisfy a clinical prediction rule: a randomized clinical trial. *Spine*. 2009;34:2720-2729.

19. Fritz JM, Whitman JM, Childs JD. Lumbar spine segmental mobility assessment: an examination of validity for determining intervention strategies in patients with low back pain. *Arch Phys Med Rehabil*. 2005;86:1745-1752.

20. Ellison JB, Rose SJ, Sahrmann SA. Patterns of hip rotation range of motion: a comparison between healthy subjects and patients with low back pain. *Phys Ther*.1990;70:537-541.

21. Mintken PE, DeRosa C, Little T, Smith B; American Academy of Orthopaedic Manual Physical Therapists. AAOMPT clinical guidelines: a model for standardizing manipulation terminology in physical therapy practice. *J Orthop Sports Phys Ther*. 2008;38:A1-6.

22. Mintken PE, DeRosa C, Little T, Smith B. A model for standardizing manipulation terminology in physical therapy practice. *J Man Manip Ther*. 2008;16:50-56.

23. Rasmussen-Barr E, Ang B, Arvidsson I, Nilsson-Wikmar L. Graded exercise for recurrent low-back pain: a randomized controlled trial with 6-, 12-, and 36-month follow-ups. *Spine*. 2009;34:221-228.

24. Kilpikoski S, Airaksinen O, Kankaanpaa M, Leminen P, Videman T, Alen M. Interexaminer reliability of low back pain assessment using the McKenzie method. *Spine*. 2002;27:E207-214.

25. Macedo LG, Maher CG, Latimer J, McAuley JH. Motor control exercise for persistent, nonspecific low back pain: a systematic review. *Phys Ther*. 2009;89:9-25.

26. Macedo LG, Smeets RJ, Maher CG, Latimer J, McAuley JH. Graded activity and graded exposure for persistent nonspecific low back pain: a systematic review. *Phys Ther*. 2010;90:860-879.

27. Rainville J, Jouve CA, Hartigan C, Martinez E, Hipona M. Comparison of short- and long-term outcomes for aggressive spine rehabilitation delivered two versus three times per week. *Spine J*. 2002;2:402-407.

28. Smith C, Grimmer-Sommers K. The treatment effect of exercise programmes for chronic low back pain. *J Eval Clin Practice*. 2010;16:484-491.

Lumbar Spine: Herniated Disc—*Muscle Energy Technique (MET) Approach*

Jason Brumitt
Melissa Murray
Jandra Mueller

CASE 15

A 36-year-old male construction worker self-referred to an outpatient physical therapy clinic with a complaint of low back pain and pain radiating from his posterior left hip all the way to his lateral foot. He first experienced pain 3 weeks ago while doing a home maintenance project. The onset of pain occurred when he attempted to lift an air conditioning unit. He reports that as he bent over to lift the unit, he experienced an intense, stabbing pain and immediately fell to the ground. He required assistance from his wife to walk back into the house. For the first 24 hours after the incident, he rested prone on a couch or on his bed. Over the past 3 days, he reports an improved tolerance to walking and standing for short periods. However, he rates his current pain level 5 out of 10 on the visual analog scale and he continues to experience radiating pain distal to his knee. Signs and symptoms are consistent with a lumbar herniated disc. His goal is to return to work as soon as possible.

▶ Based on the patient's suspected diagnosis, what do you anticipate may be the contributing factors to his condition?
▶ What examination signs may be associated with this diagnosis?
▶ What are the most appropriate physical therapy interventions?
▶ What are possible complications that may limit the effectiveness of physical therapy?

KEY DEFINITIONS

MUSCLE ENERGY TECHNIQUE (MET): Manual therapy technique in which a muscular contraction (*i.e.*, "muscle energy") by the patient is matched by a physical therapist's unyielding force applied in the opposing direction

PASSIVE INTERVERTEBRAL MOTION (PIVM) ASSESSMENT: Manual technique used to assess passive physiologic segmental motion between vertebrae

Objectives

1. Understand the anatomy, biomechanics, and function of the lumbar intervertebral discs.
2. Describe signs and symptoms associated with a herniated lumbar disc and identify potential risk factors associated with this diagnosis.
3. Describe muscle energy technique and its proposed clinical indications.
4. Describe the evidence for the efficacy of using muscle energy technique as an intervention for treating an individual with a herniated nucleus pulposus (HNP) in the lumbar spine.

Physical Therapy Considerations

PT considerations during management of the individual with a diagnosis of a herniated lumbar disc:

▶ **General physical therapy plan of care/goals:** Decrease pain; increase muscular flexibility; increase lower quadrant strength; increase muscular endurance of the core; prevent or minimize loss of aerobic fitness capacity

▶ **Physical therapy interventions:** Patient education regarding functional anatomy and injury pathomechanics; muscle energy technique; modalities and manual therapy to decrease pain; muscular flexibility exercises; resistance exercises to increase muscular endurance capacity of the core and to increase strength of lower extremity muscles; aerobic exercise program

▶ **Precautions during physical therapy:** Monitor vital signs; address precautions or contraindications for exercise, based on patient's pre-existing condition(s)

▶ **Complications interfering with physical therapy:** Occupational duties that require the patient to assume a flexed lumbar spine

Understanding the Health Condition

The functional anatomy of the lumbar spine consists of five lumbar vertebrae, the intervertebral joints, the intervertebral discs, and the regional ligaments and muscles. Each intervertebral (IV) disc (Fig. 15-1) is positioned between two adjacent

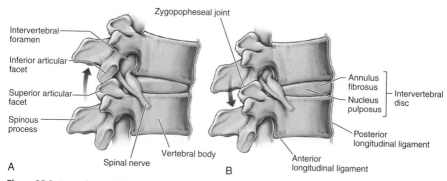

Figure 15-1. Lateral view of lumbar vertebrae and intervertebral disc. A. Spinal flexion. B. Spinal extension (Reproduced with permission from Morton DA, Foreman KB, Albertine KH, eds. *The Big Picture: Gross Anatomy.* New York: McGraw-Hill; 2011. Figure 1-4.)

vertebrae and consists of the annulus fibrosus, the nucleus pulposus, and the cartilaginous endplates (also known as vertebral endplates). The cartilaginous endplates (fibrocartilage and hyaline cartilage) are positioned on both the superior and inferior portions of the disc. Intervertebral discs lack a blood supply, and the inner two-thirds of the annulus lacks innervation as well.[1-3] The outer portion of the IV disc is the annulus fibrosus that consists of collagen fibers arranged in concentric layers oriented at a 65° angle from the vertical.[1] These collagen fibers are angled in opposite directions in each layer (lamella). The inner portion of the IV disc is the nucleus pulposus—a jelly-like structure comprised water, proteoglycans, and collagen.[1,2] In young individuals, upward of 90% of the nucleus pulposus consists of water.[2] The proteoglycans help to attract a significant amount of water.[3] As individuals age, the IV discs lose water, elastin, and proteoglycans, and gain collagen.[2]

The intervertebral disc serves several functions.[1-3] The annulus fibrosus resists and transmits forces through the spine.[2,3] The orientation of the fibers in the annulus helps to resist torsional loads.[2,3] The nucleus pulposus acts like a shock absorber that transmits loads throughout the disc in response to compressive forces.[2,3] The disc also contributes to segmental flexibility in the spine.[1-3]

Herniation of the nucleus pulposus may occur in the presence of disc degeneration and exposure to repeated pathomechanical loading. In the spine of a healthy, younger individual, a compressive load (either external or internal) deforms the nucleus pulposus and increases intradiscal pressure. The increased intradiscal pressure in response to the load is distributed radially to the annulus fibrosus or to the adjacent endplates.[3,4] Degeneration of the IV discs—due to loss of water in the nucleus pulposus and/or degeneration or tears of the annular fibers—changes the ability of the discs to accept loads and forces in various postures.

Flexion of the lumbar spine creates a compressive load through the anterior portion of the lumbar discs (Fig. 15-1A). This compressive load can cause the nucleus pulposus to migrate posteriorly and increased tensile forces are imparted onto the posterior portion of the disc. The posterior aspect of the annulus fibrosus is the portion of the IV disc at highest risk for damage. Anatomically, this region is thinner relative to the centrally located lamellae. Pathomechanically, spinal flexion and/or

Table 15-1	CLASSIFICATIONS OF HERNIATED NUCLEUS PULPOSUS
Name	Description
Protruded	Nucleus pulposus material migrates into area of damaged annular fibers. There is a bulging of the disc, but peripheral annular fibers are intact.
Extruded	Nucleus pulposus material migrates through peripheral annular fibers.
Sequestered	Herniated nucleus pulposus material disconnects from the disc.

flexion with rotation generates increased tensile loads that may contribute to annular tears. The degree of migration of the nucleus pulposus depends on the extent of damaged annular fibers. Table 15-1 lists classifications for herniated nucleus pulposus (HNP) based on degree of injury to the disc.

Physical Therapy Patient/Client Management

Multiple conservative interventions are used to treat individuals with a herniated nucleus pulposus.[5-8] Common interventions include manual therapy, mechanical traction, exercise, and modalities.[5-13] Muscle energy technique (MET) is a manual therapy technique most commonly utilized by physical therapists, osteopathic physicians, and other rehabilitation professionals.[14,15] It has been suggested that MET may increase the length of a shortened muscle, improve joint mobility, and increase muscular strength.[16] If a vertebral motion restriction or an area of muscular inflexibility in the thoracic or lumbar spine is identified during the physical therapy examination, the physical therapist may decide that MET is indicated. To use this technique, the physical therapist applies a manual force directed toward "correcting" the vertebral segment dysfunction or lengthening the shortened muscle. The patient counters the therapist's applied force with an equal force in the opposite direction. This MET technique is performed as needed to address vertebral movement dysfunction. In addition to MET, a physical therapist may utilize modalities, perform additional manual therapy techniques (joint mobilizations), and/or prescribe therapeutic exercise. The purpose of this case is to describe the use of MET for a patient with a suspected HNP.

Examination, Evaluation, and Diagnosis

A physical therapy examination for the patient with a suspected (or confirmed) HNP consists of postural and gait observation, active and passive range of motion (ROM) testing, muscle flexibility testing, neurologic screening (lumbar dermatomes, myotomes, and reflexes), muscular strength and endurance tests, passive intervertebral motion testing, and a peripheral joint scan ("clearing" examination for adjacent joints).

A patient with a HNP may present with pain (centralized and/or peripheralized to a lower extremity), lower extremity paresthesias, decreased lumbar active range of motion, paraspinal muscle spasm, and spinal segmental hypomobility.[17] A patient that presents with muscular weakness in a myotomal distribution should be referred to a spine surgeon (either an orthopaedist or a neurosurgeon) for an examination.

Passive intervertebral motion (PIVM) testing has been advocated by physical therapists as a method to assess segmental motion.[18-21] When spinal segments with restricted physiologic motion are identified, manual therapy techniques can be directed toward hypomobile segments. Improving segmental motion may improve active range of motion in the lumbar spine and may help decrease symptoms.[19] However, the reliability of PIVM testing varies depending on the region assessed.[18-21] In particular, **PIVM testing in the lumbar spine** has low reliability.[20,21] Hicks et al.[20] reported the inter-rater reliability (of 4 raters) for identifying intersegmental mobility in the lumbar spine. Raters performed a posterior to anterior test (PA; a type of PIVM) to each subject's lumbar spinous processes. Each rater was asked to describe the motion at a segment as either hypermobile, normal, or hypomobile. The inter-rater reliability for assessing motion at each segment was poor. Reliability measures ranged from a kappa value of −0.02 (95% CI, −0.25-0.28) at L3 to 0.26 (95% CI, −0.01-0.53) at L1. The investigators also calculated the inter-rater reliability of segmental motion testing based on if a subject was deemed to have had at least one hypermobile segment or if a subject was deemed to have had at least one hypomobile segment. Even with the use of this broader classification scenario, inter-rater reliability was still poor. The reliability for identifying "any hypomobile" segment was poor (kappa = 0.18; 95% CI, 0.05-0.32) and the reliability of identifying "any hypermobile" segment was also poor (kappa = 0.30; 95% CI, 0.13-0.47). More recently, Landel et al.[21] assessed the validity and inter-rater reliability of segmental motion testing at the lumbar spine. One physical therapist (reported as having 15 years of manual therapy experience) performed central PA tests in the lumbar spine on a subject *while* magnetic resonance imaging (MRI) scans (in an open MRI machine) were collected. The physical therapist noted the lumbar segments that were the "most mobile" and "least mobile." From the MRI scan, the intervertebral angle delineated by adjacent vertebral endplates was measured and the difference in intervertebral angles was used to identify and quantify segmental lumbar motion.[21,22] A second physical therapist (reported as having 16 years of manual therapy experience) performed central PA tests to the lumbar spine *outside* of the MRI machine and was also asked to report what he determined to be the most and least mobile segments. The two physical therapists were in close agreement on "the least mobile segment" (kappa = 0.71; 95% CI, 0.48-0.94). However, they were not in agreement on the "most mobile segment" (kappa = 0.29; 95% CI, −0.13-0.71).[21] With respect to the validity of the PA assessments, the correlation between segmental mobility as measured by anatomic movements during MRI scans and the therapists' PA assessments was poor.[21] For the least mobile segment, kappa = 0.04 (95% CI = −0.16-0.24) and for the most mobile segment, kappa = 0.00 (95% CI, −0.09-0.08).[21] Based on these findings, Landel et al.[21] suggested that a PA test may not be a valid test for assessing joint mobility. Despite poor to low inter-rater reliability and poor validity compared to an objective anatomical measurement of intervertebral movement, many physical therapists utilize PIVMs to identify dysfunctional joint mobility and to guide manual therapy interventions.

As an alternative or adjunct to the sole reliance on PIVMs to identify joint dysfunction, the physical therapist can assess a patient's overall flexibility to determine whether and how MET would be an appropriate intervention. Individuals with a suspected HNP may present with postural deviations and muscular inflexibility. When viewed from the rear, a lateral shift (appearing as if the patient is leaning to one side) associated with protective muscular spasms may be evident. These muscle spasms and/or lower extremity muscular inflexibility frequently limit lumbopelvic region active ROM. During the initial examination, the physical therapist should assess the patient's active lumbar spinal ROM in the standing position. With the patient in the prone and supine positions, the physical therapist should assess passive ROM of the lumbar spine, active and passive ROM of the hips and perform muscle length testing (flexibility) of the lumbar spine and the hips in prone and supine. When the patient presents with a lateral shift, muscular spasms and/or muscular inflexibility are frequently observed in the lumbar paraspinals (on the side that the patient leans toward). In lieu of a lateral shift, the patient may present with bilateral muscular spasms in the lumbar spine. Other muscles that may present with spasms or pre-existing muscular inflexibility (either ipsilaterally or bilaterally) include piriformis, iliopsoas, and hamstrings.

Plan of Care and Interventions

Several studies have reported improvements in ROM, pain, and/or disability outcome measures when using MET in asymptomatic and symptomatic populations (Table 15-2).[23-30] There is a lack of consistency on how long to perform each MET technique (range 5-10 seconds) and how many repetitions to perform per treatment session.[23-30]

Schenk et al.[23] reported that MET significantly increased cervical rotation active ROM in asymptomatic subjects with assessed motion restriction compared to a control group. Smith et al.[28] assessed the effect of MET on hamstring flexibility in 40 asymptomatic subjects. Subjects were randomized into two groups. The first group received a 30-second hamstring stretch after each MET isometric hamstring contraction against resistance (7- to 10-second holds at 40% maximum voluntary isometric contraction). The second group received a 3-second hamstring stretch after the MET (same MET procedure as was provided to first group). Both groups experienced significant improvements in hamstring flexibility; however, there was no difference between groups. Additional studies have reported significant increases in lumbar extension,[24] thoracic rotation,[25] mouth opening,[27] hamstring flexibility,[29,31] and cervical range of motion.[32]

The majority of investigations have assessed the effect of MET on asymptomatic individuals—few studies have assessed the **effect of MET on patients with pathology**. The studies that have assessed the effect of MET on patients with symptomatic pathology have shown positive results; however, flaws in methodological design limit the ability to extrapolate these results to larger patient populations. Additional investigations are warranted.

Wilson et al.[26] performed the first investigation to assess the effect of MET on patients with acute low back pain. Patients were treated twice per week for 4 weeks by a physical therapist. On the first day, the experimental group received 20 minutes moist heat to the low back followed by a MET procedure. Subjects in this group also received a home exercise program (HEP) with a MET-specific component. The control group received moist heat prior to receiving placebo manual therapy and were

Table 15-2   SUMMARY OF SELECTED STUDIES ASSESSING THE EFFECT OF MUSCLE ENERGY TECHNIQUE (MET)

Author (Year)	Subjects	Intervention(s)	Outcome(s)
Schenk et al. (1994)[23]	18 asymptomatic adults (9 females) with restricted cervical active ROM Randomized to 2 groups: MET group (mean age = 24 y) or control group (mean age = 27 y)	1. MET group: Procedure to address cervical restriction: a. 5-s isometric holds (resisting rotation direction) b. 3 repetitions c. 8 sessions × 4 wk	Significant improvement in active cervical rotation ROM ($p = 0.04$, respectively)
		2. Control group: No intervention	No change in cervical motion
Schenk et al. (1997)[24]	26 asymptomatic adults (13 females) with restricted lumbar active ROM Randomized to 2 groups: MET group and control group (mean age both groups = 25 y)	1. MET group: Procedure to address lumbar extension restriction at L5/S1 segment: a. 5-s isometric holds (resisting rotation direction) b. 4 repetitions c. 8 sessions × 4 wk	Significant improvement in lumbar extension range of motion ($p = 0.000$); change score = 6.9°
		2. Control group: No intervention	No change in lumbar motion
Lenehan et al. (2003)[25]	59 asymptomatic adults (37 females; mean age = 24 y) with restricted thoracic rotation active ROM Randomized to 2 groups: MET group and control group	1. MET group: Procedure to increase thoracic rotation (to one side): a. 5-s isometric holds b. 4 repetitions	Significant increase in thoracic rotation active ROM on the treated (restricted) side ($p < 0.005$)
		2. Control group: No intervention	No change in thoracic motion
Wilson et al. (2003)[26]	16 adults with acute low back pain (8 females) Randomized to 2 groups: MET group (mean age = 31 ± 9 y) and control group (mean age = 32 ± 9 y)	1. MET group: MET procedure to address flexion and side-bending restriction and neuromuscular re-education exercises. 8 sessions × 4 wk 2. Control group: Placebo manual therapy and neuromuscular re-education exercises 8 sessions × 4 wk	Significantly greater improvement in Oswestry Disability Index scores for MET group compared to control group at 4 wk ($p < 0.05$)

(Continued)

Table 15-2 SUMMARY OF SELECTED STUDIES ASSESSING THE EFFECT OF MUSCLE ENERGY TECHNIQUE (MET) (CONTINUED)

Author (Year)	Subjects	Intervention(s)	Outcome(s)

Blanco et al. (2006)[27]	90 adults (48 females; mean age 25 ± 4.3 y) with latent MTrPs in masseter muscle Randomized to 3 groups: MET group, strain-counterstrain (SCS) group, or control group	1. MET group procedure:
		  a. Open mouth to resistance followed by performing 6-s masseter contraction (close mouth against resistance at 25% "available strength")
		  b. 5-s rest period
		  c. Mouth opened (further) to resistance
		  d. 3 sets performed
		2. SCS group: technique applied to masseter MTrPs with treatment position held for 90 s
		3. Control group: No intervention
			Significant increase in active mouth opening post-MET ($p < 0.001$) Large effect size for MET treatment (1.46) MET group: Significantly better for increasing mouth opening than SCS and control groups ($p < 0.001$)

Smith et al. (2008)[28]	40 adults; mean age 22.1 ± 3.5 y with 75° of hamstring flexibility[a] Randomized to 2 groups: MET group (30-s stretch) or MET group (3-s stretch)	1. MET group #1 (2 sessions, 2 wk):
		  a. Isometric hamstring contraction against resistance, 7-10 s, 40% MVIC
		  b. Rest for 2-3 s
		  c. 30-s hamstring stretch followed by a 10-s rest with leg on table
		  d. 3 repetitions performed
		2. MET group #2 (2 sessions, 2 wk):
		  a and b. Same as other group
		  c. 3-s hamstring stretch
		  d. Passively flex hip to available (new) range
		  e. 4 repetitions performed
			Significant improvements in hamstring flexibility within session and between sessions for each group ($p < 0.01$) No difference between groups

Shadmehr et al. (2009)[29]	30 females (range 20-25 y) lacking at least 30° of knee extension (patient supine with hip flexed to 90°)[a] Randomized to 2 groups: static stretch group or MET group	1. Static hamstring stretch[b] (3 sets × 10-s holds, 10 sessions)
		2. MET procedure[b]:
		  a. Isometric hamstring contraction against resistance for 10 s at 50% MVIC
		  b. 10-s rest period
		  c. Knee extended by therapist and held for 10 s
		  d. 3 sets × 10-s holds, 10 sessions
			Significant improvement in hamstring flexibility for both groups ($p < 0.01$) No difference between groups

Selkow et al. (2009)[30]	20 subjects (4 females) with reported lumbopelvic pain Randomized to 2 groups: MET group (mean age = 24.1 ± 7.1 y) and control group (mean age = 29.7 ± 11.9 y)	1. MET group:
		  a. MET with patient in Thomas test position, 5-s hold
		  b. 5-s rest between each MET rep
		  c. 1 treatment session
		2. Control group: Sham stretch
			Significant decrease in pain over 24-h period for the MET group ($p = 0.03$) Significant increase in pain for control group ($p = 0.03$)

[a]Hamstring flexibility test position: Pt positioned in supine, hip flexed to 90°, knee extended.
[b]Static stretch and MET positions are similar to flexibility test[a] position.
MTrPs, myofascial trigger points; MVIC, maximal voluntary isometric contraction.

prescribed the same HEP as the experimental group but without the MET-specific component. The subjects in the experimental group were re-assessed each session and treated with MET if the assessed motion restriction was still present. The MET HEP was reviewed with each subject and progressed. The control group continued to receive moist heat each session, placebo manual therapy on randomly selected treatment sessions, and progression of the HEP. After 4 weeks, the MET treatment group experienced a significantly greater improvement in change scores for the Oswestry Disability Index (ODI) compared to the control group. A treatment effect size of 2.39 was calculated from the percent change in the ODI scores from pre- to post-intervention, indicating a large effect of MET on improving disability.

Muscle energy technique may be an appropriate intervention option for a patient presenting with a HNP. Figures 15-2 to 15-5 demonstrate a MET that can be used for the assessment and treatment of a restriction in a lower lumbar segment, as originally described by Wilson et al.[26] For the patient in this case with muscular spasm of bilateral lumbar erector spinae, this inflexibility of the erector spinae restricts lumbar flexion ROM and may also restrict rotation and lateral flexion in the lumbar region. First, the physical therapist identifies a spinous process in the lumbar spine. The therapist passively extends the patient's lower extremities to the point where the restricted motion is perceived at the lumbar segment (Fig. 15-2) and then the therapist flexes the patient's torso to the level of the restricted spinal segment (Fig. 15-3). To improve flexibility of the erector spinae, the physical therapist positions the patient's lumbar spine into lateral flexion by elevating her lower extremities (Figs. 15-4 and 15-5). The patient is then instructed to lower her legs toward the tabletop against the matching resistance of the physical therapist, which requires the patient to contract

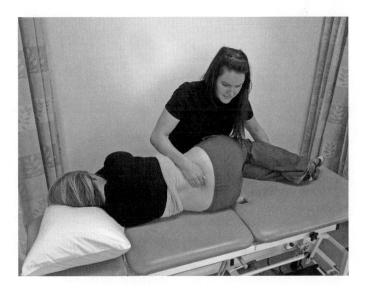

Figure 15-2. The physical therapist identifies a spinous process in the lumbar spine. The therapist passively extends the lower extremities to the point where motion is perceived at the lumbar segment (assume L5 for this example).

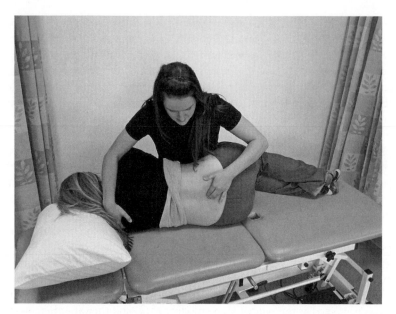

Figure 15-3. With her right upper extremity, the physical therapist flexes the patient's torso to the level of the L5 spinous process.

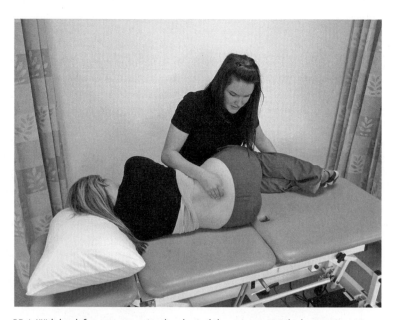

Figure 15-4. With her left upper extremity, the physical therapist moves the lower extremities toward her by flexing the hips until motion is perceived at the level of the L5 spinous process. With her right upper extremity, the therapist posteriorly rotates the patient's spine to the point that motion is perceived at L5.

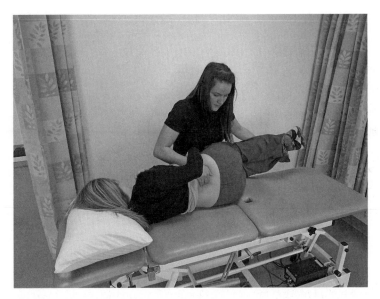

Figure 15-5. With her left upper extremity, the physical therapist creates a lateral flexion of the lumbar spine by elevating the patient's lower extremities. The patient is instructed to lower her legs toward the top of the table while the therapist resists this motion. Each repetition is held for 5 seconds. Wilson et al.[26] repeated the treatment 4 times.

the muscles of the lumbar spine on the side closest to the tabletop. Each repetition of the patient's contraction against resistance is held for 5 seconds.

A second study investigated short-term changes associated with MET after one treatment session. Selkow et al.[30] assessed the effect of one MET session on 20 adults with lumbopelvic pain during the prior 6 weeks who had not sought previous medical treatment. Those randomized to the MET treatment group were treated with 4 MET repetitions (5-second holds, 5-second rest between repetitions) with the subject in a modified Thomas test position. Patient positioning was based on findings associated with special tests for the sacroiliac (SI) joint. On the side deemed to have an anterior innominate rotation, that lower extremity was draped over the physical therapist's shoulder. The other leg rested on the edge of the table with the therapist's hand placed on the patient's thigh. The MET procedure consisted of the patient pushing one lower extremity into the therapist's shoulder and the other extremity into the hand. This technique was suggested to "correct" SI dysfunction. The authors did not describe which muscles were specifically targeted during this procedure, though it could be assumed that the MET was directed toward the hamstring group on the side presenting with the anterior innominate rotation and the iliopsoas group and/or the rectus femoris on the contralateral side.[30] Subjects randomized to the control group were treated with a sham manual therapy technique. Twenty-four hours after intervention, the MET group had a statistically significant mean decrease in worst pain (as measured on a visual analog scale) whereas the control group reported a significant mean increase in pain.

In addition to MET, other interventions (*e.g.*, therapeutic exercises, other forms of manual therapy, modalities) may be performed to decrease pain and improve function in the patient with a HNP. This case presented current evidence for use of a muscle energy technique to treat a patient with a lumbar HNP. In Cases 16, 17, and 18, the utilization of mechanical traction, the use of Mechanical Diagnosis and Therapy (MDT or McKenzie), and the use of an eclectic Norwegian manual therapy approach (Ola Grimsby) are presented.

Evidence-Based Clinical Recommendations

SORT: Strength of Recommendation Taxonomy
A: Consistent, good-quality patient-oriented evidence
B: Inconsistent or limited-quality patient-oriented evidence
C: Consensus, disease-oriented evidence, usual practice, expert opinion, or case series

1. Passive intervertebral motion (PIVM) testing of the lumbar spine has poor inter-rater reliability. **Grade B**

2. Passive intervertebral motion testing of the lumbar spine correlates poorly with intersegmental motion measured by magnetic resonance imaging. **Grade B**

3. Muscle energy technique decreases pain in patients with low back pain. **Grade B**

COMPREHENSION QUESTIONS

15.1 When applying a matching force to the patient's muscular contraction during a muscle energy technique, the physical therapist holds each repetition for how long?

A. 4 to 8 seconds

B. 5 to 10 seconds

C. 10 to 20 seconds

D. 20 to 30 seconds

15.2 How is a nucleus pulposus that has herniated through the peripheral annular fibers classified?

A. Protruded

B. Extruded

C. Sequestered

D. Intruded

ANSWERS

15.1 **B.** Five seconds is the most commonly reported hold time; however, some studies have assessed the effects of MET with 10-second holds.

15.2 **A.**

REFERENCES

1. Bogduk N. *Clinical Anatomy of the Lumbar Spine and Sacrum*. 4th ed. Edinburgh: Elseiver; 2005:11-28.

2. Moore KL, Dalley AF. *Clinically Oriented Anatomy*. 5th ed. Philadelphia, PA: Lippincott Williams & Wilkins; 2006.

3. Porterfield JA, DeRosa C. *Mechanical Low Back Pain. Perspectives in Functional Anatomy*. 2nd ed. Philadelphia, PA: WB Saunders; 1991:121-168.

4. McGill SM. *Low Back Disorders. Evidence-Based Prevention and Rehabilitation*. 2nd ed. Champaign, IL: Human Kinetics; 2007:44-47.

5. Hahne AJ, Ford JJ, McMeeken JM. Conservative management of lumbar disc herniation with associated radiculopathy: a systematic review. *Spine*. 2010;35:E488-504.

6. Chou R, Atlas SJ, Stanos SP, Rosenquist RW. Nonsurgical interventional therapies for low back pain: a review of the evidence for an American Pain Society clinical practice guideline. *Spine*. 2009;34:1078-1093.

7. Weinstein JN, Lurie JD, Tosteson TD, et al. Surgical versus nonoperative treatment for lumbar disc herniation: four-year results for the Spine Patient Outcomes Research Trial (SPORT). *Spine*. 2008;33:2789-2800.

8. Oliphant D. Safety of spinal manipulation in the treatment of lumbar disk herniations: a systematic review and risk assessment. *J Manipulative Physiol Ther*. 2004;27:197-210.

9. Donelson R, Aprill C, Medcalf R, Grant W. A prospective study of centralization of lumbar and referred pain. A predictor of symptomatic discs and anular competence. *Spine*. 1997;22:1115-1122.

10. Gillan MG, Ross JC, McLean IP, Porter RW. The natural history of trunk list, its associated disability and the influence of McKenzie management. *Eur Spine J*. 1998;7:480-483.

11. Bronfort G, Haas M, Evans RL, Bouter LM. Efficacy of spinal manipulation and mobilization for low back pain and neck pain: a systematic review and best evidence synthesis. *Spine J*. 2004;4:335-356.

12. Takasaki H, May S, Fazey PJ, Hall T. Nucleus pulposus deformation following application of mechanical diagnosis and therapy: a single case report with magnetic resonance imaging. *J Man Manip Ther*. 2010;18:153-158.

13. Gagne AR, Hasson SM. Lumbar extension exercises in conjunction with mechanical traction for the management of a patient with a lumbar herniated disc. *Physiother Theory Pract*. 2010;26:256-266.

14. Fryer G. Muscle energy technique: an evidence-informed approach. *Int J Osteopath Med*. 2011;14:3-9.

15. Fryer G, Ruszkowski W. The influence of contraction duration in muscle energy technique applied to the atlanto-axial joint. *J Osteopath Med*. 2004;7:79-84.

16. Greenman P. *Principles of Manual Therapy*. 2nd ed. Baltimore, MD: Williams & Wilkins; 1996.

17. Strayer A. Lumbar spine: common pathology and interventions. *J Neurosci Nurs*. 2005;37:181-193.

18. Brismee JM, Gipson D, Ivie D, et al. Interrater reliability of a passive physiological intervertebral motion test in the mid-thoracic spine. *J Manipulative Physiol Ther*. 2006;29:368-373.

19. Piva SR, Erhard RE, Childs JD, Browder DA. Inter-tester reliability of passive intervertebral and active movements of the cervical spine. *Man Ther*. 2006;11:321-330.

20. Hicks GE, Fritz JM, Delitto A, Mishock J. Interrater reliability of clinical examination measures for identification of lumbar segmental instability. *Arch Phys Med Rehabil*. 2003;84:1858-1864.

21. Landel R, Kulig K, Fredericson M, Li B, Powers CM. Intertester reliability and validity of motion assessments during lumbar spine accessory motion testing. *Phys Ther*. 2008;88:43-49.

22. Powers CM, Kulig K, Harrison J, Bergman G. Segmental mobility of the lumbar spine during a posterior to anterior mobilization: assessment using dynamic MRI. *Clin Biomech*. 2003;18:80-83.

23. Schenk R, Adelman K, Rousselle J. The effects of muscle energy technique on cervical range of motion. *J Man Manip Ther*. 2004;2:149-155.

24. Schenk RJ, MacDiarmid A, Rousselle J. The effects of muscle energy technique on lumbar range of motion. *J Man Manip Ther*. 1997;5:179-183.

25. Lenehan KL, Fryer G, McLaughlin P. The effect of muscle energy technique on gross trunk range of motion. *J Osteopath Med.* 2003;6:13-18.

26. Wilson E, Payton O, Donegan-Shoaf L, Dec K. Muscle energy technique in patients with acute low back pain: a pilot clinical trial. *J Orthop Sports Phys Ther.* 2003;33:502-512.

27. Rodriguez Blanco C, Fernandez de la Penas C, Hernandez Xumet JE, Pena Algaba C, Fernandez Rabadan M, Lillo de al Quintana MC. Changes in active mouth opening following a single treatment of latent myofascial trigger points in the masseter muscle involving post-isometric relaxation or strain/counterstrain. *J Bodyw Mov Ther.* 2006;10:197-205.

28. Smith M, Fryer G. A comparison of two muscle energy techniques for increasing flexibility of the hamstring muscle group. *J Bodyw Mov Ther.* 2008;12:312-317.

29. Shadmehr A, Hadian MR, Naiemi SS, Jalaie S. Hamstring flexibility in young women following passive stretch and muscle energy technique. *J Back Musculoskeletal Rehabil.* 2009;143-148.

30. Selkow NM, Grindstaff TL, Cross KM, Pugh K, Hertel J, Saliba S. Short-term effect of muscle energy technique on pain in individuals with non-specific lumbopelvic pain: a pilot study. *J Man Manip Ther.* 2009;17:E14-18.

31. Ballantyne F, Fryer G, McLaughlin P. The effect of muscle energy technique on hamstring extensibility: the mechanism of altered flexibility. *J Osteopath Med.* 2003;6:59-63.

32. Burns DK, Wells MR. Gross range of motion in the cervical spine: the effects of osteopathic muscle energy technique in asymptomatic subjects. *J Am Osteopath Assoc.* 2006;106:137-142.

Lumbar Spine: Herniated Disc—*Traction Approach*

Jason Brumitt

A 36-year-old male construction worker self-referred to an outpatient physical therapy clinic with a complaint of low back pain and pain radiating from his posterior left hip all the way to his lateral foot. He first experienced pain 3 weeks ago while doing a home maintenance project. The onset of pain occurred when he attempted to lift an air conditioning unit. He reports that as he bent over to lift the unit, he experienced an intense, stabbing pain and immediately fell to the ground. He required assistance from his wife to walk back into the house. For the first 24 hours after the incident, he rested prone on a couch or on his bed. Over the past 3 days, he reports an improved tolerance to walking and standing for short periods. However, he rates his current pain level 5 out of 10 on the visual analog scale and he continues to experience radiating pain distal to his knee. Signs and symptoms are consistent with a lumbar herniated disc. His goal is to return to work as soon as possible.

▶ Based on the patient's suspected diagnosis, what do you anticipate may be the contributing factors to his condition?
▶ What examination signs may be associated with this diagnosis?
▶ What are the most appropriate physical therapy interventions?
▶ What are possible complications that may limit the effectiveness of physical therapy?

KEY DEFINITIONS

CLINICAL PREDICTION RULE (CPR) FOR TREATMENT: Tool that has been developed from research that may help a clinician select the most effective treatment(s) based on findings from the patient's history and clinical examination

CROSSED STRAIGHT LEG RAISE: Clinical special test performed to rule in the presence of a herniated nucleus pulposus; a positive test is associated with a reproduction of a patient's symptoms when the "asymptomatic" leg (leg not experiencing radiculopathy) is passively raised[1]

LUMBOSACRAL RADICULOPATHY: Collection of signs and symptoms (*e.g.*, radiating pain, numbness, and/or weakness in the buttock or lower extremity) associated with injury to a nerve root in the lumbosacral spine

Objectives

1. Understand the anatomy, biomechanics, and function of the lumbar intervertebral discs.

2. Describe signs and symptoms associated with a herniated lumbar disc and identify potential risk factors associated with this diagnosis.

3. Describe mechanical traction and its proposed clinical indications.

4. Describe the preliminary clinical prediction rule for patients with a herniated nucleus pulposus that may benefit from treatment with mechanical traction.

Physical Therapy Considerations

PT considerations during management of the individual with a diagnosis of a herniated lumbar disc:

▶ **General physical therapy plan of care/goals:** Decrease pain; increase muscular flexibility; increase lower quadrant strength; increase muscular endurance of the core; prevent or minimize loss of aerobic fitness capacity

▶ **Physical therapy interventions:** Patient education regarding functional anatomy and injury pathomechanics; traction, modalities, and manual therapy to decrease pain; muscular flexibility exercises; resistance exercises to increase muscular endurance capacity of the core and to increase strength of lower extremity muscles; aerobic exercise program

▶ **Precautions during physical therapy:** Monitor vital signs; address precautions or contraindications for exercise, based on patient's pre-existing condition(s)

▶ **Complications interfering with physical therapy:** Occupational duties that require the patient to assume a flexed lumbar spine, contraindications associated with mechanical traction: joint instability or fracture; pregnancy, tumor, hiatal hernia, osteoporosis, acute pain, claustrophobia

Physical Therapy Patient/Client Management

Multiple conservative interventions are utilized by clinicians when treating patients with a herniated nucleus pulposus (HNP).[2-5] Common interventions include traction, exercise, manual therapy, and modalities.[2-10] The use of traction has been reported to be indicated for patients with an HNP, nerve root compression (due to foraminal stenosis, osteophyte, or HNP), joint hypomobility, or muscular spasm or tightness.[11-13] Mechanical, auto, and manual traction techniques have been developed.[14] The purpose of this case is to describe the use of mechanical traction for a patient with a suspected HNP.

Traction, a physical modality dating back to Hippocrates, has been used by physical therapists to treat dysfunction in the spine.[14] Multiple mechanisms have been proposed to explain the clinical benefits associated with mechanical traction for a patient with an HNP.[13,15] First, when the traction force is applied, a decrease in intradiscal pressure occurs that may help to reduce (via suction) herniated portions of the disc.[15] Second, tensing the posterior longitudinal ligament may provide a force against the herniation.[15] Third, traction may help decrease muscular tightness and/or help relax muscle spasms.[13,15]

Despite its widespread use, the efficacy of mechanical traction for dysfunction of the spine has been questioned in the literature. Several systematic reviews have concluded that use of **mechanical traction for patients with low back pain (LBP) secondary to an HNP** is either not supported or cannot be recommended as a treatment intervention due to a lack of high quality studies.[16-19] However, Clarke et al.[19] concluded that additional studies are still necessary to determine its efficacy for patients with LBP with or without sciatica.

A critical limitation associated with determining the efficacy of any treatment for LBP is that many studies use heterogeneous samples with respect to the *etiology* of the low back pain. It may be impossible to demonstrate significant improvement in a heterogeneous LBP population, especially if certain etiologies of back pain were unaffected (or negatively affected) by traction. A recent trend in the literature is to identify subjects who have experienced significant improvement in outcome measures and then analyze that population for similar clinical features. In other words, the secondary analysis aims to determine which etiologies of LBP were positively or negatively affected by the investigated intervention.

Fritz et al.[20] reported a **subgroup of patients** who experienced clinical improvements when treated with mechanical traction. Patients in this study were randomized into two groups. One group was prescribed extension-based exercises, treated with joint mobilizations, and educated regarding their condition. A second group received the same aforementioned treatment program plus the use of mechanical traction. The authors found that subjects who experienced peripheralization of symptoms in response to a spinal extension movement during the initial evaluation had a significantly greater mean reduction in disability (measured on the Oswestry Disability Index) after treatment with mechanical traction compared to those who did not. They also found that subjects who were treated with traction had significantly greater average improvements on the crossed straight leg raise (SLR) test. Based on their findings, Fritz et al.[11,20]

suggested that subjects "with leg symptoms (distal to buttocks), signs of nerve root compression, and either peripheralization with extension movements or a crossed straight leg raise" might be a subgroup of patients that would benefit from mechanical traction. Cai et al.[21] reported a CPR outlining discrete variables for patients with LBP who may experience improvement with the use of mechanical traction. Subjects with a diagnosis of LBP with pain and/or numbness in the low back, buttock, or lower extremity were treated with three sessions of mechanical traction (supine or prone position, traction force 30%-40% of one's body weight, 30 seconds on:10 seconds off duty cycle, 15-minute treatment session) over a 9-day period. Of the 129 subjects, 25 subjects were identified as benefiting from traction. Of those 25 subjects, four variables were associated with a successful outcome: individuals who were older than 30 years of age, low fear avoidance score (score of <21 on the Fear-Avoidance Beliefs Questionnaire work subscale), no neurologic deficits, and employment in a nonmanual labor job. Cai et al.[21] reported that if an individual presented with each of these four variables, he/she had a 69% chance of a successful outcome when treated with mechanical traction.

Examination, Evaluation, and Diagnosis

A physical therapy examination for the patient with a suspected (or confirmed) HNP may consist of observing posture and gait, active and passive range of motion (ROM) testing, muscle flexibility testing, neurologic screening (lumbar dermatomes, myotomes, and reflexes), muscular strength and endurance tests, passive intervertebral motion testing, and a peripheral joint scan (clearing examination for adjacent joints).

A patient with an HNP may present with pain (centralized to the lumbar spine or peripheralized to a lower extremity), lower extremity paresthesias, decreased lumbar active range of motion, paraspinal muscle spasm, and spinal segmental hypomobility.[22] A patient that presents with muscular weakness in a myotomal distribution should be referred to a spine surgeon (either an orthopaedist or a neurosurgeon) for an examination.

During the initial examination, the physical therapist should assess the patient's active lumbar spinal ROM in the standing position. With the patient in the prone and supine positions, the physical therapist should assess passive ROM of the lumbar spine, active and passive ROM of the hips and perform muscle length tests (flexibility testing) of the lumbar spine and the hips. When a patient presents with a lateral shift, muscular spasms and/or muscular inflexibility are frequently observed in the lumbar paraspinals (on the side that the patient leans toward). In lieu of a lateral shift, the patient may present with bilateral muscular spasms in the lumbar spine. Other muscles that may present with spasms or pre-existing muscular inflexibility (either ipsilaterally or bilaterally) include the piriformis, iliopsoas, and hamstrings.

Plan of Care and Interventions

A physical therapist has several parameters to manipulate on the mechanical traction machine prior to initiating the intervention. Table 16-1 presents published variables for traction treatment parameters (patient position, treatment frequency,

Table 16-1 TREATMENT PARAMETERS DESCRIBED FOR LUMBAR TRACTION	
Variable	**Parameters**
Patient position	Prone[20,21,23] Supine (with hips and knees both flexed up to 90°)[10,21,24-26]
Treatment frequency	1-2 times/wk[20] 2-3 times/wk[12] 5 d/wk[25]
Treatment time	10 min[12] 12 min[20] 15 min[10,21,25] 20 min[10,12,26]
Treatment duty cycle	Intermittent 30-s hold and 10-s rest[21,25] Static[12,26,27]
Traction force (% of patient's weight)	10%-60%[20,23-26]
Type of traction	Vertebral axial decompression (VAD)[14] Manual traction (pelvic harness)[24,28] Inverted traction[27] Mechanical traction[12,21,25-27]

length of treatment session, duty cycle, traction force, and type of traction). At this time, **no single set of traction treatment parameters** has been demonstrated to be superior in decreasing pain or improving functional measures.

Unlu et al.[25] evaluated the efficacy of mechanical traction compared to two other modalities for patients with acute low back pain due to HNP. The subjects (men = 18, women = 42) were similar in age (mean age 44.5 years, range 20-60 years) and had similar clinical presentations (diagnosis of HNP with pain radiating into a lower extremity) as the patient in this case. Subjects were diagnosed with an HNP by a physiatrist via a physical examination and diagnostic imaging. Subjects were randomized into one of three treatment groups: mechanical traction (5 times per week for 3 weeks, supine with hips and knees flexed to 90°, duty cycle 30 seconds on: 10 seconds off, traction force 35%-50% body weight), ultrasound (1.5 W/cm^2, continuous, 8 minutes), or low-power laser (50 mV; wavelength 830 nm). The authors reported significant improvements in pain, lateral flexion range of motion, muscular tenderness, straight leg raise motion (measured in degrees), and disability scores (measured by the Roland Disability Questionnaire and the Modified Oswestry Disability Questionnaire) between baseline and most follow-up points (3 weeks, 1 month, and 3 months) for each group. In addition, the authors reported that there was a significant decrease in the size of the HNP (measured by magnetic resonance imaging) for each group. However, the authors found no significant differences between the groups on any of the outcome measures at any follow-up time point. The authors concluded that any of the three treatment modalities could be effective for treating patients with an HNP. However, because the authors did not include a placebo (nonintervention) group, the effect of natural history or maturation cannot be excluded as a contributing factor in the mean improvements observed.

In addition to mechanical traction, other interventions (*e.g.*, therapeutic exercises, other forms of manual therapy, modalities) may be performed during a treatment session when treating a patient with an HNP. Gagne et al.[10] described the use of mechanical traction and extension-based exercises to treat a 49-year-old patient with an L5-S1 HNP. The patient was treated for 14 visits during a 5-week period. The patient was prescribed extension-based exercises during the first 5 visits. Mechanical traction was added during the final 9 visits. At the end of the fourteenth visit, the patient no longer reported tingling and numbness in the left leg.

This case presented current evidence for use of mechanical traction to treat a patient with a lumbar HNP. In Cases 15, 17, and 18, the utilization of a muscle energy technique, the use of Mechanical Diagnosis and Therapy (MDT or McKenzie), and the use of an eclectic Norwegian manual therapy approach (Ola Grimsby) are presented.

Evidence-Based Clinical Recommendations

SORT: Strength of Recommendation Taxonomy

A: Consistent, good-quality patient-oriented evidence
B: Inconsistent or limited-quality patient-oriented evidence
C: Consensus, disease-oriented evidence, usual practice, expert opinion, or case series

1. Systematic reviews do not support or refute the efficacy of mechanical traction in treating the signs and symptoms associated with a herniated nucleus pulposus. **Grade A**

2. The presence of specific criteria from the subjective history and physical examination may predict which patients with an HNP would benefit from the use of mechanical traction. **Grade B**

3. There are multiple treatment parameters for mechanical traction (*e.g.*, length of treatment, patient positions, duty cycle, etc.) that have been used for patients with an HNP. **Grade B**

COMPREHENSION QUESTIONS

16.1 Mechanical traction may be indicated for each of the following diagnoses *except*:

   A. Herniated nucleus pulposus

   B. Compression fracture

   C. Joint hypomobility

   D. Stenosis of the intervertebral foramina

16.2 Fritz et al.[20] and Cai et al.[21] have developed two preliminary clinical prediction rules to assist clinical decision making when considering the use of mechanical traction for patients with an HNP. Which of the following four statements is *most* accurate regarding these two CPRs?

A. Each CPR has three variables with one variable in common between the two studies.

B. Fritz et al. suggested that mechanical traction is indicated for patients with centralization of symptoms at baseline.

C. Cai et al. reported that mechanical traction might benefit a patient over the age of 30 years who performs primarily computer work for his employment.

D. A positive crossed straight leg raise test associated with raising the involved leg may suggest the presence of an HNP.

ANSWERS

16.1 **B.** Any type of fracture is a contraindication for the use of mechanical traction.

16.2 **C.** According to their results, Cai et al.[21] found that the two variables presented (over the age of 30 years and employment in a job that lacks manual labor) were associated with a greater chance of treatment success with mechanical traction.

REFERENCES

1. Jonsson B, Stromqvist B. Clinical appearance of sciatica due to disc herniation: a systematic review. *J Spinal Dis*. 1996;9:32-38.

2. Hahne AJ, Ford JJ, McMeeken JM. Conservative management of lumbar disc herniation with associated radiculopathy: a systematic review. Spine. 2010;35:E488-E504.

3. Chou R, Atlas SJ, Stanos SP, Rosenquist RW. Nonsurgical interventional therapies for low back pain: a review of the evidence for an American Pain Society clinical practice guideline. *Spine*. 2009;34:1078-1093.

4. Weinstein JN, Lurie JD, Tosteson TD, et al. Surgical versus nonoperative treatment for lumbar disc herniation: four-year results for the Spine Patient Outcomes Research Trial (SPORT). *Spine*. 2008;33:2789-2800.

5. Oliphant D. Safety of spinal manipulation in the treatment of lumbar disk herniations: a systematic review and risk assessment. *J Manipulative Physiol Ther*. 2004;27:197-210.

6. Donelson R, Aprill C, Medcalf R, Grant W. A prospective study of centralization of lumbar and referred pain. A predictor of symptomatic discs and anular competence. *Spine*. 1997;22:1115-1122.

7. Gillan MG, Ross JC, McLean IP, Porter RW. The natural history of trunk list, its associated disability and the influence of McKenzie management. *Eur Spine J*. 1998;7:480-483.

8. Bronfort G, Haas M, Evans RL, Bouter LM. Efficacy of spinal manipulation and mobilization for low back pain and neck pain: a systematic review and best evidence synthesis. *Spine J*. 2004;4:335-356.

9. Takasaki H, May S, Fazey PJ, Hall T. Nucleus pulposus deformation following application of mechanical diagnosis and therapy: a single case report with magnetic resonance imaging. *J Man Manip Ther*. 2010;18:153-158.

10. Gagne AR, Hasson SM. Lumbar extension exercises in conjunction with mechanical traction for the management of a patient with a lumbar herniated disc. *Physiother Theory Pract.* 2010;26:256-266.

11. Hebert J, Koppenhaver S, Fritz J, Parent E. Clinical prediction for success of interventions for managing low back pain. *Clin Sports Med.* 2008;27:463-479.

12. Harte AA, Gracey JH, Baxter GD. Current use of lumbar traction in the management of low back pain: results of a survey of physiotherapists in the United Kingdom. *Arch Phys Med Rehabil.* 2005;86:1164-1169.

13. Saunders HD. Lumbar traction. *J Orthop Sports Phys Ther.* 1979;1:36-45.

14. Beattie PF, Nelson RM, Michener LA, Cammarata J, Donley J. Outcomes after a prone lumbar traction protocol for patients with activity-limiting low back pain: a prospective case series study. *Arch Phys Med Rehabil.* 2008;89:269-274.

15. Cameron MH. *Physical Agents in Rehabilitation: From Research to Practice.* 3rd ed. St. Louis, MO: Saunders/Elsevier; 2009.

16. Philadelphia Panel. Philadelphia Panel evidence-based clinical practice guidelines on selected rehabilitation interventions for low back pain. *Phys Ther.* 2001;81:1641-1674.

17. Macario A, Pergolizzi JV. Systematic literature review of spinal decompression via motorized traction for chronic discogenic low back pain. *Pain Pract.* 2006;6:171-178.

18. Clarke JA, van Tulder MW, Blomberg SE, et al. Traction for low-back pain with or without sciatica. *Cochrane Database Syst Rev.* 2007;18:CD003010.

19. Clarke J, van Tulder M, Blomberg S, de Vet H, van der Heijden G, Bronfort G. Traction for low back pain with or without sciatica an updated systematic review within the framework of the Cochrane collaboration. *Spine.* 2006;31:1591-1599.

20. Fritz JM, Lindsay W, Matheson JW, et al. Is there a subgroup of patients with low back pain likely to benefit from mechanical traction? *Spine.* 2007;32:E793-E800.

21. Cai C, Pau YH, Lim KC. A clinical prediction rule for classifying patients with low back pain who demonstrate short-term improvement with mechanical lumbar traction. *Eur Spine J.* 2009;18:554-561.

22. Strayer A. Lumbar spine: common pathology and interventions. *J Neurosci Nurs.* 2005;37:181-193.

23. Cevik R, Bilici A, Gur A, et al. Effect of a new traction technique of prone position on distraction of lumbar vertebrae and its relation with different application of heating therapy in low back pain. *J Back Musculoskeletal Rehabil.* 2007;20:71-77.

24. Meszaros TF, Olson R, Kulig K, Creighton D, Czarnecki E. Effect of 10%, 30%, and 60% body weight traction on the straight leg raise test of symptomatic patients with low back pain. *J Orthop Sports Phys Ther.* 2000;30:595-601.

25. Unlu Z, Tasci S, Tarhan S, Pabuscu Y, Islak S. Comparison of 3 physical therapy modalities for acute pain in lumbar disc herniation measured by clinical evaluation and magnetic resonance imaging. *J Manipulative Physiol Ther.* 2008;31:191-198.

26. Borman P, Keskin D, Bodur H. The efficacy of lumbar traction in the management of patients with low back pain. *Rheumatol Int.* 2003;23:82-86.

27. Guvenol K, Tuzun C, Peker O, Goktay Y. A comparison of inverted spinal traction and conventional traction in the treatment of lumbar disc herniations. *Physiother Theory Pract.* 2000;16:151-160.

28. Corkery M. The use of lumbar harness traction to treat a patient with lumbar radicular pain: a case report. *J Man Manip Ther.* 2001;191-197.

Lumbar Spine: Herniated Disc—*Mechanical Diagnosis and Therapy (McKenzie) Approach*

Jolene Bennett
Barbara J. Hoogenboom

A 36-year-old male construction worker self-referred to an outpatient physical therapy clinic with a complaint of low back pain and pain radiating from his posterior left hip all the way to his lateral foot. He first experienced pain 3 weeks ago while doing a home maintenance project. The onset of pain occurred when he attempted to lift an air conditioning unit. He reports that as he bent over to lift the unit, he experienced an intense, stabbing pain and immediately fell to the ground. He required assistance from his wife to walk back into the house. For the first 24 hours after the incident, he rested prone on a couch or on his bed. Over the past 3 days, he reports an improved tolerance to walking and standing for short periods. However, he rates his current pain level 5 out of 10 on the visual analog scale and he continues to experience radiating pain distal to his knee. Signs and symptoms are consistent with a lumbar herniated disc. His goal is to return to work as soon as possible.

▶ Based on the patient's suspected diagnosis, what do you anticipate may be the contributing factors to his condition?
▶ What examination signs may be associated with this diagnosis?
▶ What are the most appropriate physical therapy interventions?
▶ What are possible complications that may limit the effectiveness of physical therapy?

KEY DEFINITIONS

CENTRALIZATION: Phenomenon in which distal limb pain emanating from the spine is immediately or eventually abolished in response to deliberate application of loading strategies; peripheral pain progressively retreats in a proximal direction, sometimes associated with simultaneous development or increased proximal pain; centralization is described by McKenzie[1] to occur in the derangement syndrome

DIRECTIONAL PREFERENCE/MECHANICAL DIAGNOSIS THERAPY: Preference for postures or movement in one direction (characteristic of the derangement syndrome); describes when postures or movements in one direction decrease, abolish, or centralize symptoms and postures or movements in the opposite direction often cause symptoms to worsen[1]

LOADING STRATEGIES: Dynamic or static movements, positions, or loads applied in order to stress particular structures; dynamic loads are repeated movements and static loads are sustained postures; significant loading strategies, postures, and repeated movements are those that alter symptoms[1]

Objectives

1. Understand the anatomy of the lumbar disc and its mechanical response to different directional movements of the spine.

2. Describe the McKenzie or Mechanical Diagnosis and Therapy (MDT) classification system.

3. Describe the McKenzie evaluation process and how the objective findings determine the classification system of the syndromes.

4. Describe how the objective findings from the examination determine the treatment approach for the syndromes.

5. Prescribe appropriate interventions for each phase of the condition—from acute injury to full restoration of function.

6. Describe the evidence for the efficacy of using the McKenzie approach in the treatment of lumbar spine disorders.

Physical Therapy Considerations

PT considerations during management of the individual with a diagnosis of a herniated lumbar disc:

▶ **General physical therapy plan of care/goals:** Decrease pain; centralize radicular pain; restore full trunk range of motion with no subsequent pain; return to full work duties

▶ **Physical therapy interventions:** Repeated movements with directional preference to centralize and eliminate pain in leg and lumbar spine; patient education for repeated movement exercises, posture, body mechanics for activities of daily living and work tasks

▶ **Precautions during physical therapy:** Positioning and use of arms to provide repeated movements to lumbar spine: upper extremities may not be able to handle body weight during exercises so alternative positions may need to be used

▶ **Complications interfering with physical therapy:** Irreducible derangement when peripheralization of symptoms (increase or worsening of distal symptoms) occurs in response to repeated movements or loading strategies

Physical Therapy Patient/Client Management

The McKenzie system (also known as Mechanical Diagnosis and Therapy or MDT) is a classification system for musculoskeletal injuries of the spine and extremities. It consists of **three distinct syndromes: derangement, dysfunction, and postural.** A patient's subjective history and response to active movements during the examination contribute to the classification of a syndrome and thus identify the specific treatment approach that should be taken. The physical examination consists of a series of loading stresses to the tissues of the spine or peripheral joints. Each syndrome has a unique set of responses to the loading tests. Correct identification of the syndrome helps the physical therapist define the proper mechanical treatment. Unique to the McKenzie system is the examination process in which the patient performs several different movement patterns with the therapist noting the response to each direction of movement to help determine the syndrome classification.[1]

The derangement syndrome is the most frequently observed syndrome.[1] As defined by Robin McKenzie, "internal derangement causes a disturbance in the normal resting position of the affected surfaces. Internal displacement of articular tissue of whatever origin will cause pain to remain constant until such time as the displacement is reduced. Internal displacement of articular tissue obstructs movements."[1] A meniscus tear in the knee is an example of the derangement syndrome. The tear may cause a mechanical block that can limit full knee function and the direction of mechanical forces across the knee changes the pain. An internal intervertebral disc displacement is also frequently classified as a derangement syndrome.

A "disc herniation" is a nonspecific term to indicate disc material that has displaced and/or a fissure or disruption in the annulus of the disc. The intervertebral disc is mobile and can be a source of mechanically generated pain via two avenues.[2] First, radial fissures within the annular wall disrupt the normal load-bearing properties of the annulus. This causes disproportionate weightbearing distribution and stresses the outer innervated lamellae. Second, internal displacement of the disc material can also be a potential source of pain. The position of the disc material is influenced by spinal postures and especially by prolonged spinal flexion or extension.

Such conditions cause disc material displacement according to direction.[2-9] In the current patient, uneven loading of the intervertebral disc with a heavy loaded flexion position of the trunk may cause neurogenic pain.[5]

The McKenzie approach uses repeated movements in the sagittal plane to evaluate and to treat the patient's symptom presentation. A derangement syndrome can be further labeled as reducible or irreducible based on the integrity of the hydrostatic mechanism within the disc wall. If a herniation occurs in a disc in which the outer wall is intact, it is considered reducible and repeated movements may alleviate the mechanical stresses on the disc. If the herniation occurs in a disc in which the outer wall is *not* intact, the derangement is considered irreducible and repeated movements will not improve the pain or symptoms of the patient.[1]

The clinical presentation associated with a derangement syndrome includes the centralization of any distal symptoms (*e.g.*, pain in the leg) and a decrease in pain during the application of therapeutic loading strategies. The pain associated with a derangement changes with induced directional movements as the forces change within the intervertebral disc (due to varying positions of the spine). The pain may be present during the movement and at the end-range of movement. Sagittal plane range of motion is frequently limited in flexion with a derangement that responds to extension loading strategies. As the derangement is reduced with repeated (extension) motions, the patient's range of motion into flexion should improve and return to normal. McKenzie subclassifies the derangement syndrome into central symmetrical, unilateral asymmetrical symptoms to the knee, and unilateral asymmetrical symptoms below the knee. The reader is directed to Robin McKenzie's book titled *The Lumbar Spine Mechanical Diagnosis and Therapy* for further discussion of these subclassifications.[1]

The direction of disc herniation is also important because this directs the treatment approach. More than 50% of derangements appear to start centrally in the disc and approximately 25% start posterolaterally.[1] As the derangement extends into the dura and nerve root, over 50% of them displace posterolaterally and the other 25% displace posterocentrally. Since most derangements occur in the sagittal plane, lumbar flexion and extension is part of the mechanism of injury and also the avenue for repeated movement treatment. Less than 10% of disc derangements herniate directly laterally, which would require torsional or lateral forces to be a component of the treatment. The majority of derangements occur at the L4-L5 and L5-S1 levels.[1]

The term "centralization" is associated with the derangement syndrome and is referred to extensively in the literature when discussing disc herniations.[10-15] Centralization is the response to therapeutic loading strategies. With centralization, pain is progressively abolished in a distal to proximal direction with the symptoms diminishing in intensity with each progressive movement. For example, in the individual with pain distal to the low back (*i.e.*, radicular pain), successful treatment causes the pain to move from widespread distal locations to a more central location and then, ultimately the pain is abolished.[1]

The dysfunction syndrome is characterized by pain caused by mechanical deformation of structurally impaired tissue and a limited range of motion in the affected direction. An example of a dysfunction syndrome is adhesive capsulitis of the gleno-humeral joint. This condition is a soft tissue restriction that limits range of motion. The patient reports pain primarily at the end-range of available motion. When the mechanical load is released, the pain disappears. Dysfunction syndrome is uncommon in the lumbar spine; prevalence is reported to be less than 20% of all patients with lumbar pain who have been treated by physical therapists using the MDT approach.[1] The dysfunction syndrome may be in the flexion, extension, or side gliding direction and is named for the direction that is limited. For example, if flexion is limited then the syndrome would be labeled a flexion dysfunction syndrome. The treatment for a dysfunction is to repeatedly stretch *into* the direction of limitation.

The postural syndrome is characterized by the presence of pain only when the normal tissue is deformed over a prolonged period of time (*e.g.*, sitting in a slouched position for a long period of time). The postural syndrome is treated with postural correction exercises and patient education. This syndrome is very seldom observed clinically; however, if abnormal postural loading is continued, it may lead to a derangement or a dysfunction syndrome.[1] Table 17-1 outlines the characteristics of the three syndromes defined by Robin McKenzie.

Examination, Evaluation, and Diagnosis

A key component to the McKenzie approach is the use of a structured history or subjective questioning format and follow-up with a consistent sequence of movement testing. It is imperative to test all planes of movement and repeat the movements sufficiently to get a consistent response from the patient in his symptom reaction to each movement. It is important to inform the patient that the purpose of the examination is to evaluate the response of his *chief* complaint or pain to the movement patterns. A patient may describe experiencing a stretching sensation or other secondary physiological responses during directional movement testing. The physical therapist must differentiate between these secondary responses and those that are consistent with the patient's chief complaint.

The McKenzie evaluation process follows a very specific pathway. The key is to follow the same procedures for each patient for consistency and thoroughness in all areas of the evaluation. Based on the patient's mechanism of injury and characteristics of his pain, the physical therapist should be hypothesizing that he has a lumbar derangement. However, a complete repeated movement testing examination is required to confirm this hypothesis. The goal of the objective examination is to determine which positions and movements facilitate improvement in pain and function. The repeated movement testing applies mechanical stress to spinal tissues in different directions to expose the mechanical or nonmechanical nature of the injury. The patient's responses to this testing allows the physical therapist to determine the particular syndrome and directional preference for proper treatment. During movement testing, the physical therapist needs to know the patient's baseline pain and if pain occurs during the movement and/or at the end-range of the movement. Upon returning to the starting position of the movement,

Table 17-1 CHARACTERISTICS OF MECHANICAL DIAGNOSIS THERAPY SYNDROMES[1]

Characteristics of Patient and Clinical Presentation	Derangement	Dysfunction	Postural
Age (years)	Usually 20-55	Usually over 30, except following trauma or derangement	Usually under 30
Pain *Constancy* *Location*	Constant or intermittent Local and/or referred	Intermittent Local (referred only with adherent nerve root)	Intermittent Local
History *Onset* *Reason*	Gradual or sudden Often related to prolonged positions or repetitive movements	Gradual History of trauma	Gradual Sedentary lifestyle
Symptoms worse *Type of load* *Diurnal cycle*	Static/dynamic load at mid- or end-range Worse in morning and evening	Static/dynamic loading at end-range No diurnal cycle	Static loading at end-range Worse at end of day
Symptoms better	Opposite position of what causes pain	Positions that do not put shortened tissue at end-range	Change of position and when active
Examination findings associated with each syndrome	Acute deformity may be present Pain during movement Pain changes location and/or intensity Pain centralizes or peripheralizes Patient remains better or worse as a result of repeated loading or movements Rapid changes in pain and range of motion	Pain reported at end-range of motion only Pain stops shortly after removal of stretch Pain does not change location or intensity Patient remains no better and no worse as a result of repeated loading or movements	Movement does not produce pain Range of motion is normal Sustained end-range positions eventually produce local pain
Treatment	Correct the deformity Repeated movements in the direction that centralizes the pain Correct posture Patient education regarding prevention and self management of symptoms	Repeated movements or stretches in the direction which produces end-range pain or limited motion Correct posture Patient education regarding prevention and self management of symptoms	Correct posture Education on prevention

the therapist needs to know how the movement affected the baseline pain and/or range of motion. Potential responses include: (1) increase, decrease, or no effect on baseline pain during directional movement; (2) centralization, peripheralization, or no effect on baseline pain during or after loading; (3) pain abolished as a result of the loading; (4) better, worse, or no effect on pain after loading; (5) presence or absence of pain at end-range during loading; (6) increase, decrease, or no effect on range of motion after loading (mechanical response); (7) pain worse/not worse or better/not better after loading (pain response).[1] Table 17-2 summarizes the potential responses to repeated movement testing to determine whether the patient has a dysfunction or derangement syndrome.

The main differences between the dysfunction and derangement syndromes are whether pain is present only at the end-range of motion and whether there is an increase or decrease in range of motion after loading the tissue by repeated movements. Dysfunction syndromes generally present with no pain unless the tissue is loaded at end-range and when the mechanical stress is unloaded, the pain resolves quickly. In contrast, the **derangement syndrome presents with a directional preference and loading into this direction decreases and centralizes the pain**. The key is to determine *which* repeated movement in the sagittal plane (flexion or extension) centralizes the distal pain. With a derangement, repeated movements produce a mechanical response and increase the range in motion that was limited at baseline. If the patient presents with a lateral trunk shift, the physical therapist should test lateral side gliding range of motion in both directions to determine if a lateral component is involved in the mechanical blocking of lumbar range of motion. If a lateral component is suspected and confirmed, that component must be treated *prior* to performing repeated sagittal movements. Testing for a lateral component is performed in the standing position with the patient's feet shoulder width apart. To perform a right side gliding motion, the patient moves his hips to the left while his trunk remains in neutral. The physical therapist may assist with this motion by placing one hand on the left shoulder and the opposite hand on the right iliac crest and applying force toward the midline. The shoulders should remain parallel to the ground. Because this movement pattern is a difficult concept for many patients to understand, demonstration by the physical therapist and tactile guides for the movement are often needed for proper execution. The movement is a side glide and not a side bending movement. The patient is asked to perform one repetition of the side gliding movement and the response to the movement is noted by physical therapist. Repeated movements are then performed and symptom response and range of motion limitations are noted. If restrictions and symptoms are noted, the treatment sequence should start with determining the directional preference and follow with repeated movements to centralize the distal symptoms.[1]

Based on the repeated movement testing performed on the patient in this case study, he has a derangement syndrome with an extension direction preference. The MDT approach to examination requires that the physical therapist not be hesitant to ask the patient to perform repeated movements even if he experiences pain during movement and at the end-range of motion. It is important to get the patient to the available end-range on each repeated movement and monitor symptom behavior such as centralization.

Table 17-2 SPINAL PHYSICAL EXAMINATION USING REPEATED MOVEMENT TESTING

Physical Test	Dysfunction				Derangement			
	Pain During	Centralization or Peripheralization	End-Range Pain	ROM Response	Pain During	Centralization or Peripheralization	End-Range Pain	ROM Response
Flexion in standing	No	No effect	Yes—with every repetition	No effect	Increase	Peripheralization	Yes	No effect
Extension in standing	No	No effect	No	No effect	Decrease	Centralization	Yes	Increased extension/ increased flexion
Flexion in supine	No	No effect	Yes—with every repetition	No effect	Increase	Peripheralization	Yes	No effect
Extension in prone	No	No effect	No	No effect	Decrease	Centralization	Yes	Increased extension/ increased flexion

Plan of Care and Interventions

According to McKenzie, passive or "chemical" treatments (*e.g.*, electrical stimulation, ultrasound, ice) will not diminish pain caused by a mechanical deformation.[1] In addition, no mechanical treatment such as mobilization or repeated movements will totally resolve pain arising from a majority of chemical stresses (*e.g.*, inflammation). These principles are the basis for the McKenzie approach to treating any type of musculoskeletal pain with repeated movements.[2]

The degree of chemical and mechanical pain present with each individual injury must be determined during the subjective and objective examination and subsequent evaluation.[1] Characteristics of chemical pain include constancy, appearance shortly after injury, presence of cardinal signs of inflammation, lasting pain aggravation by all repeated movements, and pain that is not responsive to any movement (*i.e.*, movement does not reduce, abolish, or centralize pain). In contrast, mechanical pain is characterized by intermittency, lasting reduction, abolition or centralization of pain induced by repeated movements, and a directional preference in which one direction of movement decreases the pain while the opposite direction increases the pain. This patient presented with both chemical and mechanical pain and the pain is starting to subside slightly. This is indicated by his improved tolerance to walking and standing for short periods of time.

The McKenzie treatment approach is tailored to each of three stages of healing.[1] The first stage is inflammation, which lasts a maximum of 1 week if treated promptly and correctly. The most important treatment principles during this phase are to minimize inflammation by chemical means and eliminate mechanical stresses with proper body positioning and/or movements within pain-free range of motion. For the current patient with a disc injury at L4-5, chemical treatment includes ice. Proper body positioning or movements includes prone lying with progression to prone on elbows static lying for 5-minute intervals, or as tolerated. Aggressive repeated movements applied during the inflammation stage may delay healing.[1] Two to four weeks postinjury, the patient enters the repair and healing stage. In this phase, repeated stress should be applied to the spinal tissues and more specifically to the disc in order to facilitate tissue repair along functional stress lines and to increase tensile strength of healing tissues. The patient should move into the edge of stiffness, but the movements should not cause lasting pain after completion of the movements. For this patient, the treatment includes progression from prone lying to prone press-ups (Fig. 17-1) with the goal of regaining full available trunk extension. During this stage, movements should work into the edge of stiffness and pain and the patient should be in control of the force production at the end-range of movement (Fig. 17-2). The area should not be over-stressed, which can cause a new onset of inflammation that can delay the patient's recovery. The final stage is remodeling, which starts approximately 5 weeks after injury. At this stage, regular stresses sufficient to provide tension without damage must be applied so that collagen elongates and strengthens. During remodeling, more force may be necessary to create these stresses; these stresses may include physical therapist-provided overpressure (Fig. 17-3), mobilization (Fig. 17-4), or manipulation if centralization and symptoms are not totally resolved. Return to full

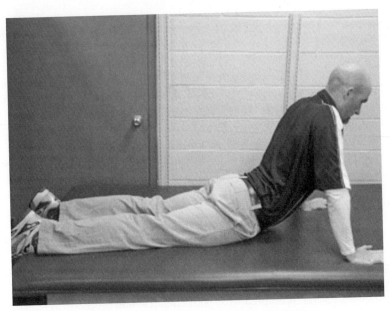

Figure 17-1. Dynamic patient-generated forces: lumbar extension at end-range.

range of motion in all directions is the goal so return to full function can be achieved. Table 17-3 outlines sample interventions for this patient during each stage of healing.

In the MDT approach, static postures are used but dynamic movements are more often utilized to determine which syndrome is present and then dynamic or repeated

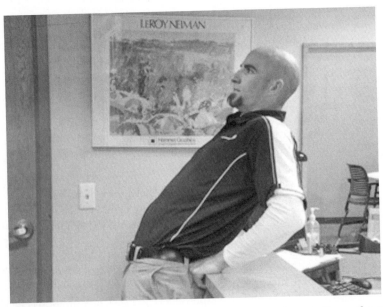

Figure 17-2. Dynamic patient-generated forces: lumbar extension at end-range with use of counter top for overpressure.

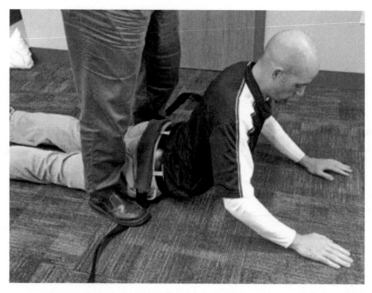

Figure 17-3. Dynamic patient-generated forces: lumbar extension at end-range with belt fixation for overpressure.

movements are used to treat the syndrome. The general guideline for the number of movements is 10 to 15 repetitions per set. The number of sets used for treatment depends on the acuity of the symptoms and usually varies from 2 to 4 sets per exercise session. A minimum of 4 to 5 exercise sessions per day is necessary to produce a clinical change in symptoms. The repeated movements should include a

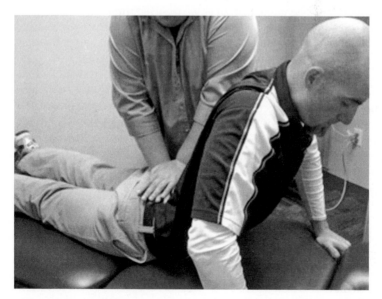

Figure 17-4. Dynamic motion: lumbar extension at end-range with therapist-generated overpressure mobilization.

Table 17-3 INTERVENTIONS ACCORDING TO STAGES OF HEALING		
Injury and Inflammation (Week 1)	Repair and Healing (Weeks 2-4)	Remodeling (Weeks 5 and beyond)
Relative rest Prone lying Prone on elbows: static positioning in mid-range with progression to end-range position	Unweighted position in prone and progress to weightbearing in standing Prone press-ups Patient moves in mid-range Patient moves to end-range (Fig. 17-1) Patient moves to end-range with patient-applied overpressure (Fig. 17-2)	Prone position: patient moves to end-range with physical therapist-provided overpressure using a belt for fixation (Fig. 17-3) Physical therapist-provided mobilization (Fig. 17-4) or manipulation

brief relaxation time between each repetition and the patient should try to make the movements as passive as possible. In this case, the patient should be advised to relax his buttock and lumbar muscles, using only his upper extremities to allow full trunk extension in the prone position.[1] The main guide to the number of repetitions and frequency of exercise is how the patient tolerates the physical loading and the symptom response.

The **efficacy of the Mechanical Diagnosis and Therapy (MDT) approach** has been tested as a clinical approach to treating low back pain. Petersen et al.[10] conducted a randomized controlled trial comparing thrust manipulation and patient education to a treatment program consisting of the MDT method and patient education. The study consisted of 350 patients who reported symptoms of low back pain with onset of more than 6 weeks and presented with centralization or peripheralization of symptoms. The manipulation group received thrust and non-thrust manipulations along with trigger point massage, whereas the MDT group was treated with repeated movements with directional preference without the use of mobilization or manipulation techniques. The MDT group showed significant improvement in level of disability (as measured by the 23-item modified Roland Morris Disability Questionnaire) compared to the manipulation group at 2 and 12 months follow-up.[10]

Centralization and directional preference are the key components of the McKenzie approach. Werneke et al.[11] performed a prospective, longitudinal cohort study to determine baseline prevalence of directional preference. The study consisted of 584 patients with nonspecific low back pain that centralized, did not centralize, or could not be classified. They found that the overall prevalence of directional preference and centralization was 60% and 41%, respectively. These classifications were investigated to determine if the classifications predicted functional status and pain intensity at discharge from care. The patients whose symptoms showed directional preference (DP) *with* centralization on the initial evaluation reported significantly better functional status and less pain at the end of care than patients who were classified as DP without centralization and those patients who were classified as having no DP and no centralization. Long et al.[12] also looked at directional preference and followed 312 patients with varying acuity of low back pain. Seventy-four percent of the 312 patients had a directional preference: 83% responded to extension, 7% responded to flexion and 10% were identified as lateral responders. Subjects who were identified as having a directional preference were then randomized into subgroups: directional exercises matching each patient's directional preference, directional exercises opposite the patient's directional preference, or nondirectional exercises. After 2 weeks (3 to 6 visits), the directional exercise group that performed exercise matched to their directional preference experienced significant reduction in pain, pain medication use, and disability measures compared to the other two treatment groups. One-third of the nonmatching exercise group dropped out from the study because they were either not improving or had worsening symptoms. In a follow-up study, Long et al.[13] investigated many factors that predicted a favorable outcome when patients were grouped according to presence or absence of directional preference. The results revealed that patients who performed exercises in the same direction as was determined to be appropriate in their initial evaluation had a 7.8 times greater likelihood of a good outcome at 2 weeks than subjects whose rehabilitation program was not matched to their directional preference. In this study, a minimal reduction of 30% on the Roland-Morris Disability Questionnaire was the outcome measurement used to determine a good outcome.

A 2004 systematic review by Clare et al.[14] included six randomized/quasi-randomized controlled studies investigating the efficacy of centralization and directional preference. The authors of this meta-analysis concluded that the reviewed studies suggested that the MDT approach is more effective than comparison treatments consisting of medications, educational booklet, and strengthening at short-term follow-up (less than 3 months). A multicenter randomized controlled study by Browder et al.[15] also examined the effectiveness of an extension-based treatment approach in patients with low back pain. The group of 48 patients who responded with centralization to extension movements were then randomized to two groups. The first group received exercise/mobilization promoting lumbar extension and the second group performed lumbopelvic strengthening exercises. At the 1-week, 4-week, and 6-month follow-ups, the extension-based exercise group demonstrated greater reductions in disability compared to the strengthening group.[15]

This case presented current evidence for use of MDT to manage a patient with a lumbar HNP. In Cases 15, 16, and 18, the utilization of a muscle energy technique, the use of mechanical traction, and the use of an eclectic Norwegian manual therapy approach (Ola Grimsby) are presented.

Evidence-Based Clinical Recommendations

SORT: Strength of Recommendation Taxonomy

A: Consistent, good-quality patient-oriented evidence
B: Inconsistent or limited-quality patient-oriented evidence
C: Consensus, disease-oriented evidence, usual practice, expert opinion, or case series

1. The McKenzie classification system of three distinct syndromes (derangement, dysfunction, postural) for musculoskeletal injuries of the spine and extremities outlines a systematic approach to direct patient examination and potential treatment strategies. **Grade C**

2. When the McKenzie approach determines directional preference at initial evaluation and matches repeated movement exercises with the same directional preference, pain intensity and disability are reduced. **Grade A**

3. The McKenzie treatment approach is effective at decreasing pain and improving function in adults with low back pain compared to manipulation, strengthening exercises, medication, and educational booklets. **Grade B**

COMPREHENSION QUESTIONS

17.1 The derangement syndrome consists of all of the following characteristics, *except:*

A. Reproduction of pain only at the end-range of motion

B. Reproduction of pain at the mid range and at the end-range of motion

C. A directional preference is demonstrated in response to repeated movements

D. Centralization of distal symptoms occurs in response to repeated movements

17.2 Key factors of mechanical pain consist of all of the following characteristics, *except:*

A. Centralization of distal symptoms with repeated movements

B. Directional preference to repeated movements

C. Intermittent pain

D. Constant pain

ANSWERS

17.1 **A.** The dysfunction syndrome is the only syndrome that has pain only at the end-range of motion.

17.2 **D.** Constant pain is not a feature of mechanical pain. Mechanical pain will be diminished or abolished when mechanical load is removed from the painful structure.

REFERENCES

1. McKenzie R, May S. *The Lumbar Spine: Mechanical Diagnosis and Therapy.* Waikanae, New Zealand: Spinal Publications; 2003.

2. Bogduk N. *Clinical Anatomy of the Lumbar Spine and Sacrum.* 3rd ed. New York: Churchill Livingstone; 1997.

3. Bogduk N. The anatomy and physiology of nociception. In: Crosbie J, McConnell J, eds. *Key Issues in Musculoskeletal Physiotherapy.* Oxford: Butterworth-Heineman; 1993.

4. Bogduk N. Innervation, pain patterns, and mechanism of pain production. In: Twomey LT, Taylor JR, eds. *Physical Therapy of the Low Back.* New York: Churchill Livingstone; 1994.

5. Schnebel BE, Simmons JW, Chowning J, Davidson R. A digitizing technique for the study of movement of intradiscal dye in response to flexion and extension of the lumbar spine. *Spine.* 1988;13:309-312.

6. Beattie PF, Brooks WM, Rothstein JM, et al. Effect of lordosis on the position of the nucleus pulposus in supine subjects. A study using magnetic resonance imaging. *Spine*.1994;19:2096-2102.

7. Fennell AJ, Jones AP, Hukins DW. Migration of the nucleus pulposus within the intervertebral disc during flexion and extension of the spine. *Spine*. 1996;21:2753-2757.

8. Brault JS, Driscoll DM, Laako LL, Kappler RE, Allin EF, Glonek T. Quantification of lumbar intradiscal deformation during flexion and extension, by mathematical analysis of magnetic resonance imaging pixel intensity profiles. *Spine*.1997;22:2066-2072.

9. Edmondston SJ, Song S, Bricknell RV, et al. MRI evaluation of lumbar spine flexion and extension in asymptomatic individuals. *Man Ther*. 2000;5:158-164.

10. Petersen T, Larsen K, Nordsteen J, Olsen S, Fournier G, Jacobsen S. The McKenzie method compared with manipulation when used adjunctive to information and advice in low back pain patients presenting with centralization or peripheralization: a randomized controlled trial. *Spine*. 2011;36:1999-2010.

11. Werneke MW, Hart DL, Cutrone G, et al. Association between directional preference and centralization in patients with low back pain. *J Orthop Sports Phys Ther*. 2011;41:22-31.

12. Long A, Donelson R, Fung T. Does it matter which exercise? A randomized control trial of exercise for low back pain. *Spine*. 2004;29:2593-2602.

13. Long A, May S, Fung T. The comparative prognostic value of directional preference and centralization: a useful tool for front-line clinicians? *J Man Manip Ther*. 2008;16:248-254.

14. Clare HA, Adams R, Maher CG. A systematic review of efficacy of McKenzie therapy for spinal pain. *Aust J Physiother*. 2004;50:209-216.

15. Browder DA, Childs JD, Cleland JA, Fritz JM. Effectiveness of an extension-oriented treatment approach in a subgroup of subjects with low back pain: a randomized clinical trial. *Phys Ther*. 2007;87:1608-1618.

Lumbar Spine: Herniated Disc—*Ola Grimsby Approach*

Shelly Coffman

A 36-year-old male construction worker self-referred to an outpatient physical therapy clinic with a complaint of low back pain and pain radiating from his posterior left hip all the way to his lateral foot. He first experienced pain 3 weeks ago while doing a home maintenance project. The onset of pain occurred when he attempted to lift an air conditioning unit. He reports that as he bent over to lift the unit, he experienced an intense, stabbing pain and immediately fell to the ground. He required assistance from his wife to walk back into the house. For the first 24 hours after the incident, he rested prone on a couch or on his bed. Over the past 3 days, he reports an improved tolerance to walking and standing for short periods. However, he rates his current pain level 5 out of 10 on the visual analog scale and he continues to experience radiating pain distal to his knee. Signs and symptoms are consistent with a lumbar herniated disc. His goal is to return to work as soon as possible.

► Based on the patient's suspected diagnosis, what do you anticipate may be the contributing factors to his condition?
► What examination signs may be associated with this diagnosis?
► What are the most appropriate physical therapy interventions?
► What are possible complications that may limit the effectiveness of physical therapy?

KEY DEFINITIONS

JOINT MOBILIZATION: Manual therapy technique comprised passive motions directed at a joint at varying speeds, amplitudes, and hold times

MANUAL THERAPY: Skilled, hands-on techniques designed to diagnose and treat soft tissue and joint structures

OLA GRIMSBY APPROACH: Norwegian-based orthopaedic physical therapy postgraduate training program that emphasizes manual therapy and exercise prescription

SOFT TISSUE MOBILIZATION: Manual therapy technique comprised directional manual force aimed at improving soft tissue mobility

Objectives

1. Describe the Ola Grimsby-based manual therapy approach to the diagnosis of musculoskeletal dysfunction and selection of conservative interventions.

2. Describe the evidence for the efficacy of using Ola Grimsby-based manual therapy approach to treat the patient with low back pain due to a herniated nucleus pulposus.

Physical Therapy Considerations

PT considerations during management of the individual with a diagnosis of a herniated lumbar disc:

▶ **General physical therapy plan of care/goals:** Decrease pain; increase muscular flexibility; increase lower quadrant strength; improve motor recruitment and endurance of global and local stabilizers of the core region; prevent or minimize loss of aerobic fitness capacity; restore normal joint and soft tissue mechanics; improve vascularity to increase blood flow/oxygenation to local soft tissue to aid in tissue repair

▶ **Physical therapy interventions:** Patient education regarding functional anatomy and injury pathomechanics and effective body mechanics; manual therapy techniques; neuromuscular facilitation and re-education techniques; muscular flexibility exercises; exercises to increase muscular endurance of global and local core stabilizers and to increase strength of lower extremity musculature; aerobic exercise program prescription; Scientific Therapeutic Exercise Progression (STEP)

▶ **Precautions during physical therapy:** Monitor vital signs; address precautions or contraindications for exercise, based on patient's pre-existing condition(s)

▶ **Complications interfering with physical therapy:** Occupational duties that require the patient to assume a flexed lumbar spine

Physical Therapy Patient/Client Management

Joint and soft tissue mobilization techniques are forms of manual therapy utilized by many healthcare practitioners including physical therapists. The goal of manual physical therapy is to restore mobility to hypomobile (also known as "restricted") joints and to reduce muscle tension in tight muscles in order to return the patient to more optimal movement patterns with reduced pain. Manual physical therapy may help reduce acute or chronic pain and/or other symptoms associated with joint dysfunction and soft tissue injuries in the lumbar spine.

The purpose of this case is to describe the Ola Grimsby assessment and treatment approach for a patient with a suspected herniated nucleus pulposus (HNP). The Ola Grimsby manual therapy approach arose out of the Norwegian model of diagnosis and treatment of movement dysfunction. The clinician assesses the subjective degree of joint play (passive accessory motion) using the Kaltenborn 0 to VI grading scale (0 is an ankylosed joint, III is a joint with normal passive mobility, VI is a pathologically unstable joint).[1] Joint mobilization techniques for hypomobile joints are indicated for pain and receptor inhibition, collagen deformation, joint lubrication, and/or freeing an entrapment (*e.g.*, meniscoid entrapment in which the fibroadipose pad within a facet joint becomes entrapped).[2] Treatment is directed toward the patient's current condition and specific pathology. The patient's posture and active movements inform the physical therapist which positions are the most comfortable and may promote relief of mechanical and/or chemical stresses. Thus, the decision to flex, extend, side bend, or rotate the spine depends on the tissue in which the therapist is trying to facilitate repair and healing, as well as what is most comfortable for the patient. Vascularity exercises are a key component of the Ola Grimsby approach and are often the first exercises prescribed. With an acute or chronic injury to an intervertebral disc, the concentration of glycosaminoglycans (GAGs), a diverse group of polysaccharides that are an integral component of the nucleus pulposus matrix, increases.[3,4] Because GAGs have negative charges, an increase in their concentration can induce osmotic swelling.[5] The goal of vascularity exercises is to help direct the swelling that accumulates around a herniated disc *away* from the nerve tissue.[6] In a prospective study of 21 patients with computed tomography-diagnosed lumbar HNP, Delauche-Cavallier et al.[7] demonstrated that decreased HNP size correlated with decreased nerve root pain following conservative treatment.

Exercise has always been an integral part of the treatment plan in the Norwegian manual therapy model. The STEP model of exercise originated from the Norwegian medical exercise therapy. In STEP, a specific dosage of exercise (*e.g.*, repetitions, rest periods between repetitions, amount of resistance, sets, etc.) is chosen to train for a "functional quality." Functional qualities refer to the vascularity, endurance and strength of involved tissues, muscular volume, speed of movement, and power. The selection and manipulation of exercise variables is necessary to establish the optimal stimuli for tissue repair and regeneration, pain inhibition, reduction in muscular guarding, and improved joint range of motion. For all exercise programs, it is important not to further aggravate a system that is already metabolically challenged by repairing injured tissues. The Ola Grimsby approach emphasizes starting exercises slowly for nerves that are likely ischemic due to high local GAG content and muscular guarding.[8] For example, with the current patient, his initial injury 3 weeks ago started the sequence of muscle guarding and increased GAG content around the injured disc tissue and the foramen that the nerve is exiting. Thus, pain and nerve compression are inhibiting motor function, so initial exercises should *not* be aimed at improving strength. Instead, relative rest and early general activity are encouraged to facilitate reduction in GAG concentration and improvement in neurologic signs. In this acute stage (1-7 days),[9] it is imperative not to apply heat or any modality that significantly increases circulation to the area because this will promote inflammation. Early in the acute stage, gentle vascularity exercises to promote blood flow and bring oxygen to this hypoxic tissue are ideal. As the patient emerges from the acute state, he enters a mixed state in which the nerve is less compressed and more irritated—this is the early chronic stage.[10] Articulations (*e.g.*, joint mobilization techniques) to restore joint mobility, avoid adhesions, and maintain motion should be incorporated. Spinal mobilizations should not be applied until more than 4 days after the initial injury.[11] Joint mobilizations are indicated when active and/or passive joint motions are limited, painful, or demonstrate a capsular end feel or loss of accessory motion. Joint mobilization techniques may increase available joint mobility, reduce pain, improve joint lubrication and nutrition, inhibit muscular guarding via inhibitory afferents, and improve proprioceptive awareness.[1]

Examination, Evaluation, and Diagnosis

The Ola Grimsby approach to musculoskeletal rehabilitation utilizes a **Diagnostic Pyramid** for each patient (Fig. 18-1). The Diagnostic Pyramid evolved from Dr. James Cyriax's differential evaluation method.[12] The Diagnostic Pyramid outlines a systematic approach to assess potential tissues involved to reach an accurate clinical diagnosis. It is not designed to be an all-inclusive examination method to diagnose any potential impairment. Rather, it is meant to act as a guide to direct further investigation and assessment. A clinical diagnosis must be made based on the history (comorbidities, subjective report), observations of the patient, and the physical examination findings. The elements of the Diagnostic Pyramid include: initial observation, thorough history and interview, structural inspection, active, passive, and resisted motions, examining joints proximal and distal to the involved region(s), and palpation. Each layer of tissue (from the skin to the bone) should be assessed for one or more of the following: color, temperature, pain, and quality of tissue. Assessment includes neurologic screening (dermatomes, myotomes, deep tendon reflexes), special tests to further refine working diagnoses, joint play, and segmental play (determined by assessing 3-5 oscillations per spinal segment). Available imaging information is also incorporated into the differential diagnosis. The compilation of all this information helps the physical therapist determine the involved tissue/s (referred to as "tissue/s in lesion") and arrive at a strong diagnosis.

It may be useful to walk through how a physical therapist would use the Diagnostic Pyramid to organize the physical examination. First, the physical therapist initiates the examination by observing the patient (at the bottom of the Diagnostic Pyramid, Fig. 18-1). This includes how the patient moves, the presence of an antalgic gait,

∆ The Diagnostic Pyramid ∆

Facility: _____ Date: _____
Patient: _____ Therapist: _____
Medical Diagnosis: _____

Summation of Tissue(s) in lesion	SKIN	SUB CUTANEOUS	LIGAMENT FASCIA	MUSCLE TENDON	JOINT CAPSULE	BURSA	JOINT CARTL	JOINT ENTRAP	NERVE	DISC	BONE	VASCULAR	META-BOLISM
X-RAY/LAB MR/CAT/EMG	144	145	146	147	148	149	150	151	152	153	154	155	156
SEGMENTAL PALY	131	132	133	134	135	136	137	138	139	140	141	142	143
JOINT PALY	118	119	120	121	122-extremity	123	124	125-blocked	126	127	128	129	130
SPECIAL TESTS	105	106	107	108	109	110	111	112	113	114	115	116	117
NEURO TESTS	92	93	94	95	96	97	98	99	100	101	102	103	104
PALPATION	79	80	81	82	83	84	85	86	87	88	89	90	91
RESISTED MOTION	66	67	68	69	70-Spine	71	72	73	74	75	76	77	78
PASSIVE MOTION	53	54	55	56	57	58	59	60	61	62	63	64	65
ACTIVE MOTION	40	41	42	43	44	45	46	47	48	49	50	51	52
STRUCTURAL INSPECTION	27	28	29	30	31	32	33	34	35	36	37	38	39
HISTORY INTERVIEW	14	15	16	17	18	19	20	21	22	23	24	25	26
INITIAL OBSERVATION	1	2	3	4	5	6	7	8	9	10	11	12	13
	SKIN	SUB CUTANEOUS	LIGAMENT FASCIA	MUSCLE TENDON	JOINT CAPSULE	BURSA	JOINT CARTL	JOINT ENTRAP	NERVE	DISC	BONE	VASCULAR	META-BOLISM

KEY

+	Positive means indicative of the tissue
x	Eliminated
o	More testing (or clarifying tests) required

? Test (information) does not determine the tissue
- It is not indicative of the tissue
Test does not apply to the ELIMINATION of tissue
Tissue eliminated or confirmed by this block

Figure 18-1. The Ola Grimsby Diagnostic Pyramid designed to assist the physical therapist in arriving at an accurate clinical diagnosis by providing a systematic approach to the examination of potentially involved tissues that may contribute to an individual's impairment or activity limitations. (Reproduced with permission from Grimsby O. *Clinical & Scientific Rationale for Modern Manual Therapy.* Ola Grimsby Institute. MT-1-page: EVAL7, 1998.)

speed of movement, etc. For example, when the current patient walked in the room, it was evident he had a lateral shift. In the bottom row labeled "Initial Observation," the therapist would place a "+" sign above each of the boxes labeled muscle tendon, joint capsule, bursa, joint cartilage, joint entrapment, nerve, and disc because at this point in the examination all seven of these structures are potential contributors to the observed antalgic gait. As the examination continues from the bottom of the Diagnostic Pyramid to the top, each box in each row is assessed for its potential contribution to the dysfunction and tissue in lesion. Once the therapist completes the assessment (*i.e.*, gets to the top of the Diagnostic Pyramid), the therapist can visually evaluate each column to determine the primary tissue in lesion (*i.e.*, the column with the most "+"s).

Postural assessment is performed with the patient in standing and is viewed from the front, side, and back. The patient in this case demonstrated a right lateral shift, a flattened thoracolumbar spine, and his left shoulder was positioned slightly lower than his right. With the patient still standing, lumbar spinal active range of motion can be assessed (noted as Active Motion in the leftmost column of the Diagnostic Pyramid). Flexion was decreased by 90% (limited by pain in the central low back area) and extension was decreased by 20% (with pain in the same distribution).

Neurologic assessment can be performed in sitting or supine, depending on the patient's comfort. For the current patient, his patellar reflex (L3-L4) was diminished on the left (1+) and normal on the right (2+).[13] Myotome testing performed in sitting revealed involvement of L4 and L5 myotomes indicated by weakness in the right anterior tibialis and extensor hallucis longus. There was no weakness noted during the remaining manual muscle tests in bilateral lower extremities. The patient also demonstrated diminished sensation (to light touch and pinprick) in the right L5 and S1 dermatomes.

Palpation revealed significant trigger points within the L3-L4 paravertebral musculature, right T12 facet, right quadratus lumborum, and left psoas. Pelvic imbalance was noted via palpation of the anterior superior iliac spines, posterior superior iliac spines, and the ischial tuberosities in standing, supine, and prone. Skin rolling demonstrated a significant decrease in fascial mobility in the central region from L1 to L5. Skin rolling is a manual technique that has been reported to assess fascial mobility.[14] It involves consecutively rolling the skin layers between the therapist's fingers.

Based on the patient's subjective history and positive neurologic findings (L4-L5 myotomal, dermatomal, and deep tendon reflex involvement), several special tests were performed to further elucidate the neurologic involvement. The patient had a positive straight leg raise test bilaterally at 60° with sharp central low back pain. This finding is suggestive of significant sciatic nerve irritability.[15,16] Cram's test was also performed. Cram's test is similar to a straight leg raise test. The therapist passively flexes the patient's hip to 120° with the knee flexed and provides thumb pressure to the popliteal fossa. While applying consistent pressure, the therapist passively extends the knee while maintaining the hip flexion. A positive Cram's test is pain (usually in the back) with the knee extended and consistent thumb pressure at the popliteal fossa. This patient had a positive Cram's test on the right, indicative of a disc lesion.[17] A positive Slump test (more pain with left knee extended than right knee extended) also suggested neural irritability in the lumbosacral spine.[18] Prone knee bend testing, a neural tension test for upper lumbar nerve root involvement,[19] was negative. Last, a disc shear test was performed. This is a manual test in which the patient is positioned in sidelying with his hips and knees flexed. The therapist stabilizes one lumbar segment and mobilizes the segment below in an anteroposterior direction. A positive disc shear test is indicated by the perception of increased joint mobility and potentially a reproduction of pain. The patient had a positive disc shear test at L4-L5, suggesting disc compromise.[20]

One of the hallmarks of the Ola Grimsby approach is **assessing passive spinal joint mobility** (passive intervertebral motions or PIVMs) with the patient in the sidelying position instead of prone. This position allows the therapist to have both hands on the vertebral segment being assessed and to take up tissue tension by flexing the patient's hips and lumbar spine. It has been hypothesized that this position better isolates the segment being evaluated than the prone position. The therapist applies 3 to 5 oscillations (in flexion, extension, rotation, or side bending) per segment to determine the degree of passive mobility.[21-24] While frequently performed by clinicians to identify hypo- or hypermobility, the diagnostic utility of manually assessing spinal joint mobility has been questioned. In 2005, Abbot et al.[25] had 27 physiotherapists with advanced manual therapy training assess passive accessory intervertebral motion (PAIVM) and passive physiological intervertebral motion (PPIVM) in 123 patients with recurrent chronic low back pain. The examiners scored each subject's spinal joint mobility using an ordinal scale. Flexion-extension radiographs were also performed for each subject to measure sagittal angular rotation and sagittal translation. To determine the specificity and sensitivity of manual segmental mobility assessment, each therapist's manual assessment scores were compared to a criterion standard for instability in the lumbar spine (flexion-extension radiographs). While PPIVMs were specific for both rotation (0.97-0.99) and translation (0.98-0.995) lumbar segmental instability, the sensitivity of PPIVMs for rotation (0.05-0.22) and translation (0.05-0.16) lumbar segmental instability was very low. These results revealed that PPIVM testing by experienced manual therapists accurately identified patients who did not present with a lumbar instability, but did not accurately identify patients who did present with lumbar instability. Similar results were found using PAIVMs. PAIVM tests were specific (0.88-0.89), but not sensitive (0.29-0.33). For further discussion of the accuracy of PIVM testing, see Case 15. For the patient in this case, mobility testing revealed Grade I+ (significant) hypomobility from T12 to L3 in flexion. Grade II (moderate) hypomobility was found in L3-L4 left rotation (which was also painful), T10-L4 in right rotation (assessed in left sidelying), and L4-L5 in extension. Grade IV (moderate) hypermobility was found in L4-L5 flexion testing.

Based on the history, observation, and physical findings gleaned from working through the Diagnostic Pyramid, this patient was hypothesized to have an L4-L5 annular tear with concomitant segmental instability. The identified impairments were pain, aberrant posture, altered segmental mobility (both hypo- and hypermobilities), decreased soft tissue mobility with muscular guarding, decreased work performance, and limited ability to perform activities of daily living (ADLs).

Plan of Care and Interventions

The treatment goals for the patient with a suspected L4-L5 HNP are to enhance lumbosacral dynamic stability, improve joint and soft tissue mobility, and fully restore his ability to work and perform ADLs. For this particular patient with identified upper lumbar mobility restriction, joint mobilizations are utilized to increase joint mobility and a muscle energy technique (MET) is incorporated to address the noted pelvic imbalance resulting from tight thoracolumbar and lumbopelvic musculature. In addition to using joint and soft tissue mobilizations, STEP exercise instruction and progression is incorporated to train for each functional quality (Table 18-1). Core strengthening and stabilization exercise progression are also included. The utilization of exercise as medicine is an important concept in the Ola Grimsby approach and the STEP exercise model. Exercise is specifically dosed with respect to the patient's current level of impairment. This means that the exercises should not exacerbate the patient's baseline pain. In addition, the exercises should be dosed with specific awareness of the patient's current metabolic reserve—that is, the amount of energy he has available for additional cellular processes beyond that required for normal bodily functions and tissue repair.[26]

STEP is an exercise therapy strategy combining the use of specifically designed equipment (without manual assistance) with exercises performed by the patient under the constant supervision of the physical therapist. It is important that the equipment is designed to optimally stimulate the relevant functional systems of the body (neuromuscular, joints, circulatory, respiratory) and to specifically target the affected tissue/s in lesion identified in the evaluation. To achieve this effect, the patient carries out the exercises from a defined starting position (determined by the physical therapist) in a specific movement direction in full or partial range of movement against a graded amount of resistance. The exercise program is designed specifically and individually for the patient based on muscle, joint, and functional testing, as well as the patient's specific diagnosis. STEP also includes reassessment of the program on every visit based on the objective findings for that day. Specific dosage of exercise is based upon the 1 repetition maximum (RM) principle[27] with chosen resistance based as percentages of the 1 RM. The application of exercise as outlined in STEP principles requires prior understanding of muscle and joint assessment. It has been recommended that formal training in manual therapy is necessary for utilizing STEP because its application is considered a combination of manual therapy and a sophisticated understanding of biomechanical and force loading principles.[28]

The use of STEP has been shown to increase function and reduce disability in adults with chronic low back pain and in adults postdiscectomy.[29-31] In a study of postsurgical discectomy patients assigned to an 8-week medical exercise therapy regimen starting 4 weeks after surgery, pain and disability were reduced significantly from baseline (presurgery). More patients in the medical exercise group reported better health at 6 and 12 months after surgery than those in a group that only performed gentle home exercises. The exercise program enabled patients to become independently mobile more rapidly than patients who participated in the limited

Table 18-1 SUMMARY OF STEP RESISTANCE TRAINING RECOMMENDATIONS AND PROGRESSION FOR THE PATIENT WITH A LUMBAR HNP

Functional Quality	Selection	Sequence	Resistance	Volume	Rest Intervals	Frequency
Tissue Repair Pain and Edema Reduction	Single joint	Away from pain, or not into pain	Initiate assisted, or 0% of 1RM, up to 50% of 1RM Initially, 0%-10% of 1RM, progress to 50% of 1RM	1-5 sets, 10-60 reps/set. Start with 2 sets of 10-15 reps, assess response. Increase toward 30-50 reps quickly, as tolerated.	>1 minute	1-5 times/d; 7 d/wk Attempt to do 2-5 times/d initially as pain allows
Mobilization	Single joint	First distraction, to inhibit pain and joint compression. Progress into joint gliding	Assisted up to 50% of 1RM. Initiate 0% of 1RM, progress toward 50% of 1RM	1-5 sets, 10-60 reps/set. For collagen deformation/creep, 3 to 5-sec holds. For this patient: Initiate small range of motion and high reps (2 sets of 15-20 reps) for gentle mobilization; progress to 20-50 reps	None	1-5 times/d; 7 d/wk
Coordination	Single joint and multi-joint exercise	Balance exercise first, then single plane exercise, progressing to tri-planar combined motions and PNF patterns	Assisted up to 50% of 1RM. For this patient, start approximately 30% of 1RM, progress to 50% of 1RM	2-5 sets, 10-50 reps/set. For this patient: Start 2 sets of 10 reps, progressing toward 20-30 reps/set	1 minute	1-3 times/d; 7 d/wk
Vascularity	Single joint and multi-joint exercise	Initially into guarded pattern, then progress to away from muscular guarding	55%-65% of 1RM	1-3 sets of 20-30 reps For this patient: Start 2 sets of 20 reps, progressing toward 30 reps	Acute: Until respiration returns to steady state. Subacute: > 30 s	Once a day; 7 d/wk

(Continued)

Table 18-1 SUMMARY OF STEP RESISTANCE TRAINING RECOMMENDATIONS AND PROGRESSION FOR THE PATIENT WITH A LUMBAR HNP (CONTINUED)

Functional Quality	Selection	Sequence	Resistance	Volume	Rest Intervals	Frequency
Endurance	Single joint and multi-joint exercise	For small and large muscle groups, diverse variety of sequencing	50%-70% of 1RM For this patient: Initiate 50% of 1RM and quickly progress toward 70% of 1RM.	1-3 sets, 20-30 reps/set. Start with 2 sets of 20 reps.	1-2 min for high rep sets (>20). <1min for <15 reps	2-3 times/wk for beginner/acute. Progress to 3-4 times/wk as pain reduces.
Hypertrophy	Single joint and multi-joint exercise	Small > large muscle groups Single joint > multi-joint Lower intensity > higher intensity	60%-80% of 1RM For this patient: 60%-70% of 1RM. Progress toward 80% at discharge to independent HEP.	2-3 sets of 6-12 reps	1-2 min	2-3 times/wk to start. Progress to 2-4 times/wk
Strength	Primarily multi-joint exercise	Small > large muscle groups Single joint > multi-joint Lower intensity > higher intensity	60%-80% of 1RM For this patient: 60%-70% of 1RM. Progress toward 80% at discharge to independent HEP.	1-3 sets of 6-12 reps	1-2 min except core musculature should be 2-3 min	2-3 times/wk to start. Progress to 2-4 times/wk

Reproduced with permission from Rivard J, Grimsby O. Science, Theory and Clinical Application in Orthopaedic Manual Physical Therapy. The Academy of Graduate Physical Therapy, Inc. Volume 3, page xiv, 2009.

home exercise regimen, as well as enabling them to return to work sooner than their later exercising controls.[29]

Initially, the plan of care for this patient would include treatments twice per week, decreasing to once per week as his symptoms and functional level improve. On the initial visit, it is important to focus on patient education regarding posture, pathoanatomy, body mechanics, and disc and joint mechanics. A patient's understanding of his current condition and treatment expectations can lead to better compliance and overall outcomes. Vascularity exercises to decrease local GAG concentrations may be the only exercises prescribed on the first visit. A common vascularity exercise for low back pain is to have the patient in the sidelying position and ask him to gently rotate his pelvis and low back in a small range of motion while keeping his upper body stable on the mat or floor. This exercise contracts and relaxes the paravertebral musculature, with the twofold goal of moving chemical inflammatory mediators out of the local region and moving blood flow and oxygen into the injured tissues. To avoid aggravating the current inflammatory process, the patient is advised to avoid heat modalities. To reduce inflammation, the patient is encouraged to use ice and engage in general movement.

On the second therapy visit, the focus is on neuromuscular inhibition. The therapist can use soft tissue mobilization and/or hold/relax techniques to decrease muscle spasms and normalize motor recruitment and joint mobilization techniques to decrease tonic muscular guarding. A muscle energy technique to address the noted quadratus lumborum tightness and/or spasms and pelvic imbalance may aid in restoring normal function at a more rapid rate. With the patient in the supine position, the right hip is passively flexed with the knee flexed. The patient is asked to attempt to move his hip into hip extension while the therapist provides resistance to this motion. This isometric hamstring contraction is held for roughly 10 seconds and repeated 3 times. The contraction of the hamstring muscles will pull the right hemipelvis (ilium, acetabulum, ischium, and pubis) into posterior rotation, resisting the anterior pull of the currently spasmed quadratus lumborum. Core flexion and extension stabilization exercises should also be added to the home exercise program (HEP) to enable greater functional gains and daily stimulus for repair.

Treatment qualities in the STEP program that are emphasized early are endurance and strength. On the third visit, the resisted STEP program was initiated because at this stage pain levels were diminished, movement was less guarded, and the lateral shift was decreased, all indicative of a reduction in inflammation. Three exercises were initiated: drinking bird (Fig. 18-2), incline sit-up (Fig. 18-3), and sitting rotation (Fig. 18-4). Since this patient is exiting the acute phase, the goal is for endurance and neuromuscular retraining. Each exercise is performed for 20 to 30 repetitions and 2 to 3 sets. None of these exercises should exacerbate his pain. As the patient improves and is able to tolerate some of the previously painful positions and activities for limited periods (*e.g.*, improvement in sitting tolerance, sleeping, standing, etc.), the STEP program should be progressed to include motions with combined flexion/rotation resisted exercises, with more focus on strengthening exercises.

Combined extension and rotation exercises are added on later visits, since this combined position close-packs the facet joints. Thoracolumbar extension mobilization

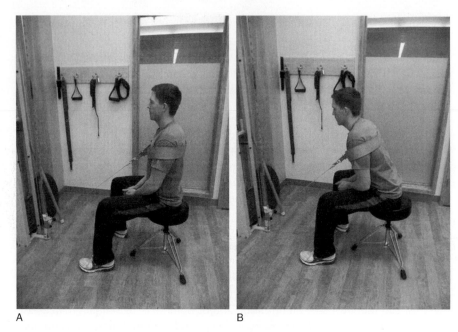

A   B

Figure 18-2. Drinking bird exercise. **A.** Patient begins exercise seated on a stool with hips and knees at 90° with a strap around his trunk at chest height, attached to the weighted pulley system, with the pull of the weight down at a 45° angle. **B.** The therapist instructs the patient to maintain an erect posture, and flex forward at the hips, bending to an approximately 45° angle. This exercise activates the erector spinae bilaterally, working eccentrically on forward bending and concentrically on return from the flexed position. In order for this movement to occur, the patient needs to slowly eccentrically contract the spinal extensors while bending forward against resistance provided by the weighted pulley system. The goal is to strengthen the erector spinae and stabilize the lower lumbar segments against the weight of the trunk and gravity, which is particularly important in ADL function. The exercise should always be performed in a pain-free range of motion; if it is painful for the patient to move the full 45° excursion, limitation of the range is indicated.

exercises can be added to facilitate improved movement availability *away* from his hypermobile lumbar region. Because this patient was stiff from T12 to L3 and hypermobile below these segments, an appropriate exercise is having the patient sit on a chair, maintaining maximal hip and lower lumbar flexion. With hands clasped behind his neck, the patient attempts to lift the trunk by pointing his elbows forward, but maintaining lower lumbar flexion. The goal of this exercise is to mobilize the upper lumbar segments while protecting the lower lumbar spine (Fig. 18-5). Overall progression of the STEP program toward strength and endurance continues with eccentric strengthening to facilitate greater stability and receptor activity around joint structures.

As the disc tissue repairs and the patient is able to initiate and progress the strengthening program, his functional abilities should vastly improve. Neural signs should be fairly resolved in this state. In the later stages of this episode of care, focus should be

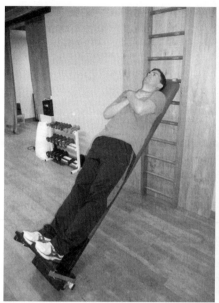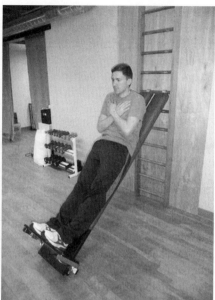

A   B

Figure 18-3. Incline sit-up exercise. **A.** The patient is supine on the inclined board with arms crossed across the chest. For initial treatments, the board is inclined more toward the vertical to ease the workload against gravity and at a level that the patient can successfully engage trunk flexors/abdominals in a slow and controlled fashion. **B.** The patient is asked to attempt to intentionally flex one vertebrae at a time up off the board, moving slowly through the range of motion until he has moved through the sacrum. He is then directed to sit tall as if being pulled toward the ceiling, then to reverse the movement, laying one vertebrae at a time back on the board, starting with the sacrum until he is again flat on the board. This exercise engages the upper and lower abdominals while minimizing psoas activation and emphasizes thoracolumbar flexion mobilization and flexion/extension joint coordination. The goal of this exercise is to self-mobilize T12-L3 segments that were found to be hypomobile in physiologic and passive flexion by actively engaging the abdominal muscles and moving through the directed range of motion over a number of repetitions.

on the identified lower thoracic and upper lumbar rotation and flexion restrictions. Joint mobilizations should be incorporated to restore normal movement patterns. For the HEP, the STEP focuses on endurance at higher weights, inclusion of power as a functional quality to be trained toward, and an overall increased level of challenge. Prior to discharge from physical therapy, the treatment plan should focus on postural strength and endurance, as well as education regarding continued self-care, ergonomics, and the incorporation of rest breaks to prevent or decrease the likelihood of recurrent bouts of back pain.

This case presented current evidence for use of the Ola Grimsby approach to manage a patient with a lumbar HNP. In Cases 15, 16, and 17, the utilization of a muscle energy technique, the use of mechanical traction, and the use of Mechanical Diagnosis and Therapy (MDT or McKenzie), are presented.

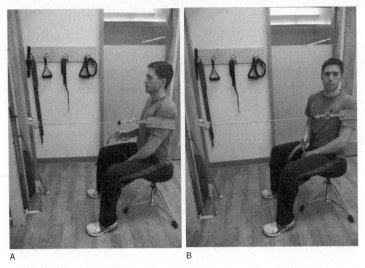

Figure 18-4. Sitting spinal rotation exercise. **A.** Patient begins exercise seated on a stool with hips and knees at 90° with a weighted strap around the outside of one shoulder and down to the opposite waist angle, where the right hand is holding the other end of the strap. The pull of the weight stack is directly in front of the patient's shoulder on which the strap rests. **B.** The patient is instructed to slowly rotate his trunk to the left against the resistance while keeping his pelvis anchored and balanced on the stool. The goal of this exercise is to enhance dynamic coordination around a thoracic and lumbar rotatory axis, engaging the multifidi concentrically and eccentrically.

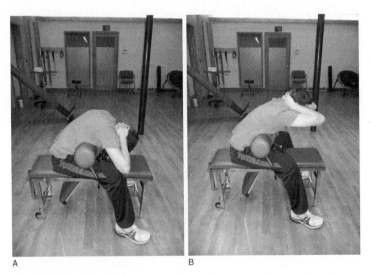

Figure 18-5. Thoracolumbar mobilization exercise. **A.** Patient begins the exercise straddling a bench with his spine flexed over a firm roll, feet in front of knees to move center of motion forward, and hands clasped gently behind his head with elbows pointing toward floor. **B.** The patient moves his elbows down toward the floor and then slowly lifts elbows parallel with the floor while maintaining lower lumbar flexion (keeping a flexion moment over the roll), which creates a mobilization moment through the lower thoracic spine, just anterior to the bolster placement. The purpose of this exercise is to self-mobilize the identified stiff thoracolumbar junction while protecting the lower lumbar spine, and therefore direct stress away from the hypermobile lower lumbar region and provide additional movement options besides the lumbar spine by creating greater thoracolumbar mobility.

Evidence-Based Clinical Recommendations

SORT: Strength of Recommendation Taxonomy

A: Consistent, good-quality patient-oriented evidence
B: Inconsistent or limited-quality patient-oriented evidence
C: Consensus, disease-oriented evidence, usual practice, expert opinion, or case series

1. The Diagnostic Pyramid outlines a systematic approach to direct the examination and the potential tissues involved in a patient's clinical presentation. **Grade C**

2. When assessed by a trained manual therapist, passive intervertebral motions have high specificity but poor sensitivity compared to intervertebral motion as measured by flexion-extension radiographs. **Grade B**

3. The Ola Grimsby STEP reduces disability, decreases pain, and improves ADL function in patients with low back pain. **Grade B**

COMPREHENSION QUESTIONS

18.1 Functional qualities to be trained for in STEP exercise program include all of the following *except:*

A. Strength

B. Endurance

C. Balance

D. Vascularity

18.2 Eccentric strengthening is an important part of the STEP training program:

A. In the beginning to improve vascularity

B. Toward the end of the program to improve receptor activity

C. Toward the end of the program to improve overall power

D. In the middle of the program to transition from endurance to strength

ANSWERS

18.1 **C.** Balance is not a functional quality trained for in STEP.

18.2 **B.** Eccentric strengthening exercises are added toward the end of a program. Eccentrics add a degree of difficulty and aid in receptor training that helps joint stability, not power (option C). Eccentric training would be too aggressive to incorporate in the beginning of a therapeutic exercise program (option A).

REFERENCES

1. Kaltenborn F. *Manual Mobilization of the Joints. Volume 11: The Spine*. 4th ed. Oslo: Olaf Norlis Bokhandel; 2002.

2. Fryer G. Intervertebral dysfunction: a discussion of the manipulable spinal lesion. *J Osteopath Med*. 2003;6:64-73.

3. Hendry NG. The hydration of the nucleus pulposus and its relation to intervertebral disc derangement. *J Bone Joint Surg Br*. 1958;40-B:132-144.

4. Ishihara H, Warensjo K, Roberts S, Urban JP. Proteoglycan synthesis in the intervertebral disk nucleus: the role of extracellular osmolality. *Am J Physiol*. 1997;272:C1499-C1506.

5. Roberts S, Urban JP, Evans H, Eisenstein SM. Transport properties of the human cartilage endplate in relation to its composition and calcification. *Spine*. 1996;21:415-420.

6. Castro WH, Assheuer J, Schulitz KP. Haemodynamic changes in lumbar nerve root entrapment due to stenosis and/or herniated disc of the lumbar spinal canal—a magnetic resonance imaging study. *Eur Spine J*. 1995;4:220-225

7. Delauche-Cavallier MC, Budet C, Laredo JD, et al. Lumbar disc herniation. Computed tomography scan changes after conservative treatment of nerve root compression. *Spine*. 1992;17:927-933.

8. Inkinen RI, Lammi MJ, Lehnonen S, Puustjarvi K, Kaapa E, Tammi MI. Relative increase of biglycan and decorin and altered chondroitin sulfate epitopes in the degenerating human intervertebral disc. *J Rheumatol*. 1998;25:506-514.

9. Akeson W, Woo S, Amiel D, Coutts, R, Daniel D. The connective tissue response to immobility. *Clin Orthop Rel Res*. 1973;93:356-361.

10. Grimsby O. Residency course curriculum. *Manual Therapy Part I*, Jan, 1991.

11. Grimsby O, Rivard J. *Science, Theory and Clinical Application in Orthopaedic Manual Physical Therapy*. The Academy of Graduate Physical Therapy; 2008.

12. Pettman E. A history of manipulative therapy. *JMMT*. 2007;15:165-174.

13. Hislop HJ, Montgomery J. *Daniels and Worthingham's Muscle Testing: Techniques of Manual Examination*. 8th ed. St. Louis, MO: Saunders Elsevier; 2007.

14. Sherman KJ, Dixon MW, Thompson D, Cherkin DC. Development of a taxonomy to describe massage treatments for musculoskeletal pain. *BMC Complement Altern Med*. 2006;6:24.

15. Rabin A, Gerszten PC, Karausky P, Bunker CH, Potter DM, Welch WC. The sensitivity of the seated straight-leg raise test compared with the supine straight-leg raise test in patients presenting with magnetic resonance imaging evidence of lumbar nerve root compression. *Arch Phys Med Rehabil*. 2007;88:840-843.

16. Deville WL, van der Windt DA, Dzaferagic A, Bezemer PD, Bouter LM. The test of Lasegue: systematic review of the accuracy in diagnosing herniated discs. *Spine*. 2000;25:1140-1147.

17. Solomon J, Nadler SF, Press J. Physical exam of the lumbar spine. In: Malanga GA, ed. *Musculoskeletal Physical Examination: An Evidence-based Approach*. Philadelphia, PA: Elsevier Mosby; 2006:189-226.

18. Majlesi J, Togay H, Unalan H, Toprak S. The sensitivity and specificity of the slump and the straight leg raising tests in patients with lumbar disc herniation. *J Clin Rheumatol*. 2008;14:87-91.

19. Herron LD, Pheasant HC. Prone knee-flexion provocative testing for lumbar disc protrusion. *Spine*. 1980;5:65-67.

20. Laslett M, Aprill CN, McDonald B, Young SB. Diagnosis of sacroiliac joint pain: validity of individual provocation tests and composites of tests. *Man Ther*. 2005;10:207-218.

21. Ola Grimsby Residency Course Notes, Chapter 14, Lumbar Spine, P. 100. Ola Grimsby Institute 2004.

22. Keating JC Jr, Bergmann TF, Jacobs GE, Finer BA, Larson K. Interexaminer reliability of eight evaluative dimensions of lumbar segmental abnormality. *J Manipulative Physiol Ther*. 1990;13:463-470.

23. Strender LE, Sjoblom A, Sundell K, Ludwig R, Taube A. Interexaminer reliability in physical examination of patients with low back pain. *Spine*. 1997;22:814-820.

24. Abbot JH. Lumbar segmental hypomobility: criterion-related validity of clinical examination items (a pilot study). *NZ J Physiother*. 2003;31:3-9.

25. Abbot JH, McCane B, Herbison P, Moginie G, Chapple C, Hogarty T. Lumbar segmental instability: a criterion-related validity study of manual therapy assessment. *BMC Musculoskelet Disord*. 2005;6:56.

26. Holten O, Faugli HP. *Medisinsk Treningsterapi (Medical Exercise Therapy)*. Ilniversitetsforlaaet. 0608 Oslo, Norway; 1996.

27. Delorme TL. Restoration of muscle power by heavy resistance exercises. *J Bone Joint Surg*. 1945;27:645-667.

28. Jacobsen F, Holten O, Faugli P, Leirvik R. Medical Exercise Therapy. *Fysioterapeuten*.1992;7:19-22.

29. Newsome RJ, May S, Chiverton N, Cole AA. A prospective, randomised trial of immediate exercise following lumbar microdiscectomy: a preliminary study. *Physiotherapy*. 2009;95:273-279.

30. Torstensen TA, Ljunggren AE, Meen HD, Odland E, Mowinckel P, Geijerstam S. Efficiency and costs of medical exercise therapy, conventional physiotherapy, and self exercises in patients with chronic low back pain: a pragmatic, randomized, single-blinded, controlled trial with 1-year follow-up. *Spine*.1998;23:2616-2624.

31. Danielsen JM, Johnsen R, Kibsgaard SK, Hellevik E. Early aggressive exercise for postoperative rehabilitation after disectomy. *Spine*. 2000;25:1015-1020.

Slipped Capital Femoral Epiphysis (SCFE)

Michael D. Ross
Kristi A. Greene

CASE 19

An 11-year-old female with a history of progressively worsening right knee pain for the past 5 months was referred to physical therapy. The patient has a body mass index of 24 kg/m² and her previous medical history is unremarkable. When she was evaluated by the physical therapist, the patient presented with an antalgic gait pattern with the right lower extremity in a slight externally rotated position. Her knee examination was unremarkable and testing did not reproduce her chief complaint of knee pain. However, the patient experienced anterolateral hip pain during examination of her right hip. Right hip flexion and internal rotation range of motion were limited both actively and passively and these motions reproduced her hip and knee pain. Based upon the history and physical examination findings, the physical therapist was concerned about a possible slipped capital femoral epiphysis.

▶ What examination signs may be associated with the diagnosis of a slipped capital femoral epiphysis?
▶ What are the examination priorities?
▶ Based on the patient's suspected diagnosis, what do you anticipate may be the contributing factors to her condition?
▶ What are the most appropriate physical therapy interventions?
▶ What is her rehabilitation prognosis?

KEY DEFINITIONS

IN SITU SURGICAL FIXATION: Standard treatment for a slipped capital femoral epiphysis in which a screw is placed through the physis and epiphysis to prevent further progression of the slip

KLEIN LINE: Method to assess for a slipped capital femoral epiphysis on the anterior to posterior hip radiograph by drawing a line along the superior border of the femoral neck; in a normal hip, the Klein line intersects a portion of the femoral epiphysis; in the individual with a slipped capital femoral epiphysis, the Klein line is level with, or lateral to, the epiphysis

SLIPPED CAPITAL FEMORAL EPIPHYSIS: Posterior and inferior displacement of the proximal femoral epiphysis (femoral head) on the metaphysis (femoral neck) through the proximal femoral physis (growth plate)

STABLE SLIPPED CAPITAL FEMORAL EPIPHYSIS: A slip classification in terms of mechanical stability in which the individual is able to bear weight with or without crutches but may walk with an antalgic gait

UNSTABLE SLIPPED CAPITAL FEMORAL EPIPHYSIS: A slip classification in terms of mechanical stability in which the slip is too painful and unstable to allow the individual to bear weight even with crutches

Objectives

1. Describe slipped capital femoral epiphysis and identify risk factors associated with this condition.
2. Identify appropriate diagnostic imaging that should be completed to rule in or rule out slipped capital femoral epiphysis.
3. Describe the most appropriate physical therapy interventions for a patient with a slipped capital femoral epiphysis.
4. Describe the prognosis for an individual with a slipped capital femoral epiphysis.

Physical Therapy Considerations

PT considerations during management of the individual with a suspected diagnosis of slipped capital femoral epiphysis:

▶ **General physical therapy plan of care/goals:** Prevent slip progression; avoid complications such as osteonecrosis and chondrolysis

▶ **Physical therapy interventions:** Patient education regarding functional anatomy and injury pathomechanics; instruct patient in a non-weightbearing gait pattern on the affected lower extremity; referral for radiographs; if radiographs confirm diagnosis of slipped capital femoral epiphysis, an urgent referral to an orthopaedic surgeon should be placed so appropriate surgical options can be considered in a timely manner

▶ **Precautions during physical therapy:** Avoid weightbearing on affected lower extremity

▶ **Complications interfering with physical therapy:** Slip progression, osteonecrosis, chondrolysis, development of a contralateral slipped capital femoral epiphysis

Understanding the Health Condition

Slipped capital femoral epiphysis (SCFE) occurs when there is posterior and inferior displacement of the proximal femoral epiphysis (femoral head) on the metaphysis (femoral neck).[1,2] The slip occurs through the proximal femoral physis (growth plate), usually as a result of chronic microfractures through the physis due to physiologic loading from rapid growth during adolescence.[3,4]

The overall incidence of SCFE for children between the ages of 9 and 16 years of age has been reported at 10.80 cases per 100,000 children, with a higher incidence in boys (13.35 cases per 100,000 children) versus girls (8.07 cases per 100,000 children).[5] The mean age at time of diagnosis is 12 and 13.5 years for girls and boys, respectively.[5] African American and Hispanic American children are more commonly affected than Caucasian children.[5,6]

Although the etiology is typically multifactorial, the result is an increase in shear stresses across a weakened physis. Anatomic risk factors for SCFE include retroversion of the femur, increased obliquity of the physis, and weakening of the perichondrial ring complex.[7] Biomechanical and biochemical factors are also important contributors to the development of an SCFE. The majority of affected individuals are above the 95th percentile for body mass index for their age (BMI-for-age).[8] The current patient has a BMI of 24, placing her BMI-for-age at the 94th percentile,[8] which was likely a contributing factor in the development of her SCFE. Increased body mass increases the shear forces across the physis, potentially leading to weakening and eventual displacement of the femoral epiphysis on the metaphysis. Individuals with an SCFE of one extremity are at increased risk of a contralateral SCFE as bilateral involvement may be seen in 20% to 50% of patients.[6,9] Slipped capital femoral epiphysis is occasionally associated with endocrine or metabolic disorders (e.g., hypothyroidism, hyperthyroidism, growth hormone deficiency, hypogonadism, panhypopituitarism, renal disease).[2] Therefore, individuals who do not fit the typical profile for SCFE (e.g., younger in age, low to normal BMI-for-age)[10] should be referred for evaluation for endocrine or metabolic disorders.[11]

Slipped capital femoral epiphysis is most commonly classified in terms of mechanical stability as either stable or unstable. Approximately 90% of SCFE cases are classified as stable.[10,12] Individuals with a stable SCFE are able to bear weight with or without crutches, but may walk with an antalgic gait.[13] Those individuals with an unstable SCFE are not able to bear weight even with crutches because the slip is too painful and unstable.[10] Classification of SCFE in terms of mechanical stability is important since individuals with a stable SCFE have a better prognosis in terms of achieving improved outcomes with fewer complications compared to those with an unstable SCFE.[5] All patients with a suspected SCFE require an urgent referral to an orthopaedic surgeon. However, because of the increased risk of osteonecrosis, patients with an unstable SCFE require an emergent referral to an orthopaedic surgeon. Early diagnosis of SCFE is associated with improved prognosis. Consequently, delays in diagnosis and continued weightbearing can lead to progression of the SCFE and further deformity, delayed surgical intervention, and complications such as osteonecrosis and chondrolysis.[2]

Physical Therapy Patient/Client Management

If there is concern for an SCFE based upon patient history and physical examination findings, the physical therapist should educate the patient on functional anatomy and injury pathomechanics. Since weightbearing should be avoided,[10] the physical therapist should train the patient in a non-weightbearing gait pattern on the affected lower extremity. The patient should also be referred for radiographs and if a diagnosis of an SCFE is confirmed, an urgent referral to an orthopaedic surgeon should be placed so appropriate surgical options can be considered in a timely manner.[14] The primary goal for most injured individuals is to return to pain-free activity as quickly and as safely as possible after surgery in a manner that does not overload the healing tissues.

Examination, Evaluation, and Diagnosis

The most common symptom for the young patient with an SCFE is pain that is usually localized to the hip or groin regions, or less commonly, in the distal thigh and knee regions.[1,14,15] Table 19-1 describes clinical features of hip conditions in younger individuals that can assist in the differential diagnosis.[16] The conditions are listed in descending order of frequency (i.e., more common conditions are listed first). Pain associated with an SCFE is worse with activity and patients usually report an inability to perform athletic activities. When a patient presents primarily with distal thigh and knee pain, the physical therapist may overlook SCFE as a cause and instead focus the examination and treatment on the primary area of symptoms.[15] This can delay diagnosis of the etiology of the patient's symptoms and lead to further progression of the SCFE, and potentially an adverse outcome. Therefore, in young patients with a primary complaint of distal thigh and knee pain, the hip should always be thoroughly examined.

In most cases, pain associated with an SCFE develops insidiously and progressively worsens over the course of several weeks without a clear mechanism of injury.[10,17] If this is the case, the patient may present with an antalgic gait (i.e., stable SCFE) and the lower extremity may be held in a position of abduction and external rotation (Fig. 19-1).[18] In less than 10% of cases, the pain associated with an SCFE is severe and associated with a traumatic incident such as a fall.[2] In this case, the patient may not be able to bear weight on the involved lower extremity even with the use of crutches because of severe pain and instability (i.e., unstable SCFE).

Table 19-1   DIFFERENTIAL DIAGNOSIS OF HIP PAIN IN THE YOUNG INDIVIDUAL

Condition	Age (years)	Clinical Features	Diagnosis
Groin strain	All ages	Pain after sudden or forceful movement	Radiography to rule out slipped capital femoral epiphysis
Hip apophysitis	12-25	Activity-related hip pain	History of overuse; radiography to rule out fractures
Apophyseal avulsion fractures of the hips and pelvis	12-25	Pain after sudden or forceful movement	History of trauma; radiography
Transient synovitis	< 10	Antalgic gait or hip pain	Radiography; laboratory testing; ultrasonography
Fractures	All ages	Pain after traumatic event	History of significant trauma; radiography
Stress fractures of the femoral neck and pelvis	12-25	Activity-related hip pain; insidious onset	History of overuse; hip radiography; bone scan; magnetic resonance imaging
Slipped capital femoral epiphysis	9-16	Hip, groin, thigh, or knee pain; antalgic gait	Bilateral hip radiography
Legg-Calvé-Perthes disease	4-9	Vague hip pain, decreased internal rotation of hip	Hip radiography or magnetic resonance imaging
Septic arthritis	All ages	Fever, antalgic gait, hip pain	Radiography; laboratory testing; joint aspiration

Modified with permission from Peck D. Slipped capital femoral epiphysis: diagnosis and management. Am Fam Physician. 2010;82:259-62.

For **hip range of motion (ROM)** assessment, the physical therapist should compare the findings of the involved hip with the uninvolved hip. Limited and painful internal rotation and flexion at the hip are common findings in the patient with an SCFE.[2] If the patient is able to flex the hip beyond 90°, it may move into obligatory external rotation as the prominent femoral neck contacts the acetabulum (due to posterior and inferior displacement of the proximal femoral epiphysis).[2] Examination of the knee is often normal, even if the chief complaint is pain referred to the distal thigh or knee.[15]

The **diagnosis of an SCFE should be considered** in any patient between the ages of 9 and 16 years with a primary complaint of hip, groin, thigh, and knee pain who presents with an antalgic gait.[16] **Bilateral anterior to posterior and lateral view radiographs** (lateral frog leg views for a stable SCFE; cross-table lateral views for an unstable SCFE to minimize patient discomfort and the risk of further slip progression) allow for comparison between extremities and are crucial in establishing the diagnosis of an SCFE.[1,14,18] When ordering radiographs, it is critical that the radiologist is informed that an SCFE is suspected so it can be properly confirmed

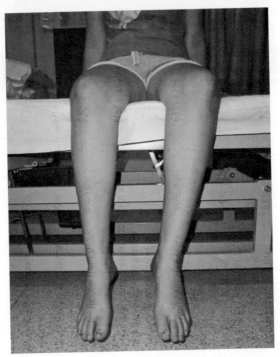

Figure 19-1. 11-year-old female with a left-sided slipped capital femoral epiphysis. Note the left hip is positioned in slight abduction and external rotation.

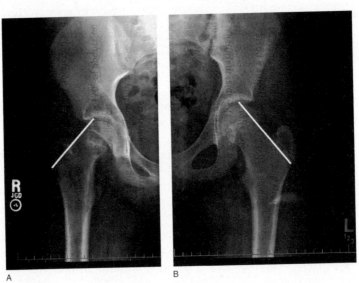

A   B

Figure 19-2. Anterior to posterior hip radiographs of an 11-year-old female with history and physical examination findings concerning for a slipped capital femoral epiphysis. **A.** The patient's involved right hip with Klein line positioned slightly lateral to the femoral epiphysis, consistent with a slipped capital femoral epiphysis. Proximal femoral osteopenia and widening of the physis are also seen. **B.** The patient's uninvolved left hip with Klein line intersecting the femoral epiphysis. (Reproduced with permission from Michael D. Ross.)

or ruled out. Since there is some risk of bilateral SCFE at initial presentation,[6,9] it is important to note that symmetric appearance of the physes does not necessarily mean both are normal.

On the anterior to posterior radiographic view, the Klein line can be used to assess for an SCFE by drawing a line along the superior border of the femoral neck.[1] In a normal hip joint, the Klein line intersects a portion of the femoral epiphysis; in the patient with an SCFE, the Klein line is level with, or lateral to, the epiphysis. Anterior to posterior (Fig. 19-2) and lateral frog leg view (Fig. 19-3) radiographs of the current patient[19] demonstrate the Klein line positioned slightly lateral to the femoral epiphysis and proximal femoral osteopenia and widening of the physis. The osteopenia correlates well with the patient's 5-month history of right knee pain and likely limited weightbearing on the right lower extremity. The widening of the physis may be seen in the early stages of the disorder before posterior and inferior displacement of the proximal femoral epiphysis is observed.

In a patient with normal or inconclusive radiographs with a high index of suspicion of an SCFE, a bone scan or magnetic resonance imaging may be helpful in confirming the diagnosis. At the "pre-slip" stage, the bone scan may demonstrate increased uptake at the proximal aspect of the femoral neck and magnetic resonance imaging may demonstrate abnormalities in the physis.

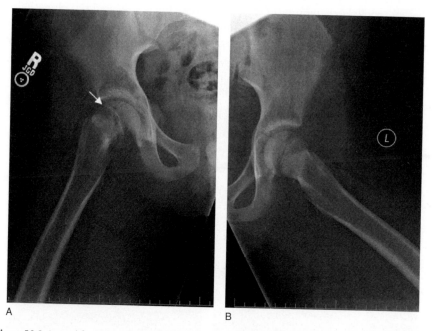

A   B

Figure 19-3. Lateral frog leg radiographs of an 11-year-old female with history and physical examination findings concerning for a slipped capital femoral epiphysis. **A.** The patient's involved right hip demonstrated inferior displacement of the femoral epiphysis consistent with a slipped capital femoral epiphysis (arrow). **B.** The patient's uninvolved left hip. (Reproduced with permission from Michael D. Ross.)

Plan of Care and Interventions

Diagnosing an SCFE can be challenging and clinicians may initially overlook the diagnosis, especially when patients present with vague symptoms that may appear to be unrelated to the hip.[19-21] The prognosis for the patient with an SCFE is often dependent upon how quickly the diagnosis is made because this influences the timing of appropriate surgical interventions.[20-23] Delays in diagnosis can lead to osteonecrosis and chondrolysis, as well as early-onset hip osteoarthritis.[24,25]

Once diagnosed, the typical management of a patient with an SCFE is preventing progression of the slip through surgical stabilization of the physis.[1,26] Due to the risk of slip progression, the patient with an SCFE should be referred to an orthopaedic surgeon and remain non-weightbearing on the involved lower extremity until surgery. Since surgery is the primary treatment for an SCFE, there is little evidence on conservative treatment approaches, including physical therapy.[2,16] The **surgical treatment approach** for a mild to moderate stable slip is *in situ* fixation of the epiphysis with a single screw, which usually provides adequate fixation (Fig. 19-4).[1,21,26-28] This technique has been shown to be effective with low rates of recurrence and complications.[21,27]

An unstable SCFE is a more severe injury than a stable SCFE.[16] There is some controversy regarding the specifics of the surgery including timing of surgical intervention, need for preoperative traction, importance of realigning the epiphysis, and whether prophylactic pinning of the contralateral hip is indicated.[14,27] Nonetheless, the treatment for an unstable SCFE must consider the blood supply to the femoral head because the rate of osteonecrosis following surgical intervention has been

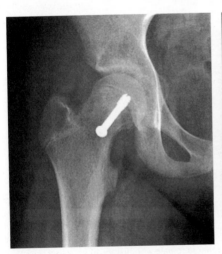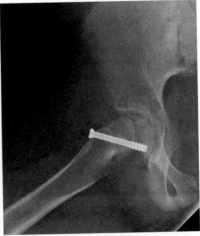

Figure 19-4. Anterior to posterior (left image) and lateral frog leg (right image) radiographs of an 11-year-old female's right hip following *in situ* fixation of a slipped capital femoral epiphysis. (Reproduced with permission from Michael D. Ross.)

reported to be as high as 50%, while other studies have reported a range between 3% and 15%.[29] The surgical treatment approach for an unstable slip commonly entails decompression of the hip joint (to reduce intra-articular pressure) with gentle closed reduction, depending on the degree of the deformity and fixation with one or two screws.[2]

Patients are typically toe-touch weightbearing (non-weightbearing for an unstable SCFE) for the first 6 weeks following surgery. Careful radiographic and clinical monitoring is necessary to ensure that appropriate closure of the proximal femoral physis occurs without progression of the slip.[2] Patients are allowed to gradually return to full weightbearing and normal daily activities after 6 weeks (although this timeframe may be longer for patients with an unstable SCFE), but athletic activities are usually restricted until the physis has closed. After closure of the physis, patients may eventually progress to athletic activities.[14]

Due to the paucity of research for rehabilitation after surgery for individuals with an SCFE, it is not clear what role the physical therapist plays following surgery. Nonetheless, if a patient is referred following surgery, the physical therapist should address findings from the musculoskeletal examination while applying precautions associated with the surgery. Specifically, the physical therapist should ensure that patients adhere to weightbearing and activity restrictions. Once the patient is able to bear weight and progress with rehabilitation activities, any increase in pain or decrease in hip range of motion should be communicated to the orthopaedic surgeon because these could be early signs that the patient may be progressing too quickly, which could potentially delay closure of the physis. Once the patient is able to begin rehabilitation, physical therapy interventions for patients following surgical stabilization for an SCFE may entail: patient education regarding functional anatomy, injury pathomechanics, and activity restrictions/modifications; gait training; hip range of motion exercises; resistance exercises to increase strength and endurance of the core and lower extremity musculature; aerobic exercise; and an appropriate functional exercise progression once the patient is cleared to return to athletic activities.

Evidence-Based Clinical Recommendations

SORT: Strength of Recommendation Taxonomy

A: Consistent, good-quality patient-oriented evidence
B: Inconsistent or limited-quality patient-oriented evidence
C: Consensus, disease-oriented evidence, usual practice, expert opinion, or case series

1. Physical examination of individuals with a slipped capital femoral epiphysis typically reveals an antalgic gait, decreased internal rotation of the hip, and obligatory external rotation as the hip flexes beyond 90°. **Grade C**

2. Physical therapists should consider the diagnosis of an SCFE when a young individual presents with an antalgic gait and groin, hip, thigh, or knee pain. **Grade C**

3. When history and physical examination findings are concerning for an SCFE, conventional radiography should include anterior to posterior and lateral views of the hips (lateral frog leg views for a stable SCFE; cross-table lateral views for an unstable SCFE). **Grade C**

4. The standard treatment of a stable SCFE is *in situ* fixation with a single screw. **Grade C**

COMPREHENSION QUESTIONS

19.1 A physical therapist is evaluating a 12-year-old male who has moderate groin and knee pain. The patient is able to bear weight, but has an antalgic gait. Hip internal rotation is limited and painful, and when the hip is passively flexed, it abducts and externally rotates. Which of the following diagnostic imaging modalities would be initially indicated to assess for a slipped capital femoral epiphysis?

A. Anterior to posterior and cross-table lateral view radiographs

B. Anterior to posterior and lateral frog leg view radiographs

C. Bone scan

D. Magnetic resonance imaging

19.2 Which of the following is the *most* appropriate treatment for a patient with a stable slipped capital femoral epiphysis?

A. Core decompression

B. Curettage and bone grafting

C. *In situ* screw fixation

D. Total hip arthroplasty

ANSWERS

19.1 **B.** Since this patient is able to bear weight, he would be classified as potentially having a stable slipped capital femoral epiphysis. Therefore, the appropriate imaging would include anterior to posterior and lateral frog leg view radiographs. Anterior to posterior and cross-table lateral view radiographs (option A) would be indicated for an unstable SCFE (*i.e.*, the patient would not be able to bear weight). Bone scan and magnetic resonance imaging are not indicated as initial imaging modalities for patients with an SCFE (options C and D). These latter modalities would be useful for a patient with normal or inconclusive radiographs with a high index of suspicion of an SCFE.

19.2 **C.** The standard treatment of stable SCFE is *in situ* fixation with a single cannulated screw.

REFERENCES

1. Aronsson DD, Loder RT, Breur GJ, Weinstein SL. Slipped capital femoral epiphysis: current concepts. *J Am Acad Orthop Surg*. 2006;14:666-679.

2. Gholve PA, Cameron DB, Millis MB. Slipped capital femoral epiphysis update. *Curr Opin Pediatr*. 2009;21:39-45.

3. Harris WR. The endocrine basis for the slipping of the femoral head. *J Bone Joint Surg Br*. 1950;32:5-10.

4. Watts HG. Fractures of the pelvis in children. *Orthop Clin North Am*. 1976;7:615-624.

5. Lehmann CL, Arons RR, Loder RT, Vitale MG. The epidemiology of slipped capital femoral epiphysis: an update. *J Pediatr Orthop*. 2006;26:286-290.

6. Loder RT. The demographics of slipped capital femoral epiphysis. An international multicenter study. *Clin Orthop Relat Res*. 1996;322:8-27.

7. Cohen M, Gelberman RH, Griffin PP, Kasser J, Emans JB, Millis MB. Slipped capital femoral epiphysis: assessment of epiphyseal displacement and angulation. *J Pediatr Orthop*. 1986;6:259-264.

8. Manoff EM, Banffy MB, Winell JJ. Relationship between body mass index and slipped capital femoral epiphysis. *J Pediatr Orthop*. 2005;25:744-746.

9. Riad J, Bajelidze G, Gabos PG. Bilateral slipped capital femoral epiphysis: predictive factors for contralateral slip. *J Pediatr Orthop*. 2007;27:411-414.

10. Loder RT, Richards BS, Shapiro PS, Reznick LR, Aronson DD. Acute slipped capital femoral epiphysis: the importance of physeal stability. *J Bone Joint Surg Am*. 1993;75:1134-1140.

11. Papavasiliou KA, Kirkos JM, Kapetanos GA, Pournaras J. Potential influence of hormones in the development of slipped capital femoral epiphysis: a preliminary study. *J Pediatr Orthop B*. 2007;16:1-5.

12. Loder RT, Starnes T, Dikos G, Aronsson DD. Demographic predictors of severity of stable slipped capital femoral epiphyses. *J Bone Joint Surg Am*. 2006;88:97-105.

13. Loder RT. Slipped capital femoral epiphysis in children. *Curr Opin Pediatr*. 1995;7:95-97.

14. Loder RT. Slipped capital femoral epiphysis. *Am Fam Physician*.1998;57:2135-2142, 2148-2150.

15. Matava MJ, Patton CM, Luhmann S, Gordon JE, Schoenecker PL. Knee pain as the initial symptom of slipped capital femoral epiphysis: an analysis of initial presentation and treatment. *J Pediatr Orthop*. 1999;19:455-460.

16. Peck D. Slipped capital femoral epiphysis: diagnosis and management. *Am Fam Physician*. 2010;82:259-262.

17. Kasper JC, Gerhardt MB, Mandelbaum BR. Stress injury leading to slipped capital femoral epiphysis in a competitive adolescent tennis player: a case report. *Clin J Sport Med*. 2007;17:72-74.

18. Houghton KM. Review for the generalist: evaluation of pediatric hip pain. *Pediatr Rheum Online J*. 2009;7:10.

19. Greene KA, Ross MD. Slipped capital femoral epiphysis in a patient referred to physical therapy for knee pain. *J Orthop Sports Phys Ther*. 2008;38:26.

20. Rahme D, Comley A, Foster B, Cundy P. Consequences of diagnostic delays in slipped capital femoral epiphysis. *J Pediatr Orthop B*. 2006;15:93-97.

21. Katz DA. Slipped capital femoral epiphysis: the importance of early diagnosis. *Pediatr Ann*. 2006;35:102-111.

22. Loder RT. Correlation of radiographic changes with disease severity and demographic variables in children with stable slipped capital femoral epiphysis. *J Pediatr Orthop*. 2008;28:284-290.

23. Carney BT, Weinstein SL, Noble J. Long-term follow-up of slipped capital femoral epiphysis. *J Bone Joint Surg Am*. 1991;73:667-674.

24. Kocher MS, Bishop JA, Weed B, Hresko MT, Kim YJ, Kasser JR. Delay in diagnosis of slipped capital femoral epiphysis. *Pediatrics*. 2004;113:e322-e325.

25. Green DW, Reynolds RA, Khan SN, Tolo V. The delay in diagnosis of slipped capital femoral epiphysis: a review of 102 patients. *HSS J*. 2005;1:103-106.

26. Givon U, Bowen JR. Chronic slipped capital femoral epiphysis: treatment by pinning in-situ. *J Pediatr Orthop B*. 1999;8:216-222.

27. Kalogrianitis S, Tan CK, Kemp GJ, Bass A, Bruce C. Does unstable slipped capital femoral epiphysis require urgent stabilization? *J Pediatr Orthop B*. 2007;16:6-9.

28. Morrissy RT. Slipped capital femoral epiphysis-natural history, etiology, and treatment. *Instr Course Lect*. 1980;29:81-86.

29. Loder RT. Unstable slipped capital femoral epiphysis. *J Pediatr Orthop*. 2001;21:694-699.

DISCLAIMER

The views expressed in this article are those of the authors and do not necessarily reflect the official policy or position of the Department of the Air Force, Department of Defense, or the U.S. Government.

Hip Osteoarthritis (OA)

Paul Reuteman

CASE 20

A 58-year-old male self-referred to an outpatient physical therapy clinic with a primary complaint of right anterolateral hip pain. The pain intensity and progression of his functional limitations prompted him to seek medical attention. Diagnostic imaging was performed that revealed signs of hip osteoarthritis (Fig. 20-1). His primary care physician referred him to an orthopaedic surgeon to discuss surgical options. However, the patient chose a conservative route to treat his symptoms and scheduled a consultation with a physical therapist. He describes experiencing intermittent hip pain that is aggravated by squatting, ascending stairs, and hip rotation during weightbearing activities. He has not been able to engage in his usual cardiovascular conditioning program or any strength training due to pain. His goal is to return to his previous level of function during his activities of daily living and resume his cardiovascular and strength training program at his local fitness club.

▶ Based on the patient's diagnosis, what are the contributing factors to his condition?
▶ What examination signs and priorities are associated with hip osteoarthritis?
▶ What are the functional limitations and assets of the patient?
▶ What are the most appropriate physical therapy interventions for a patient with hip osteoarthritis?

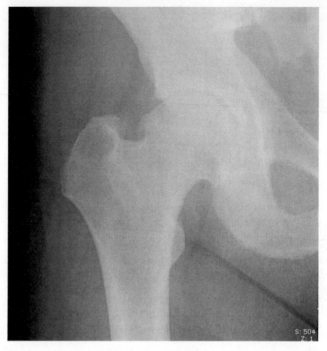

Figure 20-1. Anteroposterior (AP) radiograph of the right hip showing sclerotic changes, decreased joint space, and an osteophyte on the superior joint margin.

KEY DEFINITIONS

IMPAIRMENT-BASED PHYSICAL THERAPY: Physical therapy interventions addressing modifiable musculoskeletal impairments that are associated with decreased function and/or increased activity-related pain; the decision to utilize specific interventions is based on continual assessment of the patient's impairments and how they are affected by each intervention; as the status of the patient changes, the plan of care is modified

JOINT HYPOMOBILITY: Decrease in normal movement of a joint due to articular surface dysfunction or disease or injury that affects bone, muscle, ligament, or the joint itself; often leads to limited active and passive range of motion

JOINT MOBILIZATION: Passive movement directed at joint structures with the aim of achieving a therapeutic effect (increase in joint motion and/or decrease in pain); a high-velocity, low-amplitude thrust maneuver is a type of mobilization technique also known as a joint manipulation

OSTEOARTHRITIS: Defective integrity of articular cartilage associated with changes in the underlying bone and at joint margins; these changes often lead to pain, loss of mobility and muscle strength, impaired function, and decreased quality of life

REGIONAL INTERDEPENDENCE: Theory that dysfunction either proximally and/or distally may contribute to pain in the involved joint

Objectives

1. Utilize evidence and clinical practice guidelines for the examination and treatment of an individual with hip osteoarthritis.

2. Prescribe appropriate manual therapy and joint range of motion activities for an individual with hip osteoarthritis.

3. Prescribe appropriate therapeutic exercises, including resistance and stretching exercises, for a person with hip osteoarthritis.

Physical Therapy Considerations

PT considerations during management of the individual with a diagnosis of hip osteoarthritis:

▸ **General physical therapy plan of care/goals:** Improve joint mobility and range of motion; decrease pain and increase function; increase muscular strength; increase tolerance to daily activities; prevent or minimize loss of aerobic fitness capacity

▸ **Physical therapy interventions:** Patient education regarding functional anatomy and pathomechanics; manual therapy to the lumbopelvic region and hip joint to decrease pain and improve motion; resistance exercises to increase muscular strength and endurance of the trunk and lower extremity muscles; aerobic exercises to increase cardiovascular conditioning; primary prevention of further joint damage

▸ **Precautions during physical therapy:** Monitor vital signs, monitor symptom reproduction during treatment, address activities that are contraindicated for patients with hip osteoarthritis

Understanding the Health Condition

Hip pain associated with osteoarthritis (OA) is one of the most common causes of hip pain in older adults.[1,2] Osteoarthritis of the hip joint is a clinical syndrome with signs and symptoms associated with defective integrity of the articular cartilage and changes in the underlying bone and at the joint margins. These changes often lead to pain, loss of mobility and muscle strength, impaired function, and a decreased quality of life.[3,4] The cause of osteoarthritis is multifactorial and several risk factors have been identified. Age appears to be the most common predisposing factor as the condition mostly affects those 50 years of age and older.[1]

Radiographs are the current gold standard for diagnosing hip OA. The Kellgren Lawrence scale has defined four grades of hip OA based on joint space narrowing, sclerotic changes of subchondral bone and the presence of osteophytes.[5] For clinicians who do not have frequent access to radiographic imaging, **clinical criteria have been established by the American College of Rheumatology** to assist in identifying patients presenting with hip OA.[6] From these criteria, patients are classified as having hip OA if they report experiencing hip pain, their age is greater than 50 years, and they present with either of the following cluster of findings: (1) hip internal rotation range of motion (ROM) <15° and hip flexion ROM ≤115° or, (2) hip internal rotation ROM >15° but accompanied by pain and the duration of morning stiffness of the hip <60 minutes.[6]

A 2008 study in 72 adults identified five clinical variables to predict individuals who have confirmed OA on radiographic studies.[7] The variables included: pain aggravated with squatting, hip pain with the scour test, hip pain with active hip flexion or with active hip extension, and passive hip internal rotation ROM less than 25°. If at least four of these five variables were identified, the positive likelihood ratio was equal to 24.3 (95% confidence interval: 4.4-142.1). Thus, this preliminary clinical prediction rule increased the probability of hip OA being present on imaging studies from 29% to 91%.[7]

Total hip arthroplasty (THA) appears to be the intervention of choice for patients with hip OA. The number of THA procedures performed in the management of hip OA continues to grow. It is estimated that 231,000 THA procedures were performed in the United States during 2006.[8] An epidemiologic study of a community in a Midwestern state revealed the age- and sex-adjusted use of THA increased from 50.2 per 100,000 in 1969-1972 to 145 per 100,000 in 2005-2009. This represents almost a 300% increase in the number of THA procedures performed over an approximate 30-year span. From 1969 to 2009, the rate of THA procedures on younger individuals (up to 49 years of age) also increased more than sevenfold with almost a doubling between the 1997-2000 and 2005-2008 time period.[8] This dramatic increase likely reflects both an increased vigilance in hip OA diagnosis and earlier surgical intervention. A predictable consequence of total hip arthroplasties being performed in younger individuals is the increased likelihood that an individual will "outlive" the lifespan of the prosthesis, thus requiring subsequent THA revision surgery and rehabilitation.

In recent years, several authors have advocated conservative management involving supervised physical therapy as an alternative to surgery to prevent or delay the impact of disability associated with hip OA.[1,9-11] Physical therapy appears to offer the most appropriate multimodal conservative approach combining aerobic and strengthening exercises with directed manual therapy techniques that enhance function and decrease pain.

The current patient presented with hip OA confirmed on radiographic imaging, exhibited range of motion deficits that met the OA classification identified by the American College of Rheumatology, and satisfied four of the five variables established as a clinical prediction rule for hip OA. Because the patient met these criteria, surgical intervention was recommended by his physician. However, the patient made a personal choice to pursue physical therapy in hopes of avoiding surgery.

Physical Therapy Patient/Client Management

Appropriate conservative management of hip OA requires a multimodal approach. Physical therapy interventions of directed manual therapy techniques should be combined with aerobic and strengthening exercises to enhance function and decrease pain. Educating the patient how to modify activity to prevent or reduce pain is critical. By avoiding provocative activities, the progression of OA may be reduced. It is also important to encourage the patient to find activities that enhance general conditioning without placing undue stress or creating pain at the hip. The primary physical therapy goal for most individuals is to enhance function, decrease frequency and intensity of pain during daily activities, and prolong or avoid surgery. Due to the heterogeneity of individuals with hip OA, all management models must be tailored to the patient's current impairments, anticipated goals, and how the patient responds to the intervention.

Examination, Evaluation, and Diagnosis

The examination of a patient with hip pain involves a thorough subjective history of the patient's primary complaints, a general medical history, and a discussion about the goals for rehabilitation. Individuals presenting with hip pain due to osteoarthritic changes most commonly complain of pain in the anterior groin, buttock, and posterior thigh region.[12] Almost 50% of patients with hip OA also complain of pain in the knee or lower leg.[12] Weightbearing activities, especially those that involve twisting on the involved extremity and deep squatting, are usually painful. At times, prolonged sitting may be symptomatic, especially if the hip is flexed greater than 90°. Frequently, pain is more prevalent in the early morning or after long periods of inactivity.

A disease-specific health-related quality of life questionnaire should be administered to assess the patient's perceived level of disability. The Western Ontario and McMaster Universities Osteoarthritis (WOMAC) Index and the Harris Hip Score are two outcome assessments recommended for patients with hip osteoarthritis.[13,14] The Harris Hip Score has been frequently used in studies that assess effectiveness of conservative management of hip OA and has been found to be both reliable and valid.[15]

The physical therapist must perform a complete musculoskeletal examination to identify the impairments associated with the patient's condition. Table 20-1 outlines the components of the examination in an individual with hip OA. Assessment of these impairments serves as a baseline for subsequent visits to identify if improvements are being made.

Observational gait assessment may reveal either a compensated or noncompensated Trendelenburg gait. These gait patterns signify weakness of the ipsilateral hip abductors.[16,17]

A strong correlation between hip OA and hip ROM deficits has also been identified.[7,8] Limitations in hip extension and internal rotation are especially prevalent due to tightness of the anterior capsule that is associated with hip OA. Measuring hip internal rotation (IR) ROM is easier and more standardized than measuring hip extension ROM. Measurements of hip IR ROM have been found to be reliable with the patient in either a prone or supine position.[18]

Joint mobility assessment is difficult to perform due to the general stability associated with the hip joint. Assessment of the end feel during the application of overpressure at end motions is valuable to determine capsular restrictions. A tight capsular end feel is an indication for specific manual therapy techniques to enhance hip capsule flexibility.[19]

Table 20-1 GAIT, MOTION ASSESSMENT, AND SPECIAL TESTS ASSOCIATED WITH HIP OSTEOARTHRITIS

Clinical Assessment	Patient Position	Measurements/Observations
Observational gait assessment	The patient is asked to ambulate on a level surface.	Compensated or noncompensated Trendelenburg gait is indicative of hip abductor weakness.
Active and passive hip internal rotation (Fig. 20-2)	Patient may either be prone or sitting on the edge of the table. The patient is asked to internally rotate the hip as the therapist measures IR. The therapist prevents any compensation at the pelvis.	The number of degrees the tibia moves from the neutral vertical position is measured with an inclinometer. Motion is assessed passively to determine end feel. ROM is compared bilaterally.
FABER test (Patrick's test) (Fig. 20-3)	Patient lies supine with the symptomatic lower extremity crossed over the opposite leg so that the lateral aspect of the ankle rests proximal to the patella (if possible). The therapist stabilizes the opposite pelvis as the therapist lowers the patient's knee toward the table.	The amount the tibia (on the symptomatic lower extremity) moves from the neutral vertical position is measured with an inclinometer. Motion is compared bilaterally. Pain provocation is also documented.
Scour test (Fig. 20-4)	Patient lies supine. The therapist passively flexes the hip beyond 90° of flexion and applies a vertical compressive force to the femur. The therapist moves the femur from abduction to adduction.	Painful range is documented.
Squat test (Fig. 20-5)	The patient is standing and is asked to squat, lowering his hips to his heels. He is asked to squat as low as possible prior to experiencing pain.	The amount the tibia moves from the neutral vertical position is measured with an inclinometer.
Six-Minute Walk Test	The patient is asked to cover as much distance while walking as far as possible in 6 minutes.	The physical therapist monitors blood pressure, heart rate, and rate of perceived exertion (RPE) and any hip signs or symptoms before, during, and after the testing.

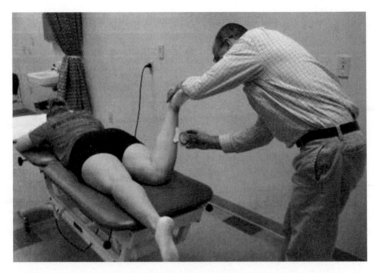

Figure 20-2. Therapist measuring hip internal rotation with the use of an inclinometer.

Manual muscle testing is performed to assess strength deficits with specific attention directed at hip abduction, external rotation, and extension since these muscles are commonly weak in the presence of hip OA.

Special tests have been described that may identify joint restrictions or reproduce pain in a patient with hip OA. These include the FABER test,[20,21] the scour test,[8,21]

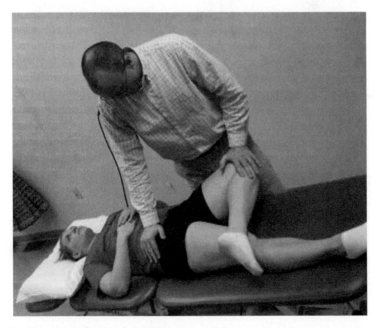

Figure 20-3. Therapist performing the FABER test.

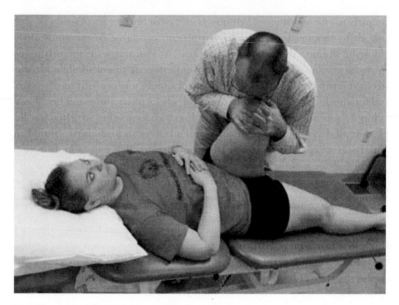

Figure 20-4. Therapist performing the scour test.

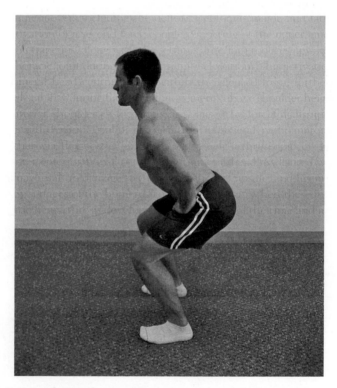

Figure 20-5. Patient performing the squat test.

and the squat test.[21,22] Little research exists on the diagnostic value of these tests; however, they can be assessed before and after physical therapy interventions to determine if a change has been achieved as a result of an intervention.

Finally, a Six-Minute Walk Test[23] should be performed to assess the patient's baseline fitness level. In addition, the physical therapist can calculate the patient's gait speed from this self-paced walk because gait speed is a prognostic variable for rehabilitation.

To establish an accurate prognosis for a patient with hip OA, multiple variables must be considered. Wright et al.[24] determined a set of five baseline variables that may be used as prognostic indicators to identify patients likely to demonstrate a *favorable* response to physical therapy intervention for primary hip OA. The variables were: (1) presence of unilateral pain, (2) age of the patient ≤ 58 years, (3) self-reported pain ≥ 6/10 on a numeric pain rating scale, (4) a 40-m self-paced walk test time ≤ 25.9 seconds and, (5) duration of symptoms ≤ 1 year. Having three or more of the five variables increased the post-test probability of success with physical therapy intervention to 99%. Failure of having any one of the five variables, decreased the post-test probability of responding favorably to physical therapy intervention from 32% to < 1% (negative likelihood ratio = 0.00; 95% CI: 0.00-0.70).[24] The current patient exhibited 4 out of 5 variables, therefore, he was considered to have a favorable prognosis to conservative care.

Plan of Care and Interventions

Interventions should follow an impairment-based physical therapy approach. Patient education, manual therapy techniques, muscle and joint capsule stretching, exercises to address hip muscle strength and endurance, and general conditioning activities are recommended. The decision to utilize specific interventions is based on the continual assessment of the patient's impairments and how these impairments are affected by the intervention. As the status of the patient changes, the treatment is modified.

An important consideration in managing hip pain is educating the patient on ways to reduce muscle-generated hip joint forces during ambulation. The therapist should explain the biomechanical rationale of **joint protection strategies** such as using a cane or a walking stick on the uninvolved side and carrying items on the involved side. These techniques are based primarily on reducing the magnitude of hip abductor muscle forces during walking.[16] In simple terms, by using these techniques, the patient may decrease loading to the hip joint which results in less stress to the joint. Educating the patient on these concepts may decrease hip joint pain, normalize gait pattern, and increase walking tolerance.

The inclusion of **manual therapy techniques** in the plan of care is valuable in enhancing outcomes for patients hip OA.[10,11] In a case series, seven patients (median age 62 years old) were prescribed manual therapy that included five different hip joint mobilization techniques (long axis distraction, lateral glides, inferior glides, caudal glides, and posterior-anterior glides) followed by exercise deemed appropriate by the treating physical therapist.[10] The median number of physical therapy sessions attended was five (range, 4-12). The median increase in total hip passive ROM at the end of treatment was 82° (range, 70°-86°). The median improvement on the Harris Hip Score was 25 points (range, 15-38 points) and the numeric pain rating scores decreased by a mean of 5 points (range, 2-7 points) on a 0-10-point scale. Many of the subjects in the study maintained improvement at a 6-month follow-up.[10]

In a larger randomized clinical trial of patients with hip OA, two different groups were studied: those that received manual therapy and exercise and those that received exercise alone over a 5-week period. The inclusion of manual therapy was found to enhance treatment outcomes assessed by the Harris Hip Score, walking speed, pain, and range of motion. At a 5-week follow-up, effect sizes favoring the manual therapy and exercise group were greatest for the Harris Hip Score (mean between-group difference 11.2; 95% CI: 6.1-16.3) and hip range of motion (mean between-group difference 16.0°; 95% CI: 8.1-22.6). Similar results were noted at a 9-month follow-up.[11]

Recommended joint mobilization techniques for managing hip OA include: long axis joint traction with a high-velocity low-amplitude thrust to address general hip capsule mobility, posterior-anterior (PA) joint mobilizations to address anterior capsule tightness, and anterior-posterior (AP) joint mobilizations to address posterior capsule tightness (Figs. 20-6 to 20-8). Based on the theory of regional interdependence[25] and the association between back pain and hip pain,[13,26] it is also recommended to include mobilization techniques to the lumbopelvic region, if hypomobility was determined during the examination. Following any joint mobilization technique, it is advisable to instruct the patient in exercises to maintain the newly gained motion. Common **stretching exercises** include anterior hip, adductor and piriformis stretching (Figs. 20-9 to 20-11).

Weakness of hip and knee muscles has been demonstrated in patients with hip OA.[27] **Strengthening exercises** to address these strength deficits are advocated in

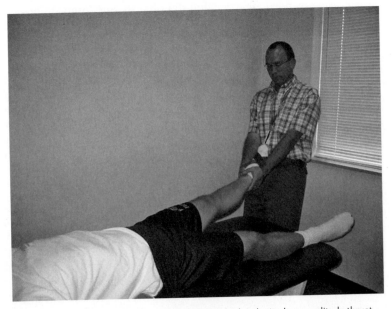

Figure 20-6. Therapist performing long axis traction with high-velocity, low-amplitude thrust.

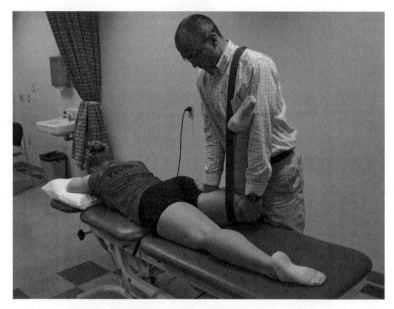

Figure 20-7. Therapist performing posterior-anterior (PA) hip joint mobilization.

the management of symptoms associated with hip OA.[27] With the most pain-provocative positions of the hip being adduction, flexion and internal rotation, exercises that target the hip abductors, extensors, and external rotators are emphasized. Exercises are progressed from a non-weightbearing position to a weightbearing position as tolerated. Initial exercises include sidelying hip abduction/external rotation

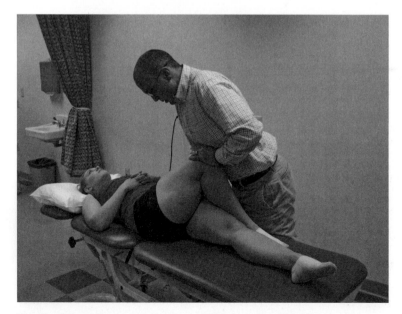

Figure 20-8. Therapist performing anterior-posterior (AP) hip joint mobilization.

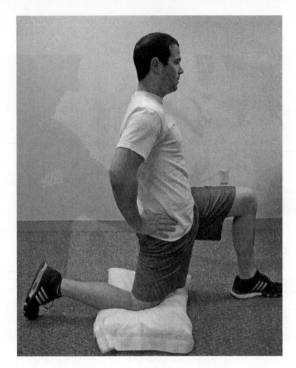

Figure 20-9. Patient performing right anterior hip stretch.

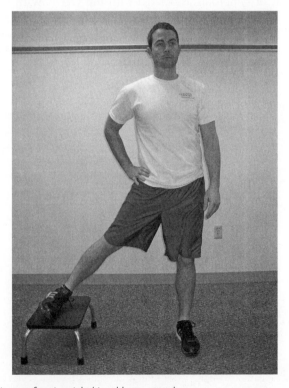

Figure 20-10. Patient performing right hip adductor stretch.

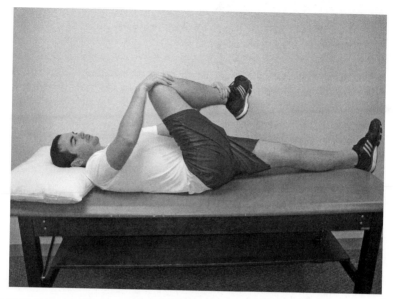

Figure 20-11. Patient performing right piriformis stretch.

and supine bridging activities. Based on electromyography (EMG) data, progression to single limb activity such as single limb squats and dead lifts achieve optimal recruitment of the hip muscles.[28] Strengthening exercises should be modified to avoid symptom provocation and to improve patient tolerance.

Little evidence exists regarding the benefit of **cardiovascular training** for individuals with hip OA. Regardless, cardiovascular training has other positive effects especially related to the potential of weight loss that may reduce stress on the hip joint. A structured stationary cycling or walking program focusing on duration, intensity, and frequency has been recommended for individuals of this age group.[29,30]

Evidence-Based Clinical Recommendations

SORT: Strength of Recommendation Taxonomy

A: Consistent, good-quality patient-oriented evidence
B: Inconsistent or limited-quality patient-oriented evidence
C: Consensus, disease-oriented evidence, usual practice, expert opinion, or case series

1. Hip osteoarthritis can be diagnosed with clusters of signs and symptoms as outlined by the American College of Rheumatology. **Grade B**

2. Education and implementation of joint protection strategies (*e.g.*, ambulation with a cane in the hand opposite the involved hip) is effective in managing symptoms associated with hip OA. **Grade B**

3. Manual therapy techniques addressed at the lumbopelvic and hip joints improve hip pain and short-term and long-term function in individuals with hip OA. **Grade B**

4. Exercise interventions focusing on self-ROM, stretching, and strengthening of muscles surrounding the hip may improve hip strength and tolerance to activity. **Grade C**

5. Cardiovascular training, including a cycling or walking program, benefits individuals with hip OA. **Grade C**

COMPREHENSION QUESTIONS

20.1 Which of the following sets of motion deficits are *most* commonly associated with hip OA?

A. Hip abduction, hip flexion

B. Hip internal rotation, hip extension

C. Hip flexion, hip external rotation

D. Hip abduction, hip internal rotation

20.2 Which of the following statements is *most* accurate regarding the use of manual therapy in the treatment of hip OA?

A. The use of manual therapy has been found to have a positive effect on pain, but does not have any effect on range of motion of the hip.

B. The use of manual therapy has been found to have a short-term positive effect on patient outcomes, but has no effect in the long term (6-9 months following discharge from physical therapy).

C. The use of manual therapy has been found to have both positive short-and long-term effects on patient outcomes (6-9 months following discharge from physical therapy).

D. The use of manual therapy does not have a positive effect on patients with hip OA.

ANSWERS

20.1 **B.** Hip internal rotation limitation is a specific variable identified in the American College of Rheumatology classification of OA. Individuals are classified as having hip OA if they experience hip pain, age is greater than 50 years, and they present with either of the following cluster of findings: (1) Hip internal rotation < 15°, hip flexion ≤ 115°, or (2) hip internal rotation > 15° but accompanied by pain and duration of morning hip stiffness < 60 minutes.[6] Also, because of tightness of the anterior capsule associated with hip OA, patients frequently have limitations in hip extension ROM.

20.2 **C.** Hoeksma and colleagues[10] published a randomized clinical trial comparing the use of manual therapy plus exercise to exercise alone in patients with hip OA. The group that received both manual therapy and exercise demonstrated significant improvement in Harris Hip Scores, walking speed, pain, and range of motion at 5 weeks after initiating treatment and at a 9-month follow-up.

REFERENCES

1. Cibulka MT, White DM, Woehrle J, et al. Hip pain and mobility deficits—hip osteoarthritis: clinical practice guidelines linked to the international classification of functioning, disability and health from the orthopaedic section of the American Physical Therapy Association. *J Orthop Sports Phys Ther*. 2009;39:A1-A25.

2. Dagenais S, Garbedian S, Wai EK. Systematic review of the prevalence of radiographic primary hip osteoarthritis. *Clin Orthop Relat Res*. 2009;467:623-637.

3. Robertsson O, Wingstrand H, Onnerfalt O. Intracapsular pressure and pain in coxarthrosis. *J Arthroplasty*. 1995;10:632-635.

4. Rosemann T, Laux G, Szecsenyi J. Osteoarthritis: quality of life, comorbidities, medication and health service utilization assessed in a large sample of primary care patients. *J Orthop Surg Res*. 2007;2:12.

5. Kellgren JH, Lawrence JS. Radiological assessment of osteo-arthrosis. *Ann Rheum Dis*. 1957;16:494-502.

6. Altman R, Alarcon G, Appelrouth D, et al. The American College of Rheumatology criteria for the classification and reporting of osteoarthritis of the hip. *Arthritis Rheum*.1991;34:505-514.

7. Sutlive TG, Lopez HP, Schnitker DE, et al. Development of a clinical prediction rule for diagnosing hip osteoarthritis in individuals with unilateral hip pain. *J Orthop Sports Phys Ther*. 2008; 38:542-550.

8. Singh JA, Vessely MB, Harmsen WS, et al. A population-based study of trends in the use of total hip and total knee arthroplasty, 1969-2008. *Mayo Clin Proc*. 2010;85:898-904.

9. MacDonald CW, Whitman JM, Cleland JA, Smith M, Hoeksma HL. Clinical outcomes following manual physical therapy and exercise for hip osteoarthritis: a case series. *J Orthop Sports Phys Ther*. 2006;36:588-599.

10. Hoeksma HL, Dekker J, Ronday HK, et al. Comparison of manual therapy and exercise therapy in osteoarthritis of the hip: a randomized clinical trial. *Arthritis Rheum*. 2004;51:722-729.

11. Wainner RS, Whitman JM. First-line interventions for hip pain: is it surgery, drugs, or us? *J Orthop Sports Phys Ther*. 2007;37:511-513.

12. Khan AM, McLoughlin E, Giannakas K, Hutchinson C, Andrew JG. Hip osteoarthritis: where is the pain? *Ann R Coll Surg Eng*. 2004;86:119-121.

13. Bellamy N, Buchanan WW, Goldsmith CH, Campbell J, Stitt LW. Validation study of WOMAC: a health status instrument for measuring clinically important patient relevant outcomes to antirheumatic drug therapy in patients with osteoarthritis of the hip or knee. *J Rheumatol*. 1988;15:1833-1844.

14. Harris WH. Traumatic arthritis of the hip after dislocation and acetabular fractures: treatment by mold arthroplasty. An end-result study using a new method of result evaluation. *J Bone Joint Surg Am*. 1969;51:737-755.

15. Hoeksma HL, Van Den Ende CH, Ronday HK, Heering A, Breedveld FC. Comparison of the responsiveness of the Harris Hip Score with generic measures for hip function in osteoarthritis of the hip. *Ann Rheum Dis*. 2003;62:935-938.

16. Neumann DA. Biomechanical analysis of selected principles of hip joint protection. *Arthritis Care Res*.1989;2:146-155.

17. Neumann DA. An electromyographic study of the hip abductor muscles as subjects with a hip prosthesis walked with different methods of using a cane and carrying a load. *Phys Ther*. 1999;79:1163-1176.

18. Simoneau GG, Hoenig KJ, Lepley JE, Papanek PE. Influence of hip position and gender on active hip internal and external rotation. *J Orthop Sports Phys Ther*. 1998;28:158-164.

19. Cyriax J. *Textbook of Orthopaedic Medicine Volume 1. Diagnosis of Soft Tissue Lesions*. 8th ed. London, UK: Bailliere Tindall; 1982.

20. Kenna C, Murtagh J. Patrick or fabere test to test hip and sacroiliac joint disorders. *Aust Fam Physician*.1989;18:375.

21. Cibere J, Thorne A, Bellamy N, et al. Reliability of the hip examination in osteoarthritis: effect of standardization. *Arthritis Rheum*. 2008;59:373-381.

22. Cliborne AV, Wainner RS, Rhon DI, et al. Clinical hip tests and a functional squat test in patients with knee osteoarthritis: reliability, prevalence of positive findings, and short-term response to hip mobilization. *J Orthop Sports Phys Ther*. 2004;34:676-685.

23. Enright PL, Sherrill DL. Reference equations for the six-minute walk in healthy adults. *Am J Respir Crit Care Med*. 1998;158(5 Pt 1):1384-1387.

24. Wright AA, Cook CE, Flynn TW, Baxter GD, Abbott JH. Predictors of response to physical therapy intervention in patients with primary hip osteoarthritis. *Phys Ther*. 2011;91:510-524.

25. Wainner RS, Whitman JM, Cleland JA, Flynn TW. Regional interdependence: a musculoskeletal examination model whose time has come. *J Orthop Sports Phys Ther*. 2007;37:658-660.

26. Ben-Galim P, Ben-Galim T, Rand N, et al. Hip-spine syndrome: the effect of total hip replacement surgery on low back pain in severe osteoarthritis of the hip. *Spine*. 2007;32:2099-2102.

27. Pelland L, Brosseau L, Wells G, et al. Efficacy of strengthening exercises for osteoarthritis (part I): a meta-analysis. *Phys Ther Rev*. 2004;9:77-108.

28. DiStefano LJ, Blackburn JT, Marshall SW, Padua DA. Gluteal muscle activation during common therapeutic exercises. *J Orthop Sports Phys Ther*. 2009;39:532-540.

29. Blumenthal JA, Emery CF, Madden DJ, et al. Effects of exercise training on cardiorespiratory function in men and women older than 60 years of age. *Amer J Cardiol*. 1991;67:633-639.

30. Stewart KJ, Bacher AC, Turner KL, et al. Effect of exercise on blood pressure in older persons: a randomized controlled trial. *Arch Intern Med*. 2005;16:756-762.

Hip Femoral Acetabular Impingement (FAI)

Erik P. Meira

A 24-year-old recreational soccer player is referred to physical therapy by a general practitioner with a diagnosis of "hip pain." The patient reports that she has had left hip pain which has been progressively increasing over the past 4 years. She reports the primary location of pain has been in the front of the hip with an occasional "piercing sensation deep inside." She cannot recall a specific injury to the joint, although her pain worsened approximately 2 months ago during a soccer game when her hip went into extreme flexion. She now has pain especially when lifting her leg to get out of bed or out of a car. In addition to an intensification of her hip pain, she now notices a "catching" sensation as she moves her hip around. She has been unable to play soccer for 2 months and there has been no improvement in her symptoms. When asked to point to the location of the pain, she makes a "C" with her thumb and fingers and grabs her hip, digging her fingers into her anterior hip. Based on the patient's history, the physical therapist suspects femoroacetabular impingement with an acetabular labral tear.

▶ What examination signs may be associated with this suspected diagnosis?
▶ What are the most appropriate examination tests?
▶ What is her rehabilitation prognosis?
▶ What are possible complications that may limit the effectiveness of physical therapy?

KEY DEFINITIONS

ACETABULAR LABRUM: Fibrocartilaginous ring around the rim of the acetabulum that can become damaged during femoroacetabular impingement; often the source of pain in symptomatic patients with femoroacetabular impingement[1,2]

CAM IMPINGEMENT: Femoroacetabular impingement caused by a cam or egg-shaped deformity of the femoral head

COMBINATION IMPINGEMENT: Femoroacetabular impingement caused by a combination of cam and pincer impingements

FEMOROACETABULAR IMPINGEMENT (FAI): Condition in which the femoral head and/or neck makes excessive contact with the acetabulum

PINCER IMPINGEMENT: Femoroacetabular impingement caused by a retroverted acetabulum that creates excessive anterior coverage of the femoral head

Objectives

1. Describe femoroacetabular impingement and identify potential risk factors associated with this diagnosis.
2. Describe the clinical examination for the patient with suspected FAI, including special tests and their associated diagnostic accuracy.
3. Prescribe appropriate joint range of motion and/or strengthening exercises for a patient with FAI.
4. Provide appropriate medical referral for the patient with suspected FAI.

Physical Therapy Considerations

PT considerations during management of the individual with a suspected diagnosis of femoroacetabular impingement:

▶ **General physical therapy plan of care/goals:** Decrease pain; increase lower quadrant strength; increase hip range of motion as tolerated; prevent or minimize loss of aerobic fitness capacity

▶ **Physical therapy interventions:** Patient education regarding functional anatomy and injury pathomechanics; modalities and manual therapy to decrease pain; resistance exercises to increase muscular endurance capacity of the core and to increase strength of lower extremity muscles; gentle stretching as tolerated to increase range of motion; aerobic exercise program

▶ **Precautions during physical therapy:** Monitor vital signs; address precautions or contraindications for exercise, based on patient's pre-exisiting condition(s); avoid activities/positions that exacerbate symptoms

▶ **Differential diagnoses:** Extra-articular pathology such as external coxa saltans, internal coxa saltans, iliopsoas strain, athletic pubalgia, or stress fracture

Understanding the Health Condition

Femoroacetabular impingement (FAI) is a condition in which there is an incongruence of the femoral head with the acetabulum, leading to abnormal contact between these two bones at the end ranges of hip motion. FAI generally presents as a cam impingement, pincer impingement, or a combination of the two. In a cam impingement, the femoral head does not have a normal spherical shape; instead, it has more of a cam or egg shape (Fig. 21-1). As the femoral head articulates in the acetabulum, a cam shape of the femoral head applies increased stress at the edges of the joint. In a pincer impingement, it is the shape of the acetabulum that causes the impingement. In this case, the acetabulum is retroverted, which causes the anterior wall of the acetabulum to cover an excessive amount of the femoral head (Fig. 21-2). As the hip joint articulates, the femoral neck makes contact with the acetabular rim earlier in the range of motion, causing increased stress to the joint that can damage the acetabular labrum, the articular cartilage, or both. This damage results in the pain that causes the patient to seek medical services.[1,2]

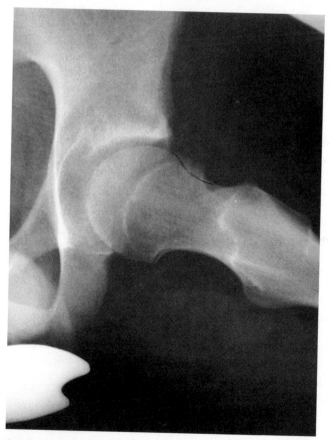

Figure 21-1. Radiograph showing a cam- or egg-shaped femoral head. The portion of the bone inside the darkened line represents a normal shape of the femoral head. (Reproduced with permission from Mark B. Wagner, MD.)

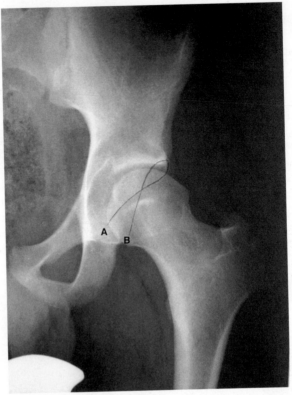

Figure 21-2. Pincer impingement with crossover sign on an anteroposterior radiograph. The darkened line demonstrates the "crossing over" of **A** (anterior rim of acetabulum) and **B** (posterior rim of acetabulum). (Reproduced with permission from Mark B. Wagner, MD.)

The incidence of FAI in the general population is relatively high. Recent studies have shown that roughly 20% of asymptomatic individuals have some kind of FAI.[3-6] FAI usually affects people between 20 and 40 years of age. Cam impingement is more common in males, whereas pincer impingement is slightly more common in females. In one study of 200 asymptomatic adults, 14% had at least one hip with cam morphology and 79% of those were male.[4] A retrospective study reported close to 30% of asymptomatic males have evidence of a cam deformity.[5] In a radiographic database of over 4000 individuals, pincer deformity was seen in 19% of asymptomatic females and 15% of asymptomatic males.[3] A recent study of 39 asymptomatic collegiate and professional hockey players reported that 64% had abnormal magnetic resonance imaging findings.[6] Because hip pathologies are common, it is essential to determine whether a patient's pain is caused by FAI, which can result in damage to the acetabular labrum and/or articular cartilage.

Over time, FAI can damage the hip joint through repetitive contact between the two incongruent joint surfaces. Since many sports require extensive hip mobility, individuals with FAI often become symptomatic through repeated athletic activities.[1,2] Because the individual with FAI experiences pain with deep squatting and end-range internal and external rotation activities, these motions should be avoided when FAI is suspected.[1,2] Athletes often mistake their limited comfortable hip range of motion as an indication of poor flexibility and try to resolve the problem through stretching. This can exacerbate the pain and potentially cause more damage to the joint.[1,2] It is common for patients to present with increasing pain over time that becomes significantly exacerbated and intolerable after one "final" event.[1,2]

Pain from the hip usually refers to the anterior hip and into the groin. Without prompting, patients often make the shape of a "C" with their thumb and fingers and grab the hip when asked to point to the painful area to demonstrate that the pain is deep. This is known as the "C-sign."[1] Since patients who have hip joint pathology frequently have guarding and irritation in the hip flexors and adductors, it can be difficult to differentiate between muscle and joint pathology.

It has been suggested that radiographic evidence of FAI and even damage to the acetabular labrum *without* the presence of pain should not be corrected.[6,7] However, in symptomatic patients, **arthroscopic surgical correction of FAI** is very effective for reducing pain and increasing function.[8]

Physical Therapy Patient/Client Management

A primary role for the physical therapist is in differentially diagnosing the etiology of hip pain. If FAI is a suspected cause of a patient's pain, involving an orthopaedic surgeon for assistance with case management and further diagnostics is appropriate. Since FAI is a condition involving the shape of the bone, therapy interventions cannot alter the bony anatomy. Interventions should focus on pain management and improving function. Increasing strength and teaching the patient to avoid painful positions may be enough to allow her to return to desired activities. There is some low-level evidence supporting that correcting faulty movement mechanics may be beneficial in reducing pain and increasing function.[9] There is stronger evidence supporting the benefits of surgical correction of FAI.[8]

Examination, Evaluation, and Diagnosis

The physical therapist must take a thorough patient history. The patient with suspected FAI often complains of pain deep in the anterior hip. The pain often increases with activities that create resistance to the iliopsoas muscle group such as raising the leg to get out of bed or a car because this increases the stress to the hip joint and the anterior-superior labrum. The patient may also complain of mechanical signs such as a sporadic "catching" in the joint with subsequent pain. The pain often improves with rest. However, the pain usually returns when more athletic activities are resumed.[1,2,7]

On deep palpation, the patient may present with tenderness in the anterior hip while positioned in supine. Resisted straight leg raise is often painful because it places increased load to the iliopsoas and therefore the anterior joint.[1,2] Passive rotation of the involved leg with the patient in supine may reproduce symptoms. Symptoms are diminished if passive hip rotation is repeated while applying distraction to the joint.[1,2] The FABER (femoral

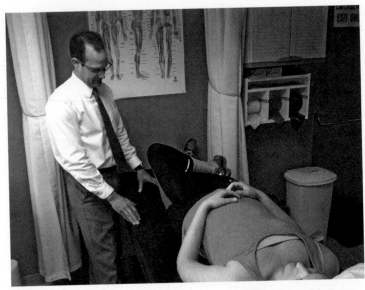

Figure 21-3. Patient's left lower extremity in the FABER (femoral abduction external rotation) position. This position is often restricted and uncomfortable when compared to the uninvolved side.

abduction external rotation) position (Fig. 21-3) is often restricted and uncomfortable when compared to the uninvolved side. If there is significant damage to the articular surfaces, a hip scour test is painful. Placing the hip into combined end-range flexion, adduction, and internal rotation (Fig. 21-4) recreates the abnormal contact

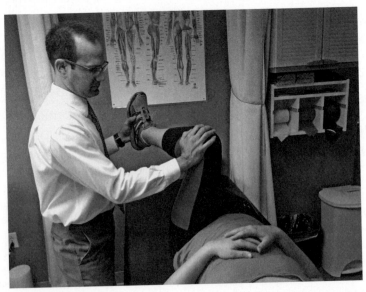

Figure 21-4. Therapist performing hip scour test on the left lower extremity. Placement of the hip into combined end-range flexion, adduction, and internal rotation recreates the abnormal contact in FAI and reproduces the patient's symptoms.

Table 21-1   SPECIAL TESTS FOR INTRA-ARTICULAR HIP JOINT PATHOLOGY AND THEIR REPORTED SENSITIVITY AND SPECIFICITY[7]

Signs/Symptoms	Sensitivity (%)	Specificity (%)
+ Groin pain	59	14
+ Catching	63	54
+ Pinching pain in sitting	48	54
– Lateral thigh pain	78	36
+ FABER	60	18
+ Impingement	78	10
– Trochanteric tenderness	57	45

"+" indicates that pain is present or elicited; "–" indicates that pain is absent

in FAI and reproduces the patient's symptoms.[1,7] Table 21-1 shows **special tests for the hip joint.** The reported diagnostic accuracy of each test was based on comparison to the criterion standard of > 50% pain relief with an intra-articular anesthetic injection, which is indicative of intra-articular pathology.[7] None of the special tests have good diagnostic accuracy. That is, none of the tests was useful to identify intra-articular structures as the cause of a patient's hip pain. The especially low specificity means that many individuals *without* intra-articular pathology would be falsely diagnosed with intra-articular hip pathology with these tests.

If the physical therapist suspects FAI and/or a possible acetabular labral tear after completing the evaluation, the therapist should refer the patient to an orthopaedic surgeon experienced in the management of intra-articular hip pathology. Radiographs will show the presence of FAI and whether the impingement is caused by a cam or pincer deformity. Confirmation of an acetabular labral tear can be achieved via a magnetic resonance arthrogram with gadolinium contrast followed by an injection of an anesthetic such as lidocaine into the hip joint.[7] A significant reduction in symptoms after the anesthetic injection indicates that the pain is coming from the joint itself and not surrounding tissues.[7]

Plan of Care and Interventions

Patients with confirmed and painful FAI may respond to **conservative management.**[9] Since range of motion limitations may be restricted by bony morphology, attempts to increase flexibility and range of motion should be performed with caution. Focus should be placed on increasing muscular strength and coordination while avoiding any positions that exacerbate pain such as end-range hip flexion, internal rotation, and abduction. Currently, only one case series of four patients with acetabular labral tears has been published suggesting the efficacy of nonsurgical rehabilitation with only a 3-month follow-up.[9] These authors suggest that controlling functional knee valgus by emphasizing hip and lumbopelvic stabilization may reduce symptoms caused by an acetabular labral tear. If a patient is unable to restrict the hip range of motion and be functional in sport or activities of daily living, surgical correction has been shown to be effective.[8]

Evidence-Based Clinical Recommendations

SORT: Strength of Recommendation Taxonomy

A: Consistent, good-quality patient-oriented evidence
B: Inconsistent or limited-quality patient-oriented evidence
C: Consensus, disease-oriented evidence, usual practice, expert opinion, or case series

1. Surgical correction is effective for decreasing pain and increasing function in patients with symptomatic femoroacetabular impingement. **Grade A**

2. Special tests for diagnosis of intra-articular hip pathology have better sensitivity than specificity, but have overall poor diagnostic accuracy. **Grade B**

3. A treatment program consisting of therapeutic strengthening exercises to limit knee valgus may be effective for reducing pain in patients with hip labral injuries associated with FAI. **Grade C**

COMPREHENSION QUESTIONS

21.1 Muscles around the hip may become irritated and exacerbate pre-exisiting hip pathology. Activation of which muscle consistently reproduces pain associated with a torn acetabular labrum?

A. Adductor magnus

B. Iliopsoas

C. Gluteus medius

D. Piriformis

21.2 A patient presents to an outpatient physical therapist with signs and symptoms of FAI with an acetabular labral tear. What is the *most* accurate way to confirm that his symptoms are coming from the hip joint and not surrounding soft tissue?

A. Clinical examination

B. Plain radiographs

C. Magnetic resonance arthrogram with gadolinium

D. Injection of an anesthetic into the joint that causes temporary reduction of pain

ANSWERS

21.1 **B.** Pain often increases with activities that create resistance to the iliopsoas muscle group such as raising the leg to get out of bed or a car because this increases the stress to the hip joint and the anterior-superior labrum.

21.2 **D.** The clinical examination (history and physical examination) is critical for the physical therapist to narrow down the differential diagnoses; however, the special tests have poor accuracy to diagnose intra-articular hip pathology (option A). Imaging studies (plain radiographs or magnetic resonance arthrogram with gadolinium) may demonstrate the presence of FAI. However, studies have demonstrated that *asymptomatic* subjects may present with cam or pincer deformities (options B and C).

REFERENCES

1. Byrd JW. Evaluation of the hip: history and physical examination. *N Am J Sports Phys Ther.* 2007; 2:231-240.

2. Philippon MJ, Stubbs AJ, Schenker ML, Maxwell RB, Ganz R, Leunig M. Arthroscopic management of femoroacetabular impingement: osteoplasty technique and literature review. *Am J Sports Med.* 2007;35:1571-1580.

3. Gosvig KK, Jacobsen S, Sonne-Holm S, Palm H, Troelsen A. Prevalence of malformations of the hip joint and their relationship to sex, groin pain, and risk of osteoarthritis: a population-based survey. *J Bone Joint Surg.* 2010;92:1162-1169.

4. Hack K, Di Primio G, Rakhra K, Beaule PE. Prevalence of cam-type femoroacetabular impingement morphology in asymptomatic volunteers. *J Bone Joint Surg.* 2010;92:2436-2444.

5. Jung KA, Restrepo C, Hellman M, AbdelSalam H, Morrison W, Parvizi J. The prevalence of cam-type femoroacetabular deformity in asymptomatic adults. *J Bone Joint Surg Br.* 2011;93:1303-1307.

6. Silvis ML, Mosher TJ, Smetana BS, et al. High prevalence of pelvic and hip magnetic resonance imaging findings in asymptomatic collegiate and professional hockey players. *Am J Sports Med.* 2011;39:715-721.

7. Martin RL, Irrgang JJ, Sekiya JK. The diagnostic accuracy of a clinical examination in determining intra-articular hip pain for potential hip arthroscopy candidates. *Arthroscopy.* 2008;24:1013-1018.

8. Ng VY, Arora N, Best TM, Pan X, Ellis TJ. Efficacy of surgery for femoroacetabular impingement: a systematic review. *Am J Sports Med.* 2010;38:2337-2345.

9. Yazbek PM, Ovanessian V, Martin RL, Fukuda TY. Nonsurgical treatment of acetabular labrum tears: a case series. *J Orthop Sports Phys Ther.* 2011;41:346-353.

Iliotibial Band Syndrome

Jason Brumitt

CASE 22

A 32-year-old recreational runner self-referred to an outpatient physical therapy clinic with a complaint of right lateral knee pain. He first experienced pain 6 weeks ago. Two weeks prior to symptom onset, he initiated a marathon-training program. His symptoms have gradually worsened; now, he is no longer able to run due to the immediate onset of the same pain. The patient's medical history is otherwise unremarkable. Signs and symptoms are consistent with iliotibial band syndrome (ITBS). His goal is to return to training for the upcoming marathon.

▶ Based on the patient's suspected diagnosis, what do you anticipate may be the contributing factors to his condition?
▶ What examination signs may be associated with this diagnosis?
▶ What are the most appropriate physical therapy interventions?

KEY DEFINITIONS

CORE STABILITY: Ability of muscles within the "core" region (abdomen, lumbar spine, pelvis, and hips) to protect (*i.e.*, stabilize) the lumbar spine from potentially injurious forces and to create and/or transfer forces between anatomical segments during functional movements

ILIOTIBIAL BAND SYNDROME: Overuse injury primarily experienced by distance runners, marked by lateral knee or lateral hip pain

TRIGGER POINT: Taut band of contracted muscle fibers within a skeletal muscle that may cause pain, decreased range of motion, and may be associated with muscular weakness[1]

Objectives

1. Describe iliotibial band syndrome and identify potential risk factors associated with this diagnosis.
2. Prescribe appropriate joint range of motion and/or muscular flexibility exercises for a person with iliotibial band syndrome.
3. Prescribe appropriate resistance exercises during each stage of healing for a person with iliotibial band syndrome.

Physical Therapy Considerations

PT considerations during management of the individual with a diagnosis of iliotibial band syndrome:

▶ **General physical therapy plan of care/goals:** Decrease pain; increase muscular flexibility and/or joint range of motion; increase lower quadrant strength; prevent or minimize loss of aerobic fitness capacity

▶ **Physical therapy interventions:** Patient education regarding functional anatomy and injury pathomechanics; modalities and manual therapy to decrease pain; muscular flexibility exercises; resistance exercises to increase muscular endurance capacity of the core and to increase strength of lower extremity muscles; aerobic exercise program; orthotic fabrication

▶ **Precautions during physical therapy:** Monitor vital signs; address precautions or contraindications for exercise, based on patient's pre-existing condition(s)

Understanding the Health Condition

The iliotibial band (ITB) is a thickening of the thigh's tensor fascia lata.[2,3] Proximally, the ITB originates from the iliac crest, envelops the tensor fasciae latae (TFL) muscle, and receives tendinous attachments from the gluteus maximus muscle before extending distally to attach to the lateral patella, the lateral patellar retinaculum,

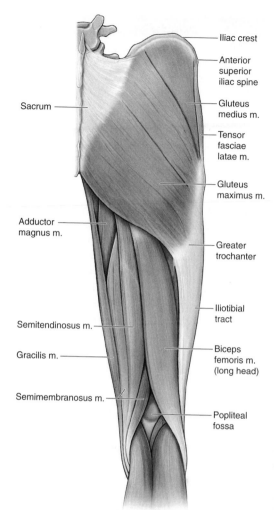

Iliac crest

Anterior superior iliac spine

Gluteus medius m.

Tensor fasciae latae m.

Gluteus maximus m.

Greater trochanter

Iliotibial tract

Biceps femoris m. (long head)

Popliteal fossa

Sacrum

Adductor magnus m.

Semitendinosus m.

Gracilis m.

Semimembranosus m.

Figure 22-1. Posterior view of hip and leg, showing tensor fasciae latae muscle and its inferior thickened extension as the iliotibial tract (band). (Reproduced with permission from Morton DA, Foreman KB, Albertine KH, eds. *The Big Picture: Gross Anatomy*. New York: McGraw-Hill; 2011. Figure 35-1B.)

and Gerdy's (lateral tibial) tubercle (Fig. 22-1).[2,4] Whiteside et al.[4] have identified three distal bands of the ITB: a broad band, a broad and dense central band, and a thin band (Table 22-1). Whiteside et al.[4] suggested that the distal anatomy of the ITB helps to increase stability on the lateral aspect of the knee.

Iliotibial band syndrome (ITBS) is an overuse injury experienced primarily by distance runners.[5] Iliotibial band syndrome has also been reported in other athletes (*e.g.*, cyclists) and active individuals (*e.g.*, hikers).[6] The primary symptom associated with ITBS is lateral knee pain.[5-7] Initial symptoms may be mild, with pain experienced at some point during one's run (or activity). If the condition worsens, pain may prevent the individual from training and pain may be present when at rest.

The onset of the syndrome is thought to be the result of repetitive friction stress, especially to the posterior portion of the distal ITB as it crosses the lateral femoral epicondyle.[5-8] It has been generally accepted that the ITB slides anterior to the lateral femoral epicondyle during knee extension and posterior to the lateral femoral epicondyle during knee flexion.[5,7] This "movement" of the ITB across the lateral

Table 22-1 DISTAL BANDS AND BONY ATTACHMENTS OF THE ITB	
Broad band	Patella Patellar tendon Quadriceps tendon
Broad and dense band	Deep fascia Gerdy's tubercle
Thin band	Fibular head Deep fascia Biceps femoris muscle and tendon

femoral epicondyle occurs at approximately 30° of knee flexion (referred to as the impingement zone).[5,7] There has been a lack of consensus as to which structures are actually impinged between the ITB and the femoral epicondyle.[2,7] Recent studies suggest that innervated fat and connective tissue are compressed between the ITB and the epicondyle.[2,3] In addition, Fairclough et al.[2] have suggested that the ITB does not slide across the epicondyle. Based on their study of 15 human cadavers (anatomical and microscopic analysis) and six asymptomatic subjects (magnetic resonance imaging), different fibers of the ITB are tensed throughout the range of knee flexion and extension. Instead of an anterior-posterior slide creating friction leading to ITBS, they propose that pain onset is due to compression of the fat between the ITB and the femur.

Iliotibial band syndrome may be the result of extrinsic and/or intrinsic risk factors. **Extrinsic factors** that have been proposed to contribute to the onset of ITBS include poor footwear, increasing weekly training distances too quickly, running too many miles in general, and running downhill.[5,8,9] Potential **intrinsic risk factors** for ITBS include hip adduction and knee internal rotation when running, weakness in the hip abductors, muscular imbalance around the hip, and muscular tightness in the lower extremity.[5,8-12]

Physical Therapy Patient/Client Management

There may be one or more appropriate interventions based on the patient's presentation. Physical therapy treatments may include modalities, soft tissue mobilization, therapeutic exercise, footwear evaluation, and/or orthotics.[5,7,11] Some patients may benefit from prescription nonsteroidal anti-inflammatory drugs (NSAIDs) or a glucocorticoid injection.[6,8] In recalcitrant cases, the patient may require a surgical consult with an orthopaedic physician.[8,13,14] The primary goal for most injured athletes/individuals is to return to pain-free sport or activity as quickly and as safely as possible in a manner that does not overload the healing tissues.

Examination, Evaluation, and Diagnosis

Individuals presenting with symptoms consistent with ITBS are likely to be distance runners.[5] The injured distance runner describes pain at the lateral knee when running. In some cases, pain may also be present at rest. During the history portion of the examination, the physical therapist should ask the patient questions regarding his medical history. In addition, the physical therapist should inquire about the patient's specific training habits, including types of surfaces the individual trains on (*e.g.*, flat terrain or hills) and which positions or activities reproduce symptoms when not running. For example, an individual with ITBS may report running on a track in only one direction or running on the crown of a road. The patient may experience pain running downhill, descending stairs, walking, or sitting with the injured leg flexed.[5]

A comprehensive musculoskeletal examination should be conducted to rule out other potential sources of lateral knee pain, including lateral collateral ligament sprain, meniscal injury, or patellofemoral pain. Musculoskeletal findings consistent with ITBS include pain with palpation to the distal ITB near the lateral femoral epicondyle, pain with palpation to trigger points in the ITB or TFL, lack of muscular flexibility in the involved lower extremity, and asymmetrical lower extremity strength.[5,15] Proximally, the muscles of the hip and thigh may present with asymmetrical tightness between the involved and uninvolved side. Wang et al.[16] found that distance runners were significantly less flexible than healthy controls in their gastrocnemius, soleus, and hamstring muscles. In addition, hamstring muscles in the runner's dominant leg were significantly less flexible than the hamstrings in the nondominant leg. Patients with ITBS often present with positive findings during either the Ober test or the Noble compression test (Table 22-2).[5,8] Manual muscle tests

Table 22-2 FLEXIBILITY AND SPECIAL TESTS ASSOCIATED WITH ITBS

Tests	Patient Position	Findings
Thomas test	Patient sits at edge of treatment table. Therapist assists patient into supine position or patient lies supine independently. Patient brings both knees to the chest. The leg to be tested is released and allowed to extend toward the table.	Asymmetrical hip extension is a positive sign of tight hip flexors (iliopsoas).
Passive straight leg raise	Patient lies supine on treatment table. The therapist passively elevates the straight leg to the point of either increased muscular tension or loss of a neutral pelvic position.	Hamstring tightness is noted with either an asymmetry between lower extremities or a general lack of flexibility.
Noble compression test	Have patient lie supine. Therapist passively flexes knee to approximately 90°. Therapist applies pressure to distal ITB near the femoral epicondyle and passively extends patient's knee.	Report of pain at approximately 30° of knee flexion is a positive sign.
Ober test	Patient assumes sidelying position on the unaffected lower extremity. Therapist passively flexes the top knee to 90°. The therapist's proximal hand (one closest to hip) stabilizes the pelvis while the distal hand abducts and extends the hip.	An inability of the hip to adduct toward the table suggests tightness in the TFL/ITB

should be performed to assess the strength of the hip and thigh muscles.[15,17] Fredericson et al.[15] identified hip abductor weakness on the involved side of 24 injured distance runners with ITBS (10 females, mean age 27 years). Niemuth et al.[17] assessed hip strength in 30 recreational runners with a unilateral lower extremity overuse injury. Injured runners (30% of whom presented with ITBS) had significantly weaker hip abductor and flexor strength compared to their uninvolved leg.

Plan of Care and Interventions

Physical therapy interventions should address findings from the musculoskeletal examination. Modalities may help reduce acute symptoms. Therapeutic exercises are prescribed to address muscular tightness and muscular weakness.[5,7,15,18,19]

A standardized 6-week (1 session per week) treatment program consisting of rest, NSAIDs, and physical therapy interventions statistically improved hip abductor strength and successfully enabled a majority (22 of 24) of injured runners with ITBS to return to running.[15] In this study, Fredericson et al.[15] performed **phonophoresis** (parameters not presented) for up to two sessions. Patients were also prescribed two stretching and two strengthening exercises. The stretching exercises (a supine ITB stretch using a rope and a standing ITB stretch) were performed 3 times per day with each stretch held for 15 seconds each. Two strengthening exercises, the sidelying hip abduction and the standing pelvic drop, were progressed from an initial dosing of one set of 15 repetitions, with the patient adding 5 repetitions per day, to a goal of performing 3 sets of 30 repetitions.

Fredericson et al.[15] have spent years investigating the most effective ITBS interventions, resulting in more precise treatment recommendations that reflect an appreciation for the different phases of tissue healing. In a 2006 review, Fredericson et al.[7] recommended that patients rest and avoid pain-provoking activities during the acute phase. Modalities are also introduced to decrease pain and inflammation in this phase. The use of NSAIDs to reduce inflammation and, if patients are experiencing intense pain, a glucocorticoid injection, were also recommended. **Stretching exercises** to address muscular inflexibility should be initiated during the subacute phase of healing. Fredericson et al.[19] reported that the position that creates the most effective stretch is the standing ITB position with an overhead arm extension (Fig. 22-2). In addition to the classic ITB stretching exercises, some individuals have reported improved flexibility and decreased pain both during and after performing the ITB **foam roll exercise**[6] (Fig. 22-3). The effectiveness of this foam roll application to increase muscular flexibility is unknown. However, the pain reduction that some patients report with this exercise may be due to the pressure applied to trigger points in the TFL or ITB.[7]

Strengthening exercises should be introduced during the subacute phase.[5,7,15] The hip abductors (especially gluteus medius) have been identified as dysfunctional in individuals diagnosed with ITBS.[5,7,15] The gluteus medius (along with gluteus minimus and TFL muscles) maintain pelvic stability during gait and eccentrically contract to resist adduction moments at the hip. Weakness in the hip abductors allows increased hip adduction and knee internal rotation, factors that may

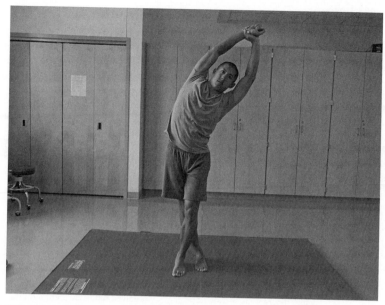

Figure 22-2. Patient performing standing ITB stretch for the right lower extremity.

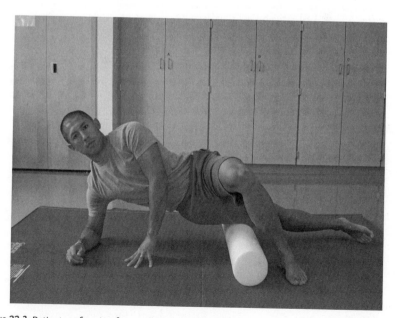

Figure 22-3. Patient performing foam roll exercise. The patient is positioned with involved right ITB on a foam roll, with the uninvolved lower extremity flexed and externally rotated to allow him to place the foot to the front of the involved leg. Both upper extremities are positioned to assist balance.

contribute to the onset of ITBS.[12] Lower extremity strengthening is progressed from open kinetic chain positions that emphasize concentric muscular contractions (e.g., sidelying hip abduction, pelvic drop exercise) to closed kinetic chain positions emphasizing eccentric muscular contractions (Table 22-3).[5,7] Fredericson et al.[5,7] recommended that each eccentric exercise should be performed bilaterally for two to three sets of 5 to 8 repetitions progressing to sets of 15 repetitions.

Table 22-3 ECCENTRIC EXERCISES FOR ILIOTIBIAL BAND SYNDROME		
Eccentric Exercise	**Starting Position**	**Exercise Technique**
Modified matrix exercise	Have the patient stand with the lower extremities positioned shoulder width apart. The involved leg (right leg) is externally rotated with the foot oriented in the 3 o'clock position. The uninvolved left leg is positioned with the foot pointing in the 12 o'clock direction (Fig. 22-4).	Instruct the patient to perform an abdominal bracing contraction prior to initiating the exercise. The movement is performed by having the patient rotate his hips toward the uninvolved (left) leg, transferring weight from the involved (right) to the uninvolved leg. As the weight-shifting occurs, the involved hip is lowered. Simultaneously, the patient reaches his upper extremity on the involved hip side across his body toward the uninvolved mid-thigh region (Fig. 22-5). Patient returns to the start position and repeats.
Wallbangers	Have the patient stand with the involved lower extremity (right) positioned 6 to 12 in from a wall (Fig. 22-6).	Have patient flex shoulders to 90° and rotate pelvis away from the wall (Fig. 22-6). As the patient rotates his anterior pelvis away from the wall, he should flex his knees and lower the involved hip (right) toward the wall (Fig. 22-7). When the involved hip contacts ("bangs") against the wall, the patient returns to the start position (Fig. 22-6).
Frontal plane lunges	Have the patient start in a standing position.	The first lunge position is performed by reaching the uninvolved lower extremity (left) to the side (Fig. 22-8). The second lunge position is performed by reaching the upper extremities toward the uninvolved side (Fig. 22-9). The third lunge is performed with the patient reaching the upper extremities toward the weightbearing leg (Fig. 22-10).

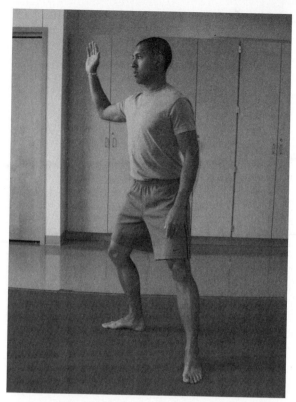

Figure 22-4. Modified matrix start position.

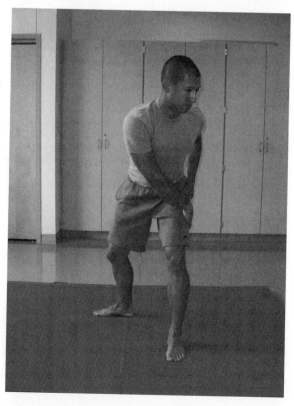

Figure 22-5. Modified matrix end position.

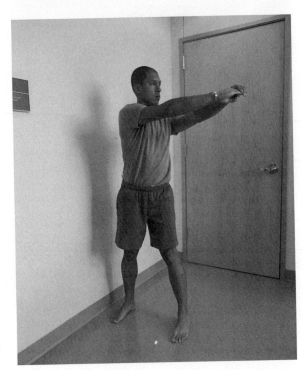

Figure 22-6. Wallbangers start position.

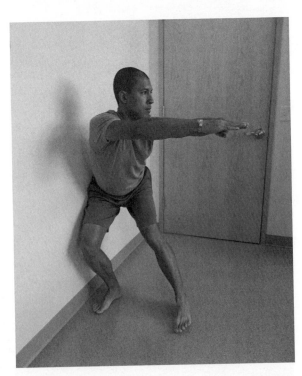

Figure 22-7. Wallbangers end position.

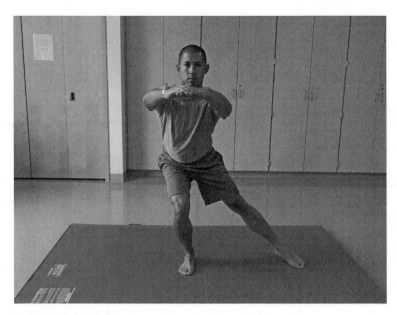

Figure 22-8. Frontal plane lunge.

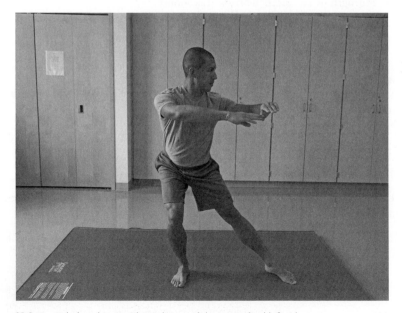

Figure 22-9. Frontal plane lunge with reach toward the uninvolved left side.

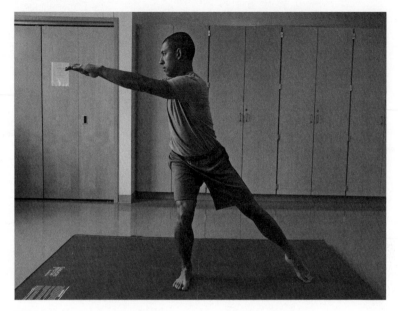

Figure 22-10. Frontal plane lunge with reach toward involved right side.

Evidence-Based Clinical Recommendations

SORT: Strength of Recommendation Taxonomy

A: Consistent, good-quality patient-oriented evidence
B: Inconsistent or limited-quality patient-oriented evidence
C: Consensus, disease-oriented evidence, usual practice, expert opinion, or case series

1. Extrinsic risk factors are associated with the onset of iliotibial band syndrome. **Grade C**

2. Intrinsic risk factors are associated with the onset of iliotibial band syndrome. **Grade B**

3. The use of phonophoresis decreases pain associated with ITBS. **Grade C**

4. Stretching and strengthening therapeutic exercises decrease pain and/or restore function in patients with ITBS. **Grade B**

5. Rolling the iliotibial band over a foam roll decreases pain and increases flexibility in patients with ITBS. **Grade C**

COMPREHENSION QUESTIONS

22.1 An outpatient physical therapist examines a distance runner suffering from ITBS in the right lower extremity. The patient presents with right hip abductor weakness. Which of the following lower extremity biomechanical dysfunctions will result from hip abduction weakness?

A. Hip abduction, knee external rotation

B. Hip abduction, knee internal rotation

C. Hip adduction, knee external rotation

D. Hip adduction, knee internal rotation

22.2 The pain associated with ITBS may not be due to repetitive friction, but rather due to compression of soft tissue. Which of the following soft tissue structures is compressed between the distal ITB and the femoral epicondyle?

A. ITB bursae

B. Lateral patellar ligament

C. Fat

D. Vastus lateralis

ANSWERS

22.1 **D.** The hip abductors are responsible for stabilizing the pelvis and eccentrically contracting to resist hip adduction. Weakness in the hip abductors (*e.g.*, gluteus medius) allows for increased hip adduction and knee internal rotation. In a prospective study of potential risk factors for ITBS, Noehren et al.[12] found that recreational runners with increased peak adduction at the hip and internal rotation at the knee were at an increased risk for ITBS.

22.2 **C.** A recent anatomical investigation by Fairclough et al.[2] identified innervated fat and connective tissue that, if compressed between the ITB and the femoral epicondyle, may contribute to the onset of ITBS.

REFERENCES

1. Simons DG, Travell JG, Simons LS. *Travell and Simons' Myofascial Pain and Dysfunction: The Trigger Point Manual. Volume 1: Upper Half of Body.* 2nd ed. Baltimore, MD: Williams & Wilkins; 1999.

2. Fairclough J, Hayashi K, Toumi H, et al. The functional anatomy of the iliotibial band during flexion and extension of the knee: implications for understanding iliotibial band syndrome. *J Anat.* 2006;208:309-316.

3. Fairclough J, Hayashi K, Toumi H, et al. Is iliotibial band syndrome really a friction syndrome? *J Sci Med Sport.* 2007;10:74-76.

4. Whiteside LA, Roy ME. Anatomy, function, and surgical access of the iliotibial band in total knee arthroplasty. *J Bone Joint Surg Am.* 2009;91:101-106.

5. Fredericson M, Wolf C. Iliotibial band syndrome in runners: innovations in treatment. *Sports Med.* 2005;35:451-459.

6. Cosca DD, Navazio F. Common problems in endurance athletes. *Am Fam Physician.* 2007;76:237-244.

7. Fredericson M, Weir A. Practical management of iliotibial band friction syndrome in runners. *Clin J Sports Med.* 2006;16:261-268.

8. Beals RK. The iliotibial tract: a review. *Curr Orthop Pract.* 2009;20:87-91.

9. Messier SP, Legault C, Schoenlank CR, Newman JJ, Martin DF, Devita P. Risk factors and mechanisms of knee injury in runners. *Med Sci Sports Exerc.* 2008;40:1873-1879.

10. Richards DP, Alan Barber F, Troop RL. Iliotibial band z-lengthening. *Arthroscopy.* 2003;19:326-329.

11. Strakowski JA, Jamil T. Management of common running injuries. *Phys Med Rehabil Clin N Am.* 2006;17:537-552.

12. Noehren B, Davis I, Hamill J. ASB clinical biomechanics award winner 2006 prospective study of the biomechanical factors associated with iliotibial band syndrome. *Clin Biomech.* 2007;22:951-956.

13. Michels F, Jambou S, Allard M, Bousquet V, Colombet P, de Lavigne C. An arthroscopic technique to treat the iliotibial band syndrome. *Knee Surg Sports Traumatol Arthrosc.* 2009;17:233-236.

14. Barber FA, Boothby MH, Troop RL. Z-plasty lengthening for iliotibial band friction syndrome. *J Knee Surg.* 2007;20:281-284.

15. Fredericson M, Cookingham CL, Chaudhari AM, Dowdell BC, Oestreicher N, Sahrmann SA. Hip abductor weakness in distance runners with iliotibial band syndrome. *Clin J Sports Med.* 2000;10:169-175.

16. Wang SS, Whitney SL, Burdett RG, Janosky JE. Lower extremity muscular flexibility in long distance runners. *J Orthop Sports Phys Ther.* 1993;17:102-107.

17. Niemuth PE, Johnson RJ, Myers MJ, Thieman TJ. Hip muscle weakness and overuse injuries in recreational runners. *Clin J Sports Med.* 2005;15:14-21.

18. Beers A, Ryan M, Kasubuchi Z, Fraser S, Taunton JE. Effects of multi-modal physiotherapy, including hip abductor strengthening, in patients with iliotibial band friction syndrome. *Physiother Can.* 2008;60:180-188.

19. Fredericson M, White JJ, Macmahon JM, Andriacchi TP. Quantitative analysis of the relative effectiveness of 3 iliotibial band stretches. *Arch Phys Med Rehabil.* 2002;83:589-592.

Patellofemoral Pain Syndrome

Robert C. Manske

A 16-year-old female competitive volleyball player with a 2-year history of intermittent anterior right knee pain and swelling is referred to physical therapy for evaluation and treatment. Six weeks ago, she had a fat pad debridement surgery and has been going to physical therapy sessions since then at another outpatient physical therapy facility. Each time she returns to volleyball, her pain and swelling return. The activities required for volleyball include running, cutting, jumping and pivoting; each of these increases her pain. During the 2 years prior to surgery, her pain was in the medial aspect of her knee. However, since surgery, she experiences the pain on both the medial and lateral sides of the knee. In the last 4 weeks, she has been experiencing pain and swelling similar to that she had prior to surgery. With either an increase in practice or game frequency, the anterior knee pain increases to 8/10 from a baseline of 1/10 on a visual analog scale (VAS). With a couple days of rest, her pain and swelling are eliminated. She has tried multiple treatments (e.g., ice, heat, compression, over-the-counter nonsteroidal anti-inflammatories), which provide symptomatic relief for short duration and are only effective if she is not playing volleyball. Although she has been in formal physical therapy for the last 6 weeks, primarily performing knee-strengthening exercises, her pain and swelling have not been effectively reduced. Her goal is to return to volleyball symptom-free now that the season has started. Her physician has not placed any restrictions on her activity.

▶ Based on her health condition, what do you anticipate may be the contributors to activity limitations?
▶ What are the examination priorities?
▶ What are the most appropriate physical therapy interventions?
▶ What precautions should be taken during physical therapy interventions?

KEY DEFINITIONS

FAT PAD: Area of highly vascularized adipose tissue directly beneath the patellar ligament that can become a source of anterior knee pain; its role is thought to help lubricate and cushion the patellar ligament from stress

LATERAL BUTTRESS EFFECT: Effect of the higher lateral patellar trochlea on the anterior surface of the distal femur; the higher lateral trochlea resists the natural lateral translation of the patella during knee flexion and extension

PATELLOFEMORAL PAIN: Also known as anterior knee pain; one of the most common forms of chronic pain in or around the anterior knee and usually has insidious onset

REGIONAL INTERDEPENDENCE: Theory that dysfunction either proximal, distal, or both from the knee joint may cause localized pain in and around the anterior knee

SCREW-HOME MECHANISM: Obligate lateral tibial rotation that occurs during the last few degrees of knee extension as the tibia glides along the longer medial femoral condyle

Objectives

1. Describe patellofemoral pain.
2. Identify methods to assess for regional interdependence.
3. Describe common muscle weaknesses that may contribute to producing patellofemoral pain.
4. Select appropriate treatment interventions for the individual with patellofemoral pain.
5. Prescribe exercises to treat patellofemoral pain that may be caused by sources other than the knee.

Physical Therapy Considerations

PT considerations during management of the individual with patellofemoral pain:

▶ **General physical therapy plan of care/goals:** Decrease pain; increase muscular flexibility; increase lower quadrant strength; prevent or minimize loss of aerobic fitness capacity

▶ **Physical therapy interventions:** Patient education regarding functional anatomy and injury pathomechanics; modalities and manual therapy to decrease pain; muscular flexibility exercises; resistance exercises to increase muscular endurance capacity of the core and to increase strength of lower extremity muscles around the hip; aerobic exercise program; home exercise program with emphasis on strengthening symptomatic lower extremity in positions that do not allow compensatory patterns

▶ **Precautions during physical therapy:** Monitor vital signs; address precautions or contraindications for exercise, based on patient's pre-existing condition(s)

Understanding the Health Condition

Patellofemoral pain, also known as anterior knee pain, is one of the most common chronic knee musculoskeletal conditions in relatively active adolescents and adults. The incidence of patellofemoral pain ranges from 9% to 15% in active young populations.[1-5] Recent evidence has concurred with the historical perspective that this **condition occurs most often in females.**[6-8] Patellofemoral pain is usually a diffuse anterior knee pain that is aggravated with activities that increase compressive forces across the knee. These types of activities include ascending and descending stairs, squatting, and prolonged sitting.[9-12]

To better understand patellofemoral pain, a basic review of normal patellofemoral anatomy is needed. The patella is a large sesamoid bone that is embedded within the tendon of the quadriceps muscles. Its shape is that of an inverted triangle with its apex directed inferior and the base superior. Both the superior and inferior aspects are roughened for the attachments of the quadriceps and the patellar ligament, respectively. The anterior surface of the patella is convex in each direction while the posterior surface has two slightly concave regions called facets. The posterior surface is covered with articular cartilage that has been shown to be anywhere from 5 to 7 mm thick in the mid-patellar region, narrowing to less than 1 mm thick along its periphery.[13-16] The lateral portion of the patella in the area of the lateral facet has increased bone mineral density, indicating a need for more bony support and possible stress shielding.[17] Within the distal portion of the femur is the patellar groove, femoral sulcus, or trochlea. This groove is a ridge that articulates with the posterior portion of the patella. Normally, the lateral trochlear facet of the patella is higher than the medial. One common form of patellofemoral pain comes from patellar instability. Patellar instability occurs when the patella cannot maintain a stable location on the anterior knee; the patient has symptoms of the knee "giving way" or a loss of control of the patella on the anterior knee. This may be caused by a trochlear dysplasia in which the lateral facet is not of optimal height. This anatomic variation leads to a decreased lateral buttress effect. The result is that the patella translates laterally (instead of directly within the patellar groove) with active quadriceps contractions.

Although the patella acts as a bony shield along the anterior knee, its other more important function is to guide the quadriceps tendon and increase the moment arm for the quadriceps muscle. Because the tendon of the quadriceps muscles inserts onto the patella, the moment arm of the quadriceps muscle is located at a further distance from the axis of knee motion. A longer moment arm facilitates knee extension by increasing the distance of the extensor mechanism from the center of knee joint. This extensor moment arm appears to provide the greatest quadriceps torque at about 20° to 60° of knee flexion.[18,19] This range of motion is also the range in which the greatest amount of patellofemoral compressive force occurs. As knee flexion motion increases during weightbearing, compressive forces increase as the angle between the femur and tibia become more acute and the lever arm between the two increases. Contact forces on the posterior patella are 0.5 to 1.5 times one's body weight with walking, three times body weight with stairs, and up to seven to eight times body weight with squatting.[18-21]

Physical Therapy Patient/Client Management

Following a thorough clinical evaluation of the patient with patellofemoral pain, a **nonsurgical approach** is advocated and usually beneficial for pain reduction and return to prior functional levels.[4,22-25] Recent evidence shows an association between patellofemoral pain and altered lower extremity kinematics caused by proximal or distal influences.[5,12,26-40] This proximal or distal influence is commonly referred to as a regional interdependence by which patellofemoral pain may be caused by etiology outside of the knee itself. For example, patellofemoral tracking abnormalities could be caused by weakness in the proximal hip musculature or from structural abnormalities distally at the foot and ankle.

Examination, Evaluation, and Diagnosis

The clinical physical examination begins with a review of the patient's current symptoms. The physical examination for the patient with patellofemoral pain begins with observation of the knee and gait analysis. The patient reports that her anterior knee pain is approximately 2-3/10 on the VAS (0 = no pain and 10 = worst pain possible) today. She reports that her pain can increase to 8/10 during and after playing volleyball. She also reports that the skin around her knee turns bluish in color following volleyball practice or competition, although the skin around the knee during the examination is of normal color and texture. She has several portal sites from her prior fat pad debridement. These incisions are well healed with no signs of redness or infection. Although no gait deviations were observed today, it is not uncommon to see excessive foot pronation during weight acceptance to mid-stance phase of gait. In patients with significant proximal hip weakness, a Trendelenburg gait pattern with contralateral hip drop during swing through and a trunk lean toward the weak side (abductor lurch) during stance may be observed.

Her knee range of motion (ROM) is not quite symmetrical. On the left side, she has 7°-0°-155°, while on the right (symptomatic) side, she has 2°-0°-155°. This notation means that on her uninvolved side, her ROM is from 7° of knee hyperextension to 155° of knee flexion. On her symptomatic side, she has a 5° deficit of knee hyperextension. She also exhibited about a 50% loss of passive and active external tibial rotation on the right side. This range was measured with the knee in 90° of knee flexion. This may be why she has lost some of her terminal knee extension due to the obligate external tibial rotation required during the screw-home mechanism at the tibiofemoral joint.

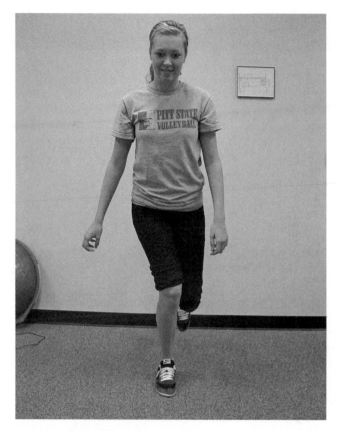

Figure 23-1. Knee valgus collapse with single-leg squat.

Her lower extremity strength was nearly normal on the uninvolved left side with the quadriceps and hamstrings graded at 5/5 and the hip abductors, extensors, and lateral rotators graded at 4+/5. On the right side, her quadriceps and hamstrings were graded at 5/5, but her hip abductors, extensors, and lateral rotators were graded at 4/5. Though the overall strength in her hip musculature was normal or good, she exhibited abnormal motor control patterns when she was asked to perform a functional test of hip strength. With both a step-down test and the single-leg squat on the right side, she demonstrated a dramatic amount of valgus collapse with concomitant hip adduction and tibial abduction (Fig. 23-1). Crossley et al.[41] have recently found that poor performance on the single-leg squat task indicates functional hip abductor muscle weakness. They made recommendations on what constitutes a poor single-leg squat so that clear objective data can be gathered clinically (Table 23-1). When the patient was asked to perform the single-leg squat task on the uninvolved side, these patterns did not occur.

To complete a thorough neurologic screen, sensation and reflexes should be tested. The patient had normal sensation to light and deep touch along the lower extremity dermatomes bilaterally. Patellar and Achilles deep tendon reflexes were

Table 23-1 POSSIBLE COMPENSATORY PATTERNS DURING SINGLE-LEG SQUAT			
Trunk/Posture	Pelvis	Hip	Knee
Lateral deviation/shift	Shunt or lateral deviation	Adduction	Valgus
Rotation	Rotation	Femoral internal	Knee not over foot
Lateral flexion	Tilt	rotation	
Forward flexion			

both normal and symmetrical (2/3 bilaterally). Deep tendon reflexes were graded as 0 = no reflex or absent; 1/3 = hypotonic reflex; 2/3 = normal reflex; 3/3 = hypertonic reflex.[42]

Plan of Care and Interventions

There are multiple interventions, each with varying levels of evidence for efficacy, available for a patient with patellofemoral pain. In general, the treatment for patellofemoral pain depends on the signs and symptoms found during the clinical examination. The current patient is unique in that she had already had surgical intervention for her current complaint and she had been treated by several physical therapists. However, none of these interventions allowed her to play volleyball pain-free.

Since the patient was unable to perform single-limb exercises without her right lower extremity falling into valgus collapse, the first exercises prescribed were on a table in supine and in standing with bilateral weightbearing. These initial exercises were chosen to strengthen the hip musculature because single-limb exercises would have been too difficult for her to perform correctly at this time. **Therapeutic exercises** to strengthen the gluteus maximus and medius were performed first with bridging performed bilaterally and then progressing to a bridge with single limb for support (Fig. 23-2). A sidelying clam exercise was done to strengthen the gluteus medius and the external hip rotators (Fig. 23-3). Resistance tubing around the knees could be added to progress the difficulty. Prone hip extension and sidelying hip abduction exercises were performed to strengthen the gluteus muscles.

Standing exercises are the next appropriate progression. An isometric hip abduction exercise can be performed in which the affected extremity is placed against the wall and the patient abducts the hip against the wall with an isometric contraction. The patient is asked to contract the core muscles (e.g., perform an abdominal bracing contraction) for stabilization while contracting the gluteus medius. No movement should occur at the pelvis during this fatiguing exercise because the purpose of this exercise is to promote endurance of hip musculature. Isotonic exercises may facilitate greater gluteus medius activity if performed in single limb stance. Even *greater* gluteus medius activity can be elicited by placing a load in the contralateral limb to that of the stance limb during exercises.[43,44] This can be done by having the patient stand on the symptomatic leg while holding a weight or applying some form

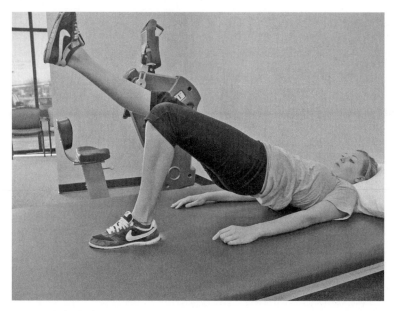

Figure 23-2. Single-leg bridge.

of resistance in the opposite arm. Distefano et al.[45] have shown high electromyographic activity in the gluteus medius during lateral band walking, single-limb squat, and the single-limb deadlift. These exercises can be incorporated as soon as the patient is able to tolerate higher-level exercises without exacerbation of symptoms or demonstration of compensatory patterns.

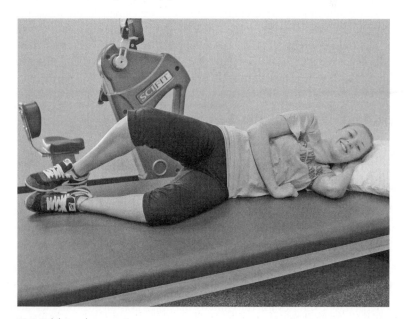

Figure 23-3. Sidelying clam exercise.

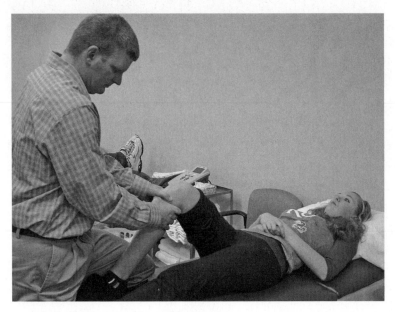

Figure 23-4. Tibial external rotation joint mobilization.

Once the strength of the gluteus muscles and external hip rotators improves to 5/5 on manual muscle testing, she can be progressed to sports-specific activities requiring jumping and hopping. Several weeks after initiation of jumping and hopping drills, the patient was formally discharged with a home exercise program of hip and trunk strengthening to maintain the strength and endurance gained during rehabilitation.

Manual therapy techniques can also be performed to gain the lost external tibial rotation identified during the initial examination. Three sessions of external tibial rotation glides of passive overpressure were needed to gain lost motion (Fig. 23-4). Anterior tibiofemoral glides were also performed to restore to 7° of knee hyperextension.

Evidence-Based Clinical Recommendations

SORT: Strength of Recommendation Taxonomy

A: Consistent, good-quality patient-oriented evidence
B: Inconsistent or limited-quality patient-oriented evidence
C: Consensus, disease-oriented evidence, usual practice, expert opinion, or case series

1. Patellofemoral pain is often associated with decreased hip strength in young, active females. **Grade B**

2. Physical therapy interventions decrease pain and disability in the majority of patients with patellofemoral pain. **Grade B**

3. Strengthening exercises for the gluteus maximus and medius muscles decrease patellofemoral pain. **Grade C**

COMPREHENSION QUESTIONS

23.1 A patient comes to a physical therapist with a 6-month history of patello-femoral pain syndrome. Patellar tendinopathy has been ruled out by the refer-ring physician. She complains of pain with squatting and descending stairs. Despite her pain, she continues to play volleyball and jog for cardiovascular conditioning. What is the *most* appropriate physical therapy intervention that should be done first for this patient?

A. Increasing quadriceps strength

B. Increasing quadriceps flexibility

C. Relative rest

D. Plyometric jump training

23.2 During examination of dynamic movement patterns of a single-leg squat and step-down test, the physical therapist notices the patient's lower extremity falls into a valgus collapse on the involved side. Which of the following mus-cle groups is *not* likely to have functional weakness?

A. Hip flexors

B. Hip extensors

C. Hip external rotators

D. Hip abductors

ANSWERS

23.1 **C.** The patient is already dealing with a chronic painful condition that she has not allowed to adequately heal. The first goal is to encourage relative rest to decrease the overuse that is occurring at the knee. Plyometric jump training would be far too aggressive for this stage of rehabilitation (option D). Without further examination, the physical therapist would be unable to ascertain yet if she needs strengthening or flexibility training (options A and B).

22.3 **A.** Although Tyler et al.[40] found the hip flexors to be significantly weak in a population of those with patellofemoral pain, this appears to be a relatively rare finding. In most instances, hip abductors, external rotators, and extensors are weak.

REFERENCES

1. Hetsroni I, Finestone A, Milgrom C, et al. A prospective biomechanical study of the association between foot pronation and the incidence of anterior knee pain among military recruits. *J Bone Joint Surg Br.* 2006;88:905-908.

2. Milgrom C, Finestone A, Eldad A, Shlamkovitch N. Patellofemoral pain caused by overactivity. A prospective study of risk factors in infantry recruits. *J Bone Joint Surg Am.* 1991;73:1041-1043.

3. Schwellnus MP, Jordaan G, Noakes TD. Prevention of common overuse injuries by the use of shock absorbing insoles. A prospective study. *Am J Sports Med.* 1990;18:636-641.

4. Wills AK, Ramasamy A, Ewins DJ, Etherington J. The incidence and occupational outcome of overuse anterior knee pain during army recruit training. *J R Army Med Corps*. 2004;150:264-269.

5. Witvrouw E, Lysens R, Bellemans J, Cambier D, Vanderstraeten G. Intrinsic risk factors for the development of anterior knee pain in an athletic population. A two-year prospective study. *Am J Sports Med*. 2000;28:480-489.

6. Boling M, Padua D, Marshall S, Guskiewicz K, Pyne S, Beutler A. Gender differences in the incidence and prevalence of patellofemoral pain syndrome. *Scan J Med Sci Sports*. 2010;20:725-730.

7. DeHaven KE, Lintner DM. Athletic injuries: comparison by age, sport, and gender. *Am J Sports Med*. 1986;14:218-224.

8. Taunton JE, Ryan MB, Clement DB, McKenzie DC, Lloyd-Smith DR, Zumbo BD. A retrospective case-control analysis of 2002 running injuries. *Br J Sports Med*. 2002;36:95-101.

9. Barton CJ, Webster KE, Menz HB. Evaluation of the scope and quality of systematic reviews on nonpharmacological conservative treatment for patellofemoral pain syndrome. *J Orthop Sports Phys Ther*. 2008;38:529-541.

10. Bohannon RW. Effect of electrical stimulation to the vastus medialis muscle in a patient with chronically dislocating patella. A case report. *Phys Ther*. 1983;63:1445-1447.

11. Powers CM. Rehabilitation of patellofemoral joint disorders: a critical review. *J Orthop Sports Phys Ther*. 1998;28:345-354.

12. Wilson T, Carter N, Thomas G. A multicenter, single-masked study of medial, neutral, and lateral patellar taping in individuals with patellofemoral pain syndrome. *J Orthop Sports Phys Ther*. 2003;33:437-448.

13. Fulkerson JP. *Disorders of the Patellofemoral Joint*. 3rd ed. Baltimore, MD: Williams & Wilkins; 1997.

14. Fulkerson JP. Diagnosis and treatment of patients with patellofemoral pain. *Am J Sports Med*. 2002;30:447-456.

15. Grelsamer RP, Weinstein CH. Applied biomechanics of the patella. *Clin Orthop Rel Res*. 2001;389:9-14.

16. Heegaard J, Leyvraz PF, Curnier A, Rakotomanana L, Huiskes R. The biomechanics of the human patella during passive knee flexion. *J Biomech*. 1995;28:1265-1279.

17. Leppala J, Kannus P, Natri A, Sievanen H, Jarvinen M, Vuori I. Bone mineral density in the chronic patellofemoral pain syndrome. *Calcif Tissue Int*. 1998;62:548-553.

18. Huberti HH, Hayes WC. Patellofemoral contact pressures. The incidence of q-angle and tendofemoral contact. *J Bone Joint Surg*. 1984;66:715-724.

19. Huberti HH, Hayes WC, Stone JL, Shybut GT. Force ratios in the quadriceps tendon and ligamentum patella. *J Orthop Res*. 1984;21:49-54.

20. Perry EC, Strother RT. Patellalgia. *Phys Sports Med*. 1985;13:43-59.

21. Reilly DT, Martens M. Experimental analysis of the quadriceps muscle force and patello-femoral joint reaction force for various activities. *Acta Orthop Scan*. 1972;43:126-137.

22. Manske RC, Davies GJ. A nonsurgical approach to examination and treatment of the patellofemoral joint, part I: examination of the patellofemoral joint. *Crit Rev Phys Rehabil Med*. 2003;15:141-166.

23. Manske RC, Davies GJ. A nonsurgical approach to examination and treatment of the patellofemoral joint, part 2: pathology and nonsurgical treatment of the patellofemoral joint. *Crit Rev Phys Rehabil Med*. 2003;15:253-294.

24. Thomee R. A comprehensive treatment approach for patellofemoral pain syndrome in young women. *Phys Ther*. 1997;77:1690-1703.

25. Wilk KE, Davies GJ, Mangine RE, Malone TR. Patellofemoral disorders: a classification system and clinical guidelines for nonoperative rehabilitation. *J Orthop Sports Phys Ther*. 1998;28:307-322.

26. Bolgla LA, Malone TR, Umberger BR, Uhl TL. Hip strength and hip and knee kinematics during stair descent in females with and without patellofemoral pain syndrome. *J Orthop Sports Phys Ther*. 2008;38:12-18.

27. Cichanowski HR, Schmitt JS, Johnson RJ, Niemuth PE. Hip strength in collegiate female athletes with patellofemoral pain. *Med Sci Sports Exer.* 2007;39:1227-1232.

28. Dierks TA, Manal KT, Hamill J, Davis IS. Proximal and distal influences on hip and knee kinematics in runners with patellofemoral pain during a prolonged run. *J Orthop Sports Phys Ther.* 2008;38: 448-456.

29. Fukuda TY, Rossetto FM, Magalhaes E, Bryk FF, Lucareli PR, de Almeida Aparecida Carvalho N. Short-term effects of hip abductors and lateral rotators strengthening in females with patellofemoral pain syndrome: a randomized controlled trial. *J Orthop Sports Phys Ther.* 2010;40:736-742.

30. Ireland ML, Willson JD, Ballantyne BT, Davis IM. Hip strength in females with and without patellofemoral pain. *J Orthop Sports Phys Ther.* 2003;33:671-676.

31. Leetun DT, Ireland ML, Willson JD, Ballantyne BT, Davis IM. Core stability measures as risk factors for lower extremity injury in athletes. *Med Sci Sports Exerc.* 2004;36:926-934.

32. Lewis CL, Sahrmann SA, Moran DW. Anterior hip joint force increases with hip extension, decreased gluteal force, or decreased iliopsoas force. *J Biomech.* 2007;40:3725-3731.

33. Magalhaes E, Fukuda TY, Sacramento SN, Forgas A, Cohen M, Abdalla RJ. A comparison of hip strength between sedentary females with and without patellofemoral pain syndrome. *J Orthop Sports Phys Ther.* 2010;40:641-647.

34. Mascal CL, Landel R, Powers C. Management of patellofemoral pain targeting hip, pelvis, and trunk muscle function: 2 case reports. *J Orthop Sports Phys Ther.* 2003;33:642-660.

35. Nakagawa TH, Muniz TB, Baldon Rde M, Dias Maciel C, de Menezes-Reiff RB, Serrao FV. The effect of additional strengthening of hip abductor and lateral rotator muscles in patellofemoral pain syndrome: a randomized controlled pilot study. *Clin Rehabil.* 2008;22:1051-1060.

36. Piva SR, Goodnite EA, Childs JD. Strength around the hip and flexibility of soft tissue in individuals with and without patellofemoral pain syndrome. *J Orthop Sports Phys Ther.* 2005;35:793-801.

37. Prins MR, van der Wurff P. Females with patellofemoral pain syndrome have weak hip muscles: a systematic review. *Aust J Physiother.* 2009;55:9-15.

38. Robinson RL, Nee RJ. Analysis of hip strength in females seeking physical therapy treatment for unilateral patellofemoral pain syndrome. *J Orthop Sports Phys Ther.* 2007;37:232-238.

39. Souza RB, Powers CM. Predictors of hip internal rotation during running: an evaluation of hip strength and femoral structure in women with and without patellofemoral pain. *Am J Sports Med.* 2009;37:579-587.

40. Tyler TF, Nicholas SJ, Mullaney MH, McHugh MP. The role of hip muscle function in the treatment of patellofemoral pain syndrome. *Am J Sports Med.* 2006;34:630-636.

41. Crossley KM, Zhang WJ, Schache AG, Bryant A, Cowan SM. Performance on the single-leg squat task indicates hip abductor muscle function. *Am J Sports Med.* 2011;39:866-873.

42. Magee DJ. *Orthopedic Physical Assessment.* 5th ed. Saunders. St. Louis, MO: Saunders Elsevier; 2008:51.

43. Hodges PW, Richardson CA. Contraction of the abdominal muscles associated with movement of the lower limb. *Phys Ther.* 1997;77:132-142.

44. Neumann DA, Cook TM. Effect of load and carrying position of the electromyographic activity of the gluteus medius muscle during walking. *Phys Ther.* 1985;65:305-311.

45. Distefano LJ, Blackburn JT, Marshall SW, Padua DA. Gluteal muscle activation during common therapeutic exercises. *J Orthop Sports Phys Ther.* 2009;39:532-540.

Patellar Tendinopathy

Luke T. O'Brien
Thomas J. Olson

CASE 24

A 17-year-old basketball player has been referred to physical therapy by his family physician for evaluation and treatment of anterior knee pain. His pain had been intermittent over the past summer. However, since the start of the fall high school sport season, his pain has increased in severity and become constant. Pain is now limiting his ability to practice and play, as well as his ability to ascend and descend stairs, and stand after long periods of sitting. His coach told him that he has "jumper's knee" and that he should "get a knee strap and he should be fine." Plain film images revealed no bony abnormalities, though his tibial and femoral epiphyseal plates are almost completely ossified. Otherwise the patient's medical history is unremarkable. Signs and symptoms are consistent with patellar tendinopathy. The patient hopes to finish his season and be ready to compete in an all-star game in the spring.

▶ Based on the patient's symptoms and history, what are the most appropriate examination tests to help confirm the diagnosis of patellar tendinopathy?
▶ What are the most appropriate physical therapy interventions?
▶ What is his rehabilitation prognosis?

KEY DEFINITIONS

APOPTOSIS: Programmed cell death in response to specific stimuli

ECCENTRIC CONTRACTION: Controlled lengthening of a muscle as it responds to an external force greater than the contractile force it is exerting

MUCOID DEGENERATION: Deterioration of collagen fibers into a nonfunctional gelatinous or mucus-like substance

NEOVASCULARIZATION: Formation of functional new microvascular networks in tissue that does not normally contain blood vessels, or blood vessels of a different type within a tissue

PROTEOGLYCANS: Mucopolysaccharides bound to protein chains in the extracellular matrix of connective tissue

TENDINITIS: Acute inflammation of a tendon, typically affecting its insertion; a type of tendinopathy[1]

TENDINOPATHY: Clinical term that encompasses all overuse conditions that affect a tendon (proximally, distally, or midsubstance) in the presence or absence of an inflammatory response; includes tendinosis[2]

TENDINOSIS: Chronic degeneration and a failed healing response within a tendon, but without the presence of characteristic inflammatory markers; a type of tendinopathy[3]

Objectives

1. Explain the distinctions between tendinitis, tendinosis, and tendinopathy.
2. Describe the pathophysiology that contributes to the development of patellar tendinosis.
3. Describe the differential diagnoses for patellar tendinopathy.
4. Prescribe the most appropriate strengthening interventions for patellar tendinopathy based on examination findings.
5. Describe additional treatment options for patients with patellar tendinopathy that have failed conservative management.

Physical Therapy Considerations

PT considerations during management of the individual with a diagnosis of patellar tendinopathy:

▶ **General physical therapy plan of care/goals:** Decrease pain and increase function; increase lower extremity strength; prevent or minimize loss of aerobic fitness capacity

▶ **Physical therapy interventions:** Patient education regarding functional anatomy and pathophysiology; modalities and manual therapy to decrease pain; management of training volume; incorporation of heavy load or eccentric-focused resistance exercises to promote tendon remodeling; general resistance exercises to increase lower extremity stability and strength; aerobic exercise program; patellar tendon straps or unloading tape

▶ **Precautions during physical therapy:** Monitor vital signs; address precautions or contraindications for exercise based on patient's pre-existing condition(s)

▶ **Complications interfering with physical therapy:** Therapist and patient must be aware that pain during therapeutic exercise is an accepted part of treating chronic patellar tendinopathy

Understanding the Health Condition

Jumper's knee, incorrectly referred to as patellar tendinitis, was first described in the early 1970s as an overuse syndrome of the knee characterized by pain at the junction of the inferior pole of the patella and the proximal patellar tendon.[4] Although "jumper's knee" seemed to be an acceptable common name for this medical condition, labeling it "tendinitis" is misleading. The suffix "-itis" refers to an inflammatory process, but the pathophysiology and pathoanatomy associated with protracted patellar tendon symptoms suggest the presence of little, if any, inflammation. As a result, the condition should be referred to as tendinopathy, with the actual degenerative process described as tendinosis.[3,5,6] In this patient case, the terms will be used in this fashion. Patellar tendinopathy is typically diagnosed in athletes who participate in sports requiring aggressive knee extension and/or repetitive eccentric knee flexion.[3,4] It most often presents with pain over the inferior pole of the patella[7] and has been shown to interfere in the normal training and competition of one in every five elite athletes.[8] Male athletes experience symptoms more frequently than their female counterparts.[8] This characteristic may be helpful in the differential diagnosis of patellar tendinopathy from more general types of anterior knee pain, like patellofemoral pain, which is more commonly seen in female athletes. The incidence of jumper's knee has been estimated to be as high as 30% to 50% in sports like basketball and volleyball where jumping is common, but it can also be widespread among soccer players and cross-country runners due to the demands of cutting, rapid acceleration/deceleration, and repetitive impact absorption on the quadriceps musculature.[7-10] Though most often described as an overuse injury, it has been suggested that a single direct trauma may also lead to tendon pathology with the same clinical presentation.[4,11,12]

The patellar tendon is a continuation of the quadriceps tendon. It aids in force transmission from the quadriceps musculature to the bones of the lower extremity, resulting in movement of the hip and knee joints (Fig. 24-1A and B). Though often referred to as the patellar ligament due to its bone-to-bone attachments, the macroscopic and microscopic appearance and function of the structure is tendinous and therefore, it should be referred to as such.[2] Generally, a tendon is composed primarily of type I collagen fibers arranged hierarchically into bundles called fascicles surrounded by connective tissue sheaths. The fascicles are then grouped and surrounded superficially by a two-layered membrane referred to as the paratenon.

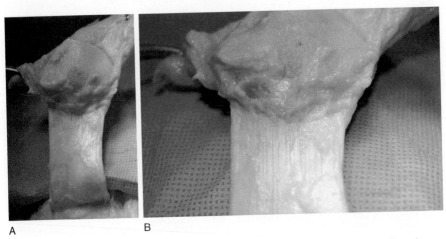

A   B

Figure 24-1. A. Posterior patellar tendon showing average length, as well as origin at patella and insertion at tibial tuberosity. **B.** Close-up of posterior patellar tendon showing normal absence of fibers over the posterior surface, as well as the standard crescent shaped fiber alignment highlighting the shortest fibers about the apex of the inferior patellar pole.

In addition to collagen, the tendon contains extracellular matrix and tenocytes. The extracellular matrix, or ground substance, is a viscous proteoglycan-rich material that provides support for the collagen fibers and regulates maturation. Tenocytes are flat, elongated cells found in small numbers in the tendon. Tenocytes control the synthesis of ground substance and collagen.[3,13]

Basso et al.[6] investigated the normal cellular structure of the patellar tendon in almost two dozen human cadaveric knees. They demonstrated that fascicles attach to the distal two-thirds of the patella in a crescent-shaped fashion, with the largest concentration found anteriorly. The anterior fascicles are longer than those that attach posteriorly. The blood supply of the patellar tendon originates from the genicular arteries and the anterior tibial artery, and it typically terminates in a network of small arterioles from the paratenon through the deeper connective tissue sheaths.[2,13] Sensory and sympathetic nerve fibers terminate in the paratenon.[3] Under a light microscope, a healthy patellar tendon appears shiny, white, and reflective (Fig. 24-1B). It consists of densely packed, parallel collagen bundles, minimally visible ground substance, and a thin distribution of tenocytes.[5] In contrast, in an individual **with a diagnosis of patellar tendinopathy, the tendon appears quite different.** When viewed macroscopically following surgical excision or under a polarized light microscope, there is a loss of reflectivity and the tissue along the posterior proximal origin adjacent to the inferior patellar pole appears yellow and disorganized.[2,5,12] This appearance is known as "mucoid degeneration."[5,12,14] Microscopically, collagen bundles appear separated secondary to the infiltration of abnormal ground substance and there is microtearing as well as necrosis of the collagen fibers themselves.[2,5,13,15,16] Changes in tenocyte nuclei and apoptosis are appreciated and fibroblast infiltration and neovascularization are also observed.[2,5,8,13,14,16] Conspicuously absent are leukocytes, neutrophils, and macrophages that would suggest an inflammatory process. Although a brief period of tendinitis cannot absolutely be ruled out during the early phases of a tendon overuse injury, by the time patients are symptomatic and seek treatment their condition may be chronic and a state of tendinosis exists.[13] By appreciating the cellular pathophysiological differences between tendinitis and tendinosis, the physical therapist will be able to prescribe appropriate interventions to address the degenerative changes associated with tendinosis.

The exact pathogenesis of patellar tendinopathy is unclear. Current evidence suggests it is likely a combination of mechanical and biochemical factors that lead to degeneration.[6,8,14,17] Degeneration seems to most commonly affect the posterior fascicles of the patellar tendon. This may be related to the fascicles' crescent alignment both coronally and longitudinally around the inferior patella.[8] The posterior fascicles are typically shorter than those attached anteriorly, and as the patellar tendon elongates during quadriceps muscle contraction and knee flexion, the shorter posterior fascicles are subject to greater strain.[6] Excessive or repeated loading may exceed a tendon's ability to repair itself. Lian and colleagues[8] have demonstrated increased tenocyte apoptosis in the patellar tendons of athletes diagnosed with jumper's knee compared to controls without a history of patellar tendinopathy. In animal models, Zhang and Wang[14] have demonstrated that the concentration of prostaglandin E2 (PGE2), a common inflammatory mediator, increases in response to repetitive mechanical loading. When tendon stem cells were then exposed to increased amounts of PGE2 in vitro, stem cell production decreased and differentiation was altered. This resulted in increased production of adipose cells and osteoclasts rather than increased production of tenocytes. Consequently, repetitive mechanical stress may actually decrease the pool of tenocytes available for the tendon repair necessitated by initial overuse of the extensor mechanism.[14] In addition, the neovascularization associated with patellar tendinosis is accompanied by an increased proliferation of substance P-receptive sensory nerve fibers in the tendon itself, not just in the paratenon.[16,17] Increased substance P concentration and nociceptive activity from the tendon increase the perception of painful stimuli in the brain and may suppress the synthesis of growth factors inhibiting tendon repair.[16,17] Together, all these processes contribute to the degeneration of the patellar tendon.

The specific combinations of risk factors that may predispose an athlete to develop patellar tendinopathy are unknown. However, several identified intrinsic factors include: male gender, quadriceps weakness, and decreased quadriceps and hamstring flexibility.[2,3,16,18,19] The extrinsic risk factors thought to contribute include: increased training volume and/or intensity, increased ground reaction forces due to activity or training surface, and poor landing mechanics.[2,3,16,18] When examining an athlete with anterior knee pain, these factors must be considered and investigated to accurately assist in the diagnosis of patellar tendinopathy.

Physical Therapy Patient/Client Management

Traditionally, treatments for patellar tendinosis emphasized reducing inflammation. This treatment philosophy was based on the inaccurate assumption that the condition was a tendinitis. Common interventions like ultrasound, cross-friction massage, cryotherapy, oral nonsteroidal anti-inflammatories (NSAIDs), and steroidal anti-inflammatory injections have not proven to be effective.[2,4,12,13,20–22] It has been suggested that the use of NSAIDs and glucocorticoid injections are contraindicated because in the absence of an inflammatory process, NSAIDs and glucocorticoids may actually exacerbate patellar tendinopathy. They do this either by masking symptoms, allowing the individual to continue activity that can cause additional tendon damage, or by increasing cellular degeneration and weakening the tendon.[2,3,13,20,22] Conservative treatments should be based on the growing body of evidence indicating that patellar tendinopathy is a failed healing response. The cornerstone of any initial plan of care should be interventions addressing the quadriceps muscle and patellar tendon unit, such as activity modification and strengthening.

Examination, Evaluation, and Diagnosis

During the acute and subacute phases, patients who demonstrate symptoms consistent with patellar tendinopathy typically complain of anterior knee pain worsened by athletic activity. As the condition progresses, pain may be experienced during activities of daily living such as stair negotiation and walking downhill. Since there are numerous pathologies that may contribute to anterior knee pain, a thorough history can be extremely valuable in the development of a differential diagnosis. Table 24-1 presents specific components of the patient's history that should be elucidated during the subjective portion of the examination.

Table 24-1 CONTENT OF QUESTIONS THAT SHOULD BE INCLUDED IN SUBJECTIVE EXAMINATION	
Question Content	Clinical Relevance
History of previous knee surgery	Scarring of the anterior interval and fat pad can cause anterior knee pain[23]
History of patella instability	Disruption of the medial patellofemoral ligament may alter patellofemoral biomechanics
Mechanism of injury	Patellar tendinosis is commonly an overuse injury; however, it may also be the result of a direct blow to the patella tendon[11]
Vocation	Some occupations may predispose the patella tendon to excessive loads (e.g., ski patrol)
Previous injury	Prior injuries to the knee, as well as to the hip and ankle (which may affect biomechanics)
Prior treatments	Athletes that have failed to improve with an eccentric loading program will have a different course of treatment compared to those that failed to improve with use of NSAIDs
Provocative movements and activities	Identifying painful movement patterns is helpful in the diagnosis and development of training modification plans
Load, volume, intensity, and duration	Important training variables manipulated incorrectly can overload a tendon resulting in the development of a tendinopathy[24]

A thorough physical assessment is essential to confirm a patellar tendinopathy diagnosis. Since the patellar tendon shares a close anatomical relationship with other potential sources of anterior knee pain, the physical therapist must make a careful examination of the surrounding bone and soft tissues to rule out other conditions. The differential diagnoses include: patellofemoral pain syndrome, patella instability, avulsion fractures, Sinding-Larsen-Johansson syndrome, Osgood-Schlatter disease, anterior interval scarring, fat pad entrapment, meniscal tear, patellar tendon tear, and infrapatellar plica.

The combined objective findings from four different examination positions (supine, seated, figure four, and prone) can be utilized to assist in developing an accurate diagnosis of patellar tendinopathy. The main assessment made in the supine position is observation of the quadriceps musculature. Obvious deficiencies in thigh girth symmetry may provide clues as to the chronicity and severity of the condition. It is also a position in which gross observations, such as a prominent tibial tubercle, can be made to determine the presence of other contributing conditions. With the patient in a seated position, the physical therapist should view the knee from directly above to assess patella tilt. It is also an ideal position to assess patellar tendon alignment. Figure 24-2 shows a patient seated with the knee in a non-weightbearing position, hanging over the edge of the treatment table. In a neutral alignment, a vertical line down the middle of the patellar tendon should bisect the second and third toes. Since the tendon is placed on tension, this is also a good position to palpate for tendon defects associated with a patellar tendon tear or rupture. Tibial tuberosity tenderness is also well assessed in this position, with reproduction of the patient's symptoms possibly indicating Osgood-Schlatter disease. In the seated figure four position, the ankle of the limb being examined is crossed over the thigh of the opposite leg. The limb is then placed into maximal external rotation. In this position, the medial collateral ligament is posterior, exposing the medial meniscus, making it an excellent position for meniscal examination as well as for palpation of the retinacular ligaments. Beginning on the medial side of the knee joint and moving from posterior to anterior, the physical therapist is able to palpate the medial collateral ligament, the medial patellofemoral ligament (Fig. 24-3A), the anterior horn of the medial meniscus (Fig. 24-3B), and the patellar tendon. The lateral joint can then be examined in a similar posterior to anterior order. Tenderness to palpation of structures other than the patellar tendon would direct the therapist to consider competing differential diagnoses. Last, the physical therapist has the patient lie in the prone position with the involved knee hanging over the edge of the treatment table. The compression provided by the edge of the bed inhibits the quadriceps, allowing for an assessment of the anterior knee free of protective guarding (Fig. 24-4). The physical therapist can first assess for patellar excursion and apprehension. Then, by placing fingers both medially and laterally to the patellar tendon and moving inferiorly, the physical therapist is able to assess the infrapatellar fat pad for size, tenderness, and sagittal mobility (Fig. 24-5). Movement of the fat pad can further be assessed by passively flexing the knee to 90°. The fat pat should be "sucked in" or disappear from underneath the therapist's fingers.[23] The patellar tendon can then be palpated. Signs consistent with patellar tendinopathy are a thickening of the tendon and tenderness with palpation. Patients typically report

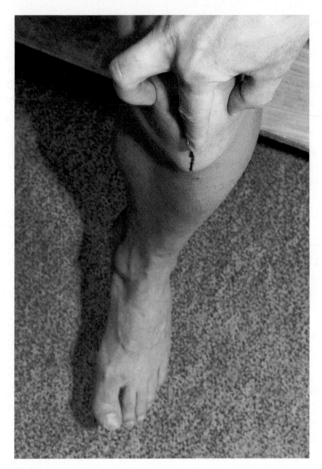

Figure 24-2. Seated knee exam position for observing patellar tendon alignment and the tibial tuberosity. Note the hypertrophied tibial tuberosity secondary to Osgood-Schlatter disease.

the greatest degree of pain to palpation at the insertion of the tendon to the inferior pole of the patella.[25] In jumping athletes (*e.g.*, volleyball players, basketball players, high jumpers), mild tenderness to palpation is considered normal.[25] As a clinical test of symptomatic tendons, tenderness to palpation has poor sensitivity (56%) and specificity (47%).[25]

Few special tests specific to patellar tendinopathy have been described. One is the flexion-extension sign. It is performed in supine by palpating the point of maximal tendon tenderness, and then passively flexing the knee to 90°. A significant reduction in tenderness in the flexed position is considered a positive test and indicative of patellar tendinopathy.[26] Although this test currently lacks published specificity or sensitivity, cadaveric dissection has shown that pressure applied anteriorly, at 90° of knee flexion, does not deform the deep fibers of the patellar tendon.[26] This shielding of the posterior fibers by the tensioned anterior fibers in flexion provides an anatomic rationale for decreased tenderness in the flexed position. Definitive diagnosis

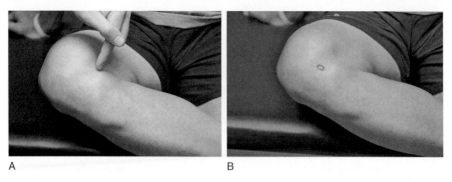

A B

Figure 24-3. Figure four knee exam position. **A.** Therapist palpates the origin of the medial patello-femoral ligament. **B.** Circle drawn on knee identifies the anterior horn of the medial meniscus.

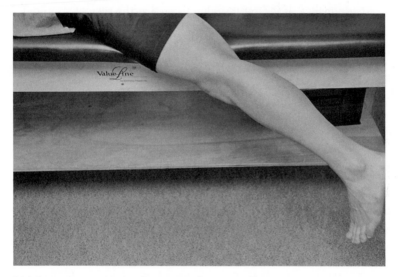

Figure 24-4. Prone exam position to eliminate quadriceps guarding.

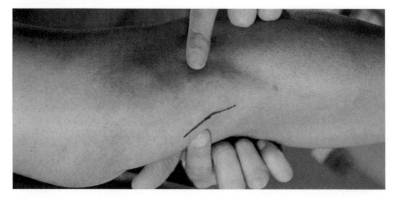

Figure 24-5. With the patient in the prone exam position, the therapist palpates the medial and lateral border of the infrapatellar fat pad.

of patellar tendinopathy is based primarily on physical examination. While MRI and ultrasonography have both been shown to be accurate in confirming the presence of patellar tendinosis, the physical therapist should keep in mind that the presence of abnormal imaging does not necessarily mean that the tendon is the source of the pain.[19,27] The best diagnostic accuracy is the confirmation of a positive clinical examination by positive imaging results.[19,27]

Outcome measures are useful to quantify clinical outcomes or to quantify progression toward therapy goals. The Victorian Institute of Sport Assessment Patellar Tendinopathy Questionnaire (VISA-P) is a reliable outcome measure designed specifically to measure the clinical outcomes of patients with patellar tendionopathy.[28] It is an eight-item questionnaire assessing symptoms, function, and the ability to play sports. The VISA-P is scored form 0-100, with 100 representing unrestricted, pain-free performance. It is typically administered at the time of an initial evaluation to establish a baseline, with reassessment conducted at 6-week intervals and at discharge.[28]

Plan of Care and Interventions

The use of eccentric exercises for the treatment of patellar tendinopathy stems from the literature that supports its use in Achilles tendiopathy.[29] While it is still uncertain exactly how eccentric exercise influences tendons, it is proposed that eccentric loading stimulates collagen fiber cross-linkage formation, facilitating tendon remodeling and overcoming the failed healing response that is the hallmark of the tendinopathy.[30]

A number of studies have sought to determine the effectiveness of **eccentric exercise** in treating patellar tendinopathy. Purdam et al.[31] investigated the effects of two different eccentric training programs on 17 subjects with painful patellar tendinopathy. One group of nine subjects performed unilateral squats in the standard foot flat position, while the second group of eight subjects performed the same exercise on a 25° decline board. Both groups performed 3 sets of 15 repetitions, twice daily for 12 weeks. Pain during performance was expected and allowed. When a subject was able to perform the repetitions without pain, load was increased via a weighted backpack to reach a new level of painful training. Good clinical results were found for the decline board training group, with a significant decrease in pain rated on the visual analog scale at 12-week and 15-month follow-ups. In contrast, the results for the standard foot-flat position training group were poor, with no significant pain improvement reported between baseline and 12-week follow-up.

Jonsson et al.[32] compared the effectiveness of an eccentric training program to a concentric training program in 15 athletes with painful patellar tendinopathy. Subjects were randomized to either an eccentric or concentric training group. The 12-week eccentric training program significantly decreased pain ratings and increased VISA-P outcome scores compared to the concentric training control program. Eccentric and concentric loading were performed using training parameters described by Purdam et al.[31] and all subjects were instructed to stop sporting activity for the first six weeks.

Visnes et al.[33] also assessed the effectiveness of eccentric exercise in 29 elite male and female volleyball players between 19 and 35 years old. The experimental group participated in an eccentric exercise program while continuing regular training and competitions. The eccentric exercise program consisted of unilateral squats on a 25° decline board. Subjects completed 3 sets of 15 repetitions, twice daily. Loaded backpacks were added when unilateral squat pain decreased. The control group continued to train, but did not perform the eccentric exercise program. No differences in VISA-P scores were identified at the 6-week or 6-month follow-ups in either group. The results of the combined eccentric exercise and participation group in this study suggest that there may be a dose-response to tendon loading. While conventional exercises may not place enough load on the tendon to stimulate remodeling (foot-flat eccentric squats as performed in the study by Purdam et al.[31] or concentric squats), too *much* total load may result in increased tendon soreness (which may have occurred in the study by Visnes et al.[33]).

Heavy, slow resistance training has shown promise in patellar tendinopathy management. A randomized controlled trial showed this was as effective as eccentric training and more effective than glucocorticoid injections.[34] This suggests that other, so far unevaluated exercises, that place high loads on the patellar tendon may be equally effective in treating tendinopathy. Table 24-2 shows sample strength training protocols for treating patellar tendinopathy. Figure 24-6 shows single leg decline squats on the involved knee from the starting (Fig. 24-6A) to the ending position (Fig. 24-6B).

Strengthening programs are designed to influence tendon remodeling to address the degenerative changes associated with tendinopathy. Excessive training volume has been identified as a key element in the development of athletic-related patellar tendinopathy.[26] Therefore, the physical therapist should modify and monitor the training volume that contributed to the development of the condition. One suggested way of addressing this is to identify the training threshold (time, load, etc.) when symptoms first occur. Training volume should then be set below this established

Table 24-2   TWO DIFFERENT STRENGTH TRAINING PROTOCOLS FOR TREATMENT OF PATELLAR TENDINOPATHY

Training Type	Exercise	Frequency	Load	Pain
Eccentric loading training[33]	Single leg squat on 25° decline board (Fig. 24-6)	Twice daily, 7 days/wk for 12 wk	3 sets × 15 reps; load in backpack increased so that exercise is always performed with discomfort	Expected
Heavy slow resistance training[36]	1. Bilateral leg press 2. Squat 3. Sled hack squat	3 times/wk for 12 wk 2-3 min rest between sets	Wk 1: 4 sets of 15 reps of progressively increasing fraction of the repetition maximum (RM) Wk 2-3: 12 RM Wk 4-5: 10 RM Wk 6-8: 8 RM Wk 9-12: 6 RM	Acceptable, but pain not to increase 24 h after cessation of training

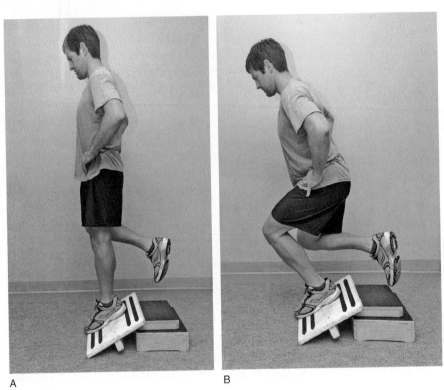

Figure 24-6. A. Start position for single leg squat on 25° decline board. **B.** Final position single leg squat on 25° decline board.

symptomatic threshold, with incremental increases in volume made at regular intervals. While pain during the performance of an exercise may be expected, an increase in baseline tendon pain 24 hours following a loading activity may indicate tendon overload. In this situation, load should be reduced to a previously tolerated load volume.

Other nonexercise treatments have been used in the treatment of patellar tendinosis. The use of unloading tape or patellar tendon straps has been advocated in the management of the condition.[35] While some clinical evidence suggests that these devices may be useful in decreasing symptoms, limited evidence exists to support this practice.[36]

Other adjuncts used in the treatment of tendinopathy are **injection therapies.** One example is the use of dry needling. Dry needling involves repeatedly passing a needle (ranging in size from 0.20 × 40 mm to 0.30 × 60 mm) through an abnormal tendon with the goal of stimulating an inflammatory response to promote normal tendon self-repair.[20] Due to the technique's invasive nature, its inclusion as a component of physical therapy practice varies by individual state regulatory boards. As of 2011, 18 states and the District of Columbia have affirmed that dry needling should be included in the physical therapist scope of practice.[37] However, the American Physical Therapy Association's description of dry needling emphasizes its use to address myofascial pain by releasing or inactivating trigger points.[37] Therefore, the use of dry needling in isolation or in conjunction with another injection therapy to promote tendon healing should be approved and supervised by a licensed physician. In an investigation by James et al.[38] dry needling combined with an injection of autologous blood and a standardized protocol of eccentric strengthening resulted in an 86% improvement in VISA-P scores and a normalization of tendon appearance during post-treatment ultrasound imaging in 47 knees of 44 athletes diagnosed with refractory patellar tendinopathy. Unfortunately, the use of simultaneous therapies in this study makes it impossible to identify which technique or techniques contributed to the reported improvements. However, several studies have investigated dry needling together with autologous blood injection to treat recalcitrant tendinopathy and demonstrated decreased pain and increased function, suggesting that the combination is indeed effective.[39,40] Connell et al.[40] estimated that ultrasound-guided dry needling alone resulted in positive outcomes for two-thirds of 35 patients with lateral epicondylalgia. However, the authors stated that further study is warranted to examine its effects in isolation and in conjunction with autologous blood therapy to address other types of tendinopathy.

Other injection therapies that require referral to a physician have also shown promise in treating patellar tendinopathy. These include ultrasound-guided polidocanol (a local anaesthetic agent) injection into areas of concentrated neovascularization along the dorsal patellar tendon[41] and protein-rich plasma injections followed by eccentric strengthening.[20] Investigations into these treatments have demonstrated significant increases in VISA-P scores at both 12- and 24-month follow-ups. Prolotherapy injection, in which a pharmacologically inert substance like dextrose is injected into the area of tendinosis, is also being investigated.[42]

Extracorporeal shockwave therapy (ESWT) is a noninvasive technique used by physiotherapists in Europe and Asia,[43,44] as well as by physicians in the United States. ESWT uses acoustic waves (similar to pulsed ultrasound) to generate high stress forces in the target tissue. The waves are generated electrohydraulically, electromagnetically, or piezoelectrically and are thought to stimulate a tissue's own repair processes.[44-46] The extracorporeal shockwave is characterized by high pressure—almost 1000 times greater than that produced by an ultrasound wave.[44,46] As a result, pain can be produced and a local anesthetic may sometimes be required. However, when delivered in low to medium energy doses, no anesthesia seems necessary.[44] How ESWT affects a degenerative tendon is not well understood, but theories include reduced concentrations of substance P-positive nerve fibers, as well as increased blood flow to promote tissue regeneration.[35,45,46] The evidence available regarding its efficacy on patellar tendinopathy is mixed. A systematic review by van Leeuwen et al.[47] concluded that ESWT is an effective treatment for patellar tendinopathy, but cautions that the methodological quality of the existing studies is variable, with most studies using small sample populations with short-term follow-ups. However, a recent blinded, randomized controlled trial conducted by Zwerver et al.[48] indicated that ESWT applied during a competitive season provided no benefit over placebo in the treatment of 18 to 35-year-old competitive, recreational volleyball, basketball, and handball athletes.[48]

It is widely accepted that conservative care is the first treatment option for patellar tendinopathy. However, only 50% of patients with severe cases may be able to return to pain-free activity after a rehabilitation program.[20] In cases where 6 months of conservative management has failed to eliminate symptoms and restore unrestricted function, referral for **surgical intervention** may be warranted.[7] Several different techniques have been proposed to address intractable patellar tendinopathy from open and arthroscopic debridement of the proximal tendon, to drilling and excision of the inferior pole of the patella. Results from all these techniques appear positive.[7,49] Approximately 80% of postoperative patients are able to return to their previous level or lower level of athletic participation with minimal to no symptoms, in 4 to 6 months.[7,49,50] Pascarella et al.[50] promote the initiation of rehabilitation the day following surgery with a progressive range of motion emphasis for the first 2 weeks. This includes the use of a continuous passive motion machine for 4 hours/day for the first week. Isometric quadriceps exercises are also advocated during this immediate postoperative phase, along with a transition from partial to full weightbearing. Aquatic therapy and low resistance closed kinetic chain exercises are introduced starting during the third postoperative week and resistance loads are then increased based on symptom-free activity. A running progression is allowed beginning in the sixth postoperative week, with a return to sports-specific training anticipated at 12 weeks.[50] Other details regarding postoperative rehabilitation are limited, but early mobilization seems to produce improved clinical outcomes.[49]

Evidence-Based Clinical Recommendations

SORT: Strength of Recommendation Taxonomy

A: Consistent, good-quality patient-oriented evidence
B: Inconsistent or limited-quality patient-oriented evidence
C: Consensus, disease-oriented evidence, usual practice, expert opinion, or case series

1. Jumper's knee is a patellar tendinosis characterized by tendon degeneration rather than a cellular inflammatory response. **Grade A**

2. Eccentric strength training decreases pain and restores function in athletes with patellar tendinopathy. **Grade B**

3. Injection therapies decrease symptoms associated with patellar tendinopathy. **Grade B**

4. Surgical intervention is an appropriate treatment option for athletes with refractory patellar tendinopathy. **Grade A**

COMPREHENSION QUESTIONS

24.1 Evidence for eccentric training treatment of patellar tendinopathy supports which of the following training parameters?

A. Decline squat, 3 sets × 15 reps, once per day for 6 weeks, with pain-free performance

B. Decline squat, 3 sets × 15 reps, once per day for 12 weeks, with pain-allowed performance

C. Decline squat, 3 sets × 10 reps, twice per day for 6 weeks, with pain-allowed performance

D. Decline squat, 3 sets × 15 reps, twice per day for 12 weeks, with pain-allowed performance

24.2 Which of the following does *not* accurately describe the tendon pathology associated with symptoms described as patellar tendinosis?

A. Mucoid degeneration

B. Increased concentration of macrophages

C. Tenocyte proliferation and apoptosis

D. Disorganized orientation of collagen fibers

ANSWERS

24.1 **D.** Purdam et al.[31] compared the effectiveness of eccentric strengthening using a decline board to eccentric training in a foot-flat position. Their results indicated that the performance of decline squats (allowing pain during performance) twice daily for 12 weeks was superior to other test conditions in reducing pain and increasing functional level.

24.2 **B.** Pathology associated with a tendinosis can be described as mucoid degeneration (option A).[5,12,14] It is characterized by a yellow, disorganized appearance. Microscopically, collagen bundles appear separated secondary to an increased infiltration of abnormal ground substance and there is microtearing and necrosis of collagen fibers (option D).[2,5,13,15,16] Changes in tenocyte nuclei and apoptosis are appreciated and fibroblast infiltration and neovascularization are observed (option C). Inflammatory cell markers like leukocytes, neutrophils, and macrophages are absent.[2,5,13,14,16]

REFERENCES

1. *The American Heritage Medical Dictionary*. Boston, MA: Houghton Mifflin Company; 2007.

2. Peers KH, Lysens RJ. Patellar tendinopathy in athletes: current diagnostic and therapeutic recommendations. *Sports Med*. 2005;35:71-87.

3. Tan SC, Chan O. Achilles and patellar tendinopathy: current understanding of pathophysiology and management. *Disabil Rehabil*. 2008;30:1608-1615.

4. Blazina ME, Kerlan RK, Jobe FW, Carter VS, Carlson GJ. Jumper's knee. *Orthop Clin North Am.* 1973;4:665-678.

5. Khan KM, Cook JL, Bonar F, Harcourt P, Astrom M. Histopathology of common tendinopathies. Update and implications for clinical management. *Sports Med.* 1999;27:393-408.

6. Basso O, Johnson DP, Amis AA. The anatomy of the patellar tendon. *Knee Surg Sports Traumatol Arthrosc.* 2001;9:2-5.

7. Cucurulo T, Louis ML, Thaunat M, Franceschi JP. Surgical treatment of patellar tendinopathy in athletes. A retrospective multicentric study. *Orthop Traumatol Surg Res.* 2009;95:S78-S84.

8. Lian OB, Engebretsen, Bahr R. Prevalence of jumper's knee among elite athletes from different sports: a cross-sectional study. *Am J Sports Med.* 2005;33:561-567.

9. Santander J, Zarba E, Iraporda H, Puleo S. Can arthroscopically assisted treatment of chronic patellar tendinopathy reduce pain and restore function? *Clin Orthop Relat Res.* 2012;470:993-997.

10. Visnes H, Bahr R. The evolution of eccentric training as treatment for patellar tendinopathy (jumper's knee): a critical review of exercise programmes. *Br J Sports Med.* 2007;41:217-223.

11. Garau G, Rittweger J, Mallarias P, Longo UG, Maffulli N. Traumatic patellar tendinopathy. *Disabil Rehabil.* 2008;30:1616-1620.

12. Roels J, Martens M, Mulier JC, Burssens A. Patellar tendinitis: (jumper's knee). *Am J Sports Med.* 1978;6:362-368.

13. Pećina M, Bojanić I, Ivković A, Bričić L, Smoljanović T, Seiwerth S. Patellar tendinopathy: histopathological examination and follow-up of surgical treatment. *Acta Chir Orthop Traumatol Cech.* 2010;77:277-283.

14. Zhang J, Wang JH. Production of PGE(2) increases in tendons subjected to repetitive mechanical loading and induces differentiation of tendon stem cells in non-tenocytes. *J Orthop Res.* 2010;28:198-203.

15. Parkinson J, Samiric T, Ilic MZ, Cook J, Feller JA, Handley CJ. Change in proteoglycan metabolism is a characteristic of human patellar tendinopathy. *Arthritis Rheum.* 2010;62:3028-3035.

16. Lian Ø, Dahl J, Ackermann PW, Frihagen F, Engebretsen L, Bahr R. Pronociceptive and antinociceptive neuromediators in patellar tendinopathy. *Am J Sports Med.* 2006; 34:1801-1808.

17. Khan KM, Cook JL, Maffulli N, Kannus P. Where is the pain coming from in tendinopathy? It may be biochemical, not only structural, in origin. *Br J Sports Med.* 2000;34:81-83.

18. Scott A, Ashe MC. Common tendinopathies in upper and lower extremities. *Curr Sports Med Rep.* 2006;5:233-241.

19. Cook JL, Kiss ZS, Khan KM, Purdam CR, Webster KE. Anthropometry, physical performance, and ultrasound patellar tendon abnormality in elite junior basketball players: a cross-sectional study. *Br J Sports Med.* 2004;38:206-209.

20. Volpi P, Quaglia A, Schoenhuber H, et al. Growth factors in the management of sport-induced tendinopathies: results after 24 months from treatment. A pilot study. *J Sports Med Phys Fitness.* 2010;50:494-500.

21. Stasinopoulos D, Stasinopoulos I. Comparison of effects of exercise programme, pulsed ultrasound and transverse friction in the treatment of chronic patellar tendinopathy. *Clin Rehabil.* 2004;18:347-352.

22. Speed CA. Fortnightly review: corticosteroid injections in tendon lesions. *BMJ.* 2001;323: 382-386.

23. Feagin JA, Steadman JR. *The Crucial Principles in Care of the Knee.* Philadelphia, PA: Lippincott Williams & Wilkins; 2008.

24. Cook JL, Purdam C. Is compressive load a factor in the development of tendinopathy? *Br J Sports Med.* 2012;46:163-168.

25. Cook JL, Kahn KM, Kiss ZS, Purdam CR, Griffiths L. Reproducibility and clinical utility of tendon palpation to detect patellar tendinopathy in young basketball players. Victorian Institute of Sport Tendon Study Group. *Br J Sports Med.* 2001;35:65-69.

26. Rath E, Schwarzkopf R, Richmond JC. Clinical signs and anatomic correlation of patellar tendinitis. *Indian J Orthop.* 2010;44:435-437.

27. Warden SJ, Kiss ZS, Malara FA, Ooi AB, Cook JL, Crossley KM. Comparative accuracy of magnetic resonance imaging and ultrasonography in confirming clinically diagnosed patellar tendinopathy. *Am J Sports Med.* 2007;35:427-436.

28. Visentini PJ, Kahn KM, Cook JL, Kiss ZS, Harcourt PR, Wark JD. The VISA score: an index of severity of symptoms in patients with jumper's knee (patellar tendinosis). Victorian Institute of Sport Tendon Study Group. *J Sci Med Sport.* 1998;1:22-28.

29. Woodley BL, Newsham-West RJ, Baxter GD. Chronic tendinopathy: effectiveness of eccentric exercise. *Br J Sports Med.* 2007;41:188-199.

30. Jeffery R, Cronin J, Bressel E. Eccentric strengthening: clinical applications to Achilles tendinopathy. *NZ J Sports Med.* 2005;35:71-87.

31. Purdam CR, Jonsson P, Alfredson H, Lorentzon R, Cook JL, Khan KM. A pilot study of the eccentric decline squat in the management of painful chronic patellar tendinopathy. *Br J Sports Med.* 2004;38:395-397.

32. Jonsson P, Alfredson H. Superior results with eccentric compared to concentric quadriceps training in patients with jumper's knee: a prospective randomised study. *Br J Sports Med.* 2005; 39:847-850.

33. Visnes H, Hoksrud A, Cook J, Bahr R. No effect of eccentric training on jumper's knee in volleyball players during the competitive season: a randomized clinical trial. *Clin J Sport Med.* 15:227-234.

34. Kongsgaard M, Kovanen V, Aagaard KP, et al. Corticosteroid injections, eccentric decline squat training and heavy slow resistance training in patellar tendinopathy. *Scan J Med Sci Sports.* 2009;19: 790-802.

35. Wang CJ, Ko JY, Chan YS, Weng LH, Hsu SL. Extracorporeal shockwave therapy for chronic patellar tendinopathy. *Am J Sports Med.* 2007;35:972-978.

36. Struijs PA, Smidt N, Arola H, van Dijk CN, Buchbinder R, Assendelft WJ. Orthotic devices for the treatment of tennis elbow: a systematic review. *Br J Gen Pract.* 2001; 51: 924-929.

37. APTA Department of Practice and APTA State Government Affairs. Physical therapists & the performance of dry needling: an educational resource paper. 2012:1-122. Available at: http://www.apta.org/StateIssues/DryNeedling/ResourcePaper/. Accessed April 9, 2012.

38. James SL, Ali K, Pocock C, et al. Ultrasound guided dry needling and autologous blood injection for patellar tendinosis. *Br J Sports Med.* 2007;41:518-522.

39. Suresh SP, Ali KE, Jones H, Connell DA. Medial epicondylitis: is ultrasound guided autologous blood injection an effective treatment? *Br J Sports Med.* 2006;40:935-939.

40. Connell DA, Ali KE, Ahmad M, Lambert S, Corbett S, Curtis M. Ultrasound-guided autologous blood injection for tennis elbow. *Skeletal Radiol.* 2006;35:371-377.

41. Hoksrud A, Öhberg L, Alfredson H, Bahr R. Ultrasound-guided sclerosis of neovessels in painful chronic patellar tendinopathy: a randomized controlled trial. *Am J Sports Med.* 2006;34:1738-1747.

42. Ryan M, Wong A, Rabago D, Lee K, Taunton J. Ultrasound-guided injections of hyperosmolar dextrose for overuse patellar tendinopathy: a pilot study. *Br J Sports Med.* 2011;45:972-977.

43. Engebretsen K, Grotle M, Bautz-Holter E, Ekeberg OM, Juel NG, Brox JI. Supervised exercises compared with radial extracorporeal shock-wave therapy for subacromial shoulder pain: 1-year results of a single-blind randomized controlled trial. *Phys Ther.* 2011;91:37-47.

44. Cheing GL, Chang H. Extracorporeal shock wave therapy. *J Orthop Sports Phys Ther.* 2003;33:337-343.

45. Berta L, Fazzari A, Ficco AM, Enrica PM, Catalano MG, Frairia R. Extracorporeal shock waves enhance normal fibroblast proliferation in vitro and activate mRNA expression for TGF-beta1 and for collagen types I and III. *Acta Orthop.* 2009;80:612-617.

46. Wang CJ. Extracorporeal shockwave therapy in musculoskeletal disorders. *J Orthop Surg Res.* 2012;7:11.

47. van Leeuwen MT, Zwerver J, van den Akker-Scheek I. Extracorporeal shockwave therapy for patellar tendinopathy: a review of the literature. *Br J Sports Med.* 2009;43:163-168.

48. Zwerver J, Hartgens F, Verhagen E, van der Worp H, van den Akker-Scheek I, Diercks RL. No effect of extracorporeal shockwave therapy on patellar tendinopathy in jumping athletes during the competitive season: a randomized clinical trial. *Am J Sports Med.* 2011;39:1191-1199.

49. Kaeding CC, Pedroza AD, Powers BC. Surgical treatment of chronic patellar tendinosis: a systematic review. *Clin Orthop Relat Res.* 2007;455:102-106.

50. Pascarella A, Alam M, Pascarella F, Latte C, Di Salvatore MG, Maffulli N. Arthroscopic management of chronic patellar tendinopathy. *Am J Sports Med.* 2011;39:1975-1983.

Knee Anterior Cruciate Ligament (ACL) Sprain: Diagnosis

Mark V. Paterno

CASE 25

A 17-year-old competitive female athlete reported injuring her knee while partici-pating in a soccer game. On the field, she attempted to execute a cutting maneuver when an opponent collided slightly with her trunk and throwing her off balance. She felt a "pop" in her right knee and an immediate sensation of her knee "giving way." She was unable to continue playing and was removed from the game. On the sideline, you observe significant effusion in the suprapatellar region. The patient reports difficulty bearing weight on the right lower extremity due to pain and lack of muscle control.

► Based on the patient's suspected diagnosis, what do you anticipate may be the contributing factors to her condition?
► What examination signs may be associated with this diagnosis?

KEY DEFINITIONS

FUNCTIONAL INSTABILITY: Sensation of "giving way" due to excessive motion and/or translation within the knee joint or inadequate neuromuscular stability within the lower extremity

MECHANICAL INSTABILITY: Increase in translation of the knee joint due to ligamentous insufficiency

Objectives

1. Describe the anatomic structure and function of the anterior cruciate ligament (ACL).
2. Identify potential secondary injuries that may occur at the time of an ACL injury and how these could affect rehabilitation prognosis.
3. Describe clinical tests with acceptable diagnostic accuracy to identify ACL laxity.

Physical Therapy Considerations

PT considerations during examination of the individual with suspected acute anterior cruciate ligament insufficiency:

▶ **General physical therapy plan of care/goals:** Decrease pain and effusion; increase muscular strength; increase lower quadrant strength; improve functional stability; prevent or minimize loss of aerobic fitness capacity

▶ **Physical therapy tests and measures:** Lachman examination, pivot shift examination

▶ **Differential diagnoses:** Patellar dislocation, osteochondral injury

Understanding the Health Condition

Acute injury to the anterior cruciate ligament (ACL) is common in pivoting and cutting activities. As many as 200,000 to 300,000 ACL injuries occur each year in the United States.[1,2] A thorough clinical assessment and diagnosis is critical for early treatment plan development.

The primary role of the ACL is to create stability in the knee joint. The ACL attaches distally in the knee joint on the tibial plateau, anterior to the medial tibial spine.[3,4] The ACL ascends in a posterior lateral direction to its femoral attachment along the posterior inner surface of the lateral femoral condyle (Fig. 25-1).[3,4] Functionally, the ACL comprises two functional bundles that provide mechanical stability through a full arc of motion.[1] The anterior medial bundle (AMB) is taut in a flexed position, while the posterior lateral bundle (PLB) tends to be taut in full extension.[2] Some authors discuss a third intermediate bundle whose functional contribution is significantly less than the AMB and PLB.[2] Together, these bundles assist

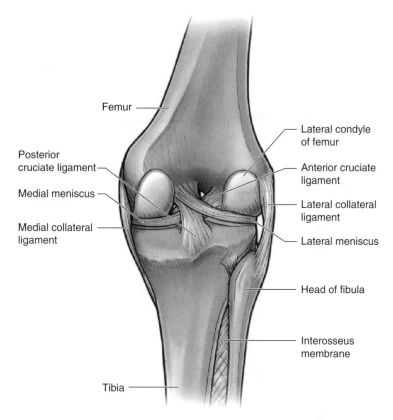

Figure 25-1. Posterior view of the lower extremity showing the attachment of the anterior cruciate ligament along the posterior inner surface of the lateral femoral condyle. (Reproduced with permission from Morton DA, Foreman KB, Albertine KH, eds. *The Big Picture: Gross Anatomy*. New York: McGraw-Hill; 2011. Figure 36-5B)

to create mechanical stability in the knee. Primarily, the ACL provides restraint to anterior tibial translation and assists in rotatory stability in the knee.[3] Injury to the ACL can result in excessive anterior translation of the tibia on the femur, often described as mechanical instability. As a result of several concurrent factors including excessive translation in the knee joint, deficits in neuromuscular control of the knee, and altered proprioception, the patient may experience episodes of giving way in the knee described as functional instability.

Treatment planning after ACL injury can follow a surgical or nonoperative route. Surgical ACL reconstruction is often recommended in an attempt to restore normal anatomy and allow the patient to return to pivoting and cutting activities.[4] Nonoperative management can be an option and is discussed in Case 26. The decision to manage operatively versus nonoperatively may be influenced by the presence of secondary pathology at the time of injury. Additional injury to the secondary stabilizers of the knee (*e.g.*, collateral ligaments and menisci) may result in additional instability at the knee.[5] Injury to the menisci or articular cartilage may also raise concern about progressive joint surface breakdown in the presence of a joint with excessive translation.[6,7] These additional pathologies may increase the likelihood of surgical management.

Short-term and long-term outcomes after ACL injury are variable. Although many patients are able to return to prior levels of function, issues with residual functional instability, pain, and a high incidence of repeat injuries have been reported following ACL injury.[8,9] Recent evidence has shown that the percentage of athletes who return to prior levels of function may be less than initially reported.[10-12] With respect to long-term outcomes after ACL injury, current evidence suggests injury to the ACL can result in a **high incidence of osteoarthritis (OA)** in as few as 10 years after the index injury.[9,13,14] These reports suggested that the incidence of OA was similar with both operative and nonoperative management of ACL injury. These limitations with both short- and long-term outcomes after ACL injury highlight the need to implement and improve injury prevention programs and postinjury management to attempt to improve outcomes for these patients.

Examination, Evaluation, and Diagnosis

Clinical assessment of potential ACL injury has evolved. Early clinical assessment of the knee focused on quantifying the amount of anterior-posterior (AP) translation in the knee as a means to assess ACL integrity. The anterior drawer examination was initially utilized to quantify this AP translation. The anterior drawer examination requires the therapist to pull the tibial plateau anteriorly while the patient's involved knee is in a position of 90° of knee flexion and 45° of hip flexion.[15] The anterior drawer has two major limitations. First, the testing position allows increased stability from the secondary restraints of the knee such as the collateral ligaments and the menisci.[3] Second, the hamstrings have a mechanical advantage to resist anterior translation at 90° of knee flexion, potentially decreasing anterior translation during the examination. The **Lachman examination** also evaluates anterior translation, but the assessment is performed with the knee in 20° to 30° of knee flexion. At this angle of knee flexion, the secondary restraints of the knee are lax and the ACL serves as the primary restraint to AP translation with little contribution from supporting structures.[3]

The **pivot shift** examination is a third clinical test to assess knee stability in the presence of suspected ACL pathology. The pivot shift examination goes beyond a simple assessment of AP translation and attempts to reproduce the "giving way" mechanism. With the patient supine, the physical therapist keeps the involved knee internally rotated and moves the knee from flexion to full extension while applying a valgus stress. This maneuver stresses the knee in AP, medial-lateral, and rotational planes. In an ACL-deficient knee, this maneuver results in a sudden reduction of a previously anteriorly subluxed lateral compartment of the knee as a result of the iliotibial band becoming taut, which simulates the "giving way" mechanism.[15,16] Unlike the anterior drawer and the Lachman examination, the pivot shift test is strongly associated with functional outcome after ACL reconstruction (*e.g.*, "giving way," activity limitation, sports participation).[17] Recent biomechanical evidence suggests that the pivot shift examination may be better suited than simple assessments of AP translation to detect a restoration of normal kinematics of the knee after

ACL reconstruction. A frequently reported limitation of the pivot shift examination is the technical difficulty to perform the test as well as the patient's potential difficulty to relax during the examination. If a patient is hesitant to experience the **"giving-way"** phenomenon reproduced by the pivot shift examination, she may recruit neuromuscular stabilizers to guard against this sensation, which significantly decreases the diagnostic accuracy of the examination.

A recent meta-analysis of 28 studies reported the diagnostic accuracy of current clinical tests for assessment of ACL injury compared to the gold standards of arthroscopy, arthrotomy, or MRI.[15] Benjaminse et al.[15] reported the Lachman examination was the most accurate test to determine ACL insufficiency with a pooled specificity of 94% and a pooled sensitivity of 85%. The pivot shift examination had even better specificity (98%), but inadequate sensitivity (24%). Finally, the anterior drawer had good specificity (91%) and sensitivity (92%) in individuals with chronic ACL insufficiency, but not in those with acute ACL injuries. The poor sensitivity of the pivot shift examination may be due to the technical difficulty of the examination as well as issues with patient relaxation during the examination. The reported poor diagnostic accuracy with the anterior drawer examination after acute disruption of the ACL may also be attributed to a patient's inability to relax the hamstrings to allow the therapist to appreciate the true AP translation.

Plan of Care and Interventions

The physical therapy plan of care and interventions for nonoperative management of ACL injury are discussed in Case 26. The patient should be referred to an orthopaedic physician while physical therapy treatment is continued if an ACL injury is suspected.

Evidence-Based Clinical Recommendations

SORT: Strength of Recommendation Taxonomy

A: Consistent, good-quality patient-oriented evidence
B: Inconsistent or limited-quality patient-oriented evidence
C: Consensus, disease-oriented evidence, usual practice, expert opinion, or case series

1. Injury to the ACL often leads to a long-term outcome of osteoarthritis. **Grade B**

2. Lachman examination is the most sensitive and specific clinical assessment to identify ACL instability in patients with both acute and chronic ACL insufficiency. **Grade A**

3. The pivot shift test has high specificity but low sensitivity to diagnose ACL ruptures. **Grade A**

4. History of a noncontact, pivoting/twisting mechanism to the knee in conjunction with patient reports of "popping," "giving way," and immediate effusion are consistent with a potential ACL injury. **Grade C**

COMPREHENSION QUESTIONS

25.1 Which of the following accurately describes the sensitivity and specificity of the Lachman examination to diagnose acute ACL rupture?

A. High sensitivity and high specificity

B. Low sensitivity and high specificity

C. Low sensitivity and low specificity

D. High sensitivity and low specificity

25.2 Which clinical test has the highest diagnostic accuracy for a *chronic* ACL injury versus an *acute* ACL injury?

A. Lachman

B. Anterior drawer

C. Pivot shift

D. None of the above

ANSWERS

25.1 **A.** The Lachman test is both highly sensitive (85%) and specific (94%) to assess acute ACL rupture.[15]

25.2 **B.** The anterior drawer is the clinical test that has the highest sensitivity (92%) and specificity (91%) for diagnosis of ACL instability in individuals with chronic ACL injuries.[15]

REFERENCES

1. Duthon VB, Barea C, Abrassart S, Fasel JH, Fritschy D, Menetrey J. Anatomy of the anterior cruciate ligament. *Knee Surg Sports Traumatol Arthrosc.* 2006;14:204-213.

2. Hollis JM, Takai S, Adams DJ, Horibe S, Woo SL. The effects of knee motion and external loading on the length of the anterior cruciate ligament (ACL): a kinematic study. *J Biomech Eng.* 1991;113:208-214.

3. Butler DL, Noyes FR, Grood ES. Ligamentous restraints to anterior-posterior drawer in the human knee. A biomechanical study. *J Bone Joint Surg Am.* 1980;62:259-270.

4. Linko E, Harilainen A, Malmivaara A, Seitsalo S. Surgical versus conservative interventions for anterior cruciate ligament ruptures in adults. *Cochrane Database Syst Rev.* 2005(2):CD001356.

5. Petrigliano FA, Musahl V, Suero EM, Citak M, Pearle AD. Effect of meniscal loss on knee stability after single-bundle anterior cruciate ligament reconstruction. *Knee Surg Sports Traumatol Arthrosc.* 2011;19 Suppl 1:86-93.

6. Dunn WR, Spindler KP, Amendola A, et al. Which preoperative factors, including bone bruise, are associated with knee pain/symptoms at index anterior cruciate ligament reconstruction (ACLR)? A Multicenter Orthopaedic Outcomes Network (MOON) ACLR Cohort Study. *Am J Sports Med.* 2010;38:1778-1787.

7. Theologis AA, Kuo D, Cheng J, et al. Evaluation of bone bruises and associated cartilage in anterior cruciate ligament-injured and -reconstructed knees using quantitative t(1rho) magnetic resonance imaging: 1-year cohort study. *Arthroscopy.* 2011;27:65-76.

8. Paterno MV, Schmitt LC, Ford KR, et al. Biomechanical measures during landing and postural stability predict second anterior cruciate ligament injury after anterior cruciate ligament reconstruction and return to sport. *Am J Sports Med.* 2010;38:1968-1978.

9. Spindler KP, Wright RW. Clinical practice. Anterior cruciate ligament tear. *N Engl J Med.* 2008;359:2135-2142.

10. Ardern CL, Taylor NF, Feller JA, Webster KE. Return-to-sport outcomes at 2 to 7 years after anterior cruciate ligament reconstruction surgery. *Am J Sports Med.* 2012;40:41-48.

11. Ardern CL, Webster KE, Taylor NF, Feller JA. Return to sport following anterior cruciate ligament reconstruction surgery: a systematic review and meta-analysis of the state of play. *Br J Sports Med.* 2011;45:596-606.

12. Ardern CL, Webster KE, Taylor NF, Feller JA. Return to the preinjury level of competitive sport after anterior cruciate ligament reconstruction surgery: two-thirds of patients have not returned by 12 months after surgery. *Am J Sports Med.* 2011;39:538-543.

13. Lohmander LS, Ostenberg A, Englund M, Roos H. High prevalence of knee osteoarthritis, pain, and functional limitations in female soccer players twelve years after anterior cruciate ligament injury. *Arthritis Rheum.* 2004;50:3145-3152.

14. von Porat A, Roos EM, Roos H. High prevalence of osteoarthritis 14 years after an anterior cruciate ligament tear in male soccer players: a study of radiographic and patient relevant outcomes. *Ann Rheum Dis.* 2004;63:269-273.

15. Benjaminse A, Gokeler A, van der Schans CP. Clinical diagnosis of an anterior cruciate ligament rupture: a meta-analysis. *J Orthop Sports Phys Ther.* 2006;36:267-288.

16. Markolf KL, Jackson SR, McAllister DR. Relationship between the pivot shift and Lachman tests: a cadaver study. *J Bone Joint Surg Am.* 2010;92:2067-2075.

17. Kocher MS, Steadman JR, Briggs KK, Sterett WI, Hawkins RJ. Relationships between objective assessment of ligament stability and subjective assessment of symptoms and function after anterior cruciate ligament reconstruction. *Am J Sports Med.* 2004;32:629-634.

Knee Anterior Cruciate Ligament (ACL) Sprain: Nonoperative Management

Mark V. Paterno

CASE 26

A 17-year-old competitive female soccer player presents to physical therapy with a diagnosis of a right acute anterior cruciate ligament (ACL) tear. She reports injuring her knee while participating in a soccer game 1 week ago. At that time, she was running down the field and attempted to execute a cutting maneuver when an opponent collided slightly with her trunk and threw her off balance. She felt a "pop" in her knee and an immediate sensation of her knee "giving way." She was unable to continue playing and sought immediate medical attention. The MRI of her right knee obtained at her medical follow-up demonstrated a complete acute ACL tear with no concomitant meniscal or articular cartilage damage. She is a senior in high school and this injury occurred in the first game of her season.

► Based on the patient's diagnosis, what factors would be appropriate to consider before choosing a nonoperative treatment plan?
► What are the most appropriate physical therapy interventions if a nonoperative treatment plan is implemented?
► What are possible complications that may limit the effectiveness of physical therapy?

KEY DEFINITIONS

COPER: Person with ACL deficiency who is able to resume all preinjury levels of activity without any episodes of the knee giving-way for at least one year[1]

NONCOPER: Person with ACL deficiency who experiences knee instability upon return to activity[1]

PERTURBATION TRAINING: Nonoperative treatment intervention for ACL-deficient individuals; training includes progressive application of disruptions to the individual's balance on unstable surfaces in an attempt to enhance dynamic neuromuscular stability in the affected knee prior to return to activity[2]

Objectives

1. Describe a decision-making algorithm to determine if an ACL-deficient individual is a candidate to pursue nonsurgical management of ACL injury.

2. Identify appropriate interventions to utilize with an individual pursuing nonsurgical management of an ACL injury.

3. Identify appropriate return-to-sport criteria for individuals pursuing conservative management of ACL injury.

Physical Therapy Considerations

PT considerations during nonoperative management of the individual with a diagnosis of acute anterior cruciate ligament tear:

▶ **General physical therapy plan of care/goals:** Decrease acute pain and effusion; increase muscular strength; increase lower quadrant strength; improve functional stability; prevent or minimize loss of aerobic fitness capacity

▶ **Physical therapy interventions:** Patient education regarding functional anatomy and injury pathomechanics; modalities and manual therapy to decrease pain and effusion; muscular flexibility exercises; resistance exercises to increase muscular strength, activation, and endurance capacity with a focus on the lower extremity and core musculature; balance and proprioceptive interventions; perturbation training

▶ **Precautions during physical therapy:** Monitor all activity to ensure no episodes of knee giving-way; address precautions or contraindications for exercise, based on patient's mechanical instability (*e.g.*, limit open kinetic chain knee extension in the range from 30° to full extension to decrease anterior shear forces at tibiofemoral joint)

▶ **Complications interfering with physical therapy:** Residual knee instability with activities of daily living (ADLs) or exercise

Understanding the Health Condition

Rupture of the anterior cruciate ligament (ACL) is a devastating injury. The primary role of the ACL is to create stability in the knee joint. The ACL is positioned obliquely in the knee joint attaching the anterior tibial plateau to the posterior portion of the inner wall of the lateral femoral condyle (Fig. 25-1).[3] In this position, the ACL provides a primary restraint to anterior tibial translation and assists in rotatory stability in the knee.[4] Therefore, injury to the ACL results in excessive anterior translation of the tibia on the femur, with subsequent mechanical instability. The sensation of the knee "giving way" is often the product of a collection of impairments, including mechanical instability, altered neuromuscular control, and altered proprioception and is referred to as functional instability. Typical management of ACL injury in the United States is surgical reconstruction—90% of patients who sustain an ACL tear pursue this course of care.[5] Despite the preponderance of patients selecting surgical management of ACL insufficiency, a percentage of patients may be able to maintain an acceptable functional level without surgical reconstruction.

The athlete attempting to participate in pivoting and cutting sports in the absence of the mechanical stability provided by an intact ACL represents a clinical challenge to rehabilitation professionals. In the early 1980s, Noyes et al.[6] discussed their theory of the "rule of thirds." The authors hypothesized that approximately one-third of ACL-deficient individuals could execute light recreational activities without repeated episodes of the knee giving-way. More recently, researchers from the University of Delaware have developed a decision-making scheme to more objectively identify individuals who may be able to participate in pivoting and cutting activity without giving-way ("copers") and those who are less likely to be able to accomplish this level of activity without surgical intervention ("noncopers").[2,7] Specific and objective criteria to identify individuals who have the potential to succeed with nonoperative intervention is critical. The consequences of experiencing repeated giving-way episodes with an ACL-deficient knee can be catastrophic. Repeated knee giving-way episodes due to mechanical and functional instability are often associated with additional meniscus injury, articular cartilage damage, and further joint degeneration.[8,9] Considering current evidence that suggests the incidence of osteoarthritis after ACL injury is between 50% and 100%,[10–12] any activity that has the potential to accelerate this negative joint cascade should be pursued with extreme caution.

Choosing nonoperative management after an ACL injury is a multifactorial decision. Ultimately, all factors under consideration must focus on a scenario that minimizes the potential for repeated giving-way of the knee. First, the patient must present with an absence of any secondary knee pathology.[2] Second, the patient must qualify via an objective algorithm that identifies candidates with the greatest likelihood for success and minimal chance of repeated giving-way. The patient's preference with a treatment plan is often driven by lifestyle choices. Some may choose to limit pivoting or cutting activity post-ACL tear as a means to decrease risk of repeated giving-way. Others may choose to delay surgical ACL reconstruction in an attempt to return to pivoting or cutting activity on a limited basis due to work-related demands or short-term athletic goals, such as in the scenario of the high school senior at the end of her competitive athletic career. Many factors including long-term joint health and short-term goals must be considered prior to selecting a treatment plan.

Physical Therapy Patient/Client Management

There may be one or more appropriate interventions for a patient who chooses nonoperative management of an ACL injury based on the patient's presentation. Once identified as a potential candidate for nonoperative management, physical therapy interventions may include resolving typical impairments such as acute effusion, limitations in range of motion (ROM) and mobility, and decreased strength. In addition, emphasis must be placed on maximizing lower extremity proprioception as a component of establishing dynamic functional stability prior to attempting to return to functional activities, such as sports. One specific intervention which has proven to increase success with ability to return to sport in a targeted population is perturbation training as described by Fitzgerald et al.[2] The primary goal for most injured athletes/individuals is to return to pain-free sport or activity as quickly and as safely as possible in a manner that optimizes functional stability in the knee and limits the potential for giving-way episodes.

Examination, Evaluation, and Diagnosis

A clinical diagnosis of an acute ACL injury is outlined in Case 25. This injury often presents with hallmark impairments. Acute hemarthrosis within the knee joint[13] with potential reflex inhibition of the quadriceps musculature is common after ACL rupture.[14] These patients may also present with a limitation in full ROM[15] and residual deficits in lower extremity muscle activation with functional weakness.[16] Collectively, these impairments may contribute to an altered gait pattern.[17] Coinciding with damage to the native ACL is a loss of proprioceptive input to the knee joint.[18] The intact ACL possesses robust mechanoreceptor innervation that allows the ACL to provide proprioceptive input to the knee joint.[14,19] Hence, injury to this structure disrupts this feedback and decreases joint position sense of the extremity. These impairments must be objectively assessed and adequately addressed prior to return to activity. Recent evidence suggests that factors such as preinjury level of function and amount of antero-posterior translation (mechanical stability) do *not* predict successful functional outcome after ACL injury.[1,20] Rather, assessments of functional movements may be a more accurate predictor of successful outcome in this population.

The ultimate selection of individuals appropriate for a nonoperative course of treatment should be the product of an objective, algorithmic assessment that can identify those with the best potential to succeed with minimal risk of repeated giving-way episodes. For individuals with acute unilateral ACL tear, Fitzgerald et al.[2,7] outlined a selection **algorithm to identify potential "copers,"** or those who had the potential to successfully return to high-level functional activity without giving-way. Those who failed the selection algorithm were described as "noncopers" and were candidates for surgical reconstruction. The selection algorithm begins with a determination of the extent of knee damage. If there is evidence of multiligamentous injuries, repairable meniscus pathology or chondral defects, the individual is already excluded as a candidate for nonoperative management. The screening assessment for nonoperative candidates consists of four single-leg hop tests,[21] a self-reported number of giving-way episodes, the Knee Outcome Survey of Activities of Daily Living (ADLs) Scale[22] and a global rating of knee function.[2] Those who demonstrate an 80% limb symmetry score on all hop tests, report no more than one episode of giving-way since initial injury, score $\geq$80% on the Knee Outcome Survey of ADLs, and have a global rating score of $\geq$60% are candidates for nonoperative rehabilitation.[2] In a recent 10-year follow-up of over 800 patients with an ACL injury, 17.5% were initially identified as potential copers. Approximately 10% of the patients chose to pursue conservative management. Within this group, 75% were able to return to sports without an ACL reconstruction. However this represents less than 8% of the initial cohort of patients who suffered an ACL injury.[1,20]

Plan of Care and Interventions

Physical therapy interventions must address findings from the musculoskeletal examination. Acute impairments including effusion, pain, loss of motion, and altered gait patterns should be initially addressed in the early phases of rehabilitation to develop an appropriate foundation. Modalities may help reduce acute signs and symptoms. Moderate to strong evidence supports the use of **supervised targeted progressive resistance exercises, neuromuscular electrical stimulation and neuromuscular re-education** for individuals with altered knee stability.[23] Targeted balance training and perturbation training should be utilized to address impaired proprioceptive function.[24,25] A return-to-sport progression should be used to ensure the individual's ability to successfully resume prior levels of function.

The development of sufficient muscle performance is critical for success on higher-level performance tests as well as for the ultimate transition to function and sport. Marked deficits in quadriceps strength and timing of quadriceps activation are common due to reflex muscle inhibition[14] as well as disuse atrophy after injury. Current evidence has shown improved quadriceps strength with the use of neuromuscular electrical stimulation in patients with an ACL injury.[26] Targeted progressive resistive exercises are also critical to increase lower extremity strength and should include a mixture of both open and closed kinetic chain interventions. However, the physical therapist must carefully choose ranges to strengthen the quadriceps that also *minimize* the anterior shear forces at the ACL-deficient tibiofemoral joint. Open kinetic chain (OKC) interventions provide an opportunity to train a specific muscle in relative isolation to target specific strength deficits that may exist. Quadriceps strengthening in an OKC (e.g., seated leg extension with foot non-weightbearing) is an effective way to increase strength. Leg extension exercises performed in a limited range (between 45° and 90° of flexion) results in minimal anterior shear at the tibiofemoral joint. In contrast, extending the knee from 45° to full extension can result in excessive anterior shear forces.[27,28] Resisted knee flexion in an OKC also improves the strength of the hamstrings, which helps in the development of functional knee stability. A complement of closed kinetic chain (CKC) interventions is appropriate to train impaired muscle groups in functional positions. Exercises such as leg presses, squatting, wall sitting and step-ups/step-downs through a knee range of motion that limits excessive shear and stress on the tibiofemoral joint (0°-60°) can progressively strengthen the lower extremity in the presence of ACL deficiency.[28] Thus, the ideal knee ranges in which to perform strengthening exercises with minimal anterior shear forces at the tibiofemoral joint are between 45° and 90° for OKC exercises and between 0° and 60° for CKC exercises.

Balance and proprioception impairments are common after ACL injury[29–31] and these deficits are thought to contribute to functional instability.[32] However, methods currently used to assess proprioceptive deficits may not provide sufficient information related to the clinical correlates of this deficit.[33] Despite limitations with assessment, consensus exists in the literature that an attempt to restore proprioceptive function in the ACL-deficient knee is necessary to enhance dynamic stability.[34] Interventions such as single-limb standing on stable and unstable surfaces are sufficient to initiate balance and proprioceptive training on the ACL-deficient limb. These interventions can be advanced from single-plane movement to more dynamic interventions that can challenge the joint in three planes of movement. A very structured proprioceptive intervention utilized in a population of patients with ACL deficiency is perturbation training.[2] Perturbation training is a progression of balance exercises in which the patient stands on unstable surfaces such as roller boards and tilt boards. The patient is progressively challenged to maintain single-limb balance on unstable surfaces as various perturbations are applied to the unstable surface. The challenge of the perturbation task advances as the patient becomes more skilled in controlling the movement and demonstrates increased stability. In theory, these interventions help improve reactive stability of the joint by developing appropriate neuromuscular responses to external stress in the absence of mechanical stability. Based on results of clinical studies with physically active individuals with ACL injuries who are appropriately selected for nonoperative management, Fitzgerald et al.[2] have suggested including perturbation training within a rehabilitation program for 2 to 3 sessions per week for a total of 10 visits to promote successful return to prior level of function.

Progression beyond the initial phases of nonoperative management of an ACL injury requires the individual to demonstrate an ability to successfully attain certain criteria directed toward return-to-sport. To participate in a dynamic functional progression (and before returning to sport), an individual must be able to demonstrate normal knee ROM and sufficient strength (>90% limb symmetry index), balance, proprioception, and neuromuscular control.[35] Failure to meet these goals prior to functional reintegration can result in the development of compensations and abnormal movement patterns with activity.[25,36] Once these goals are met, a functional progression back to activity and/or sports is recommended prior to initiation of desired sports-specific activities.[35,37] Prior to return to sport, a **functional reintegration program** should be developed to meet the unique, activity-specific goals of each patient. Emphasis should be on the development of progressive reintegration with initial interventions occurring at reduced speed and/or intensity. With the current young female soccer player, after resolution of her impairments (*i.e.*, attainment of normal knee ROM and strength), successful completion of perturbation training, and an absence of any giving-way with activity, a functional progression should begin with light pivoting and cutting activities that simulate maneuvers experienced on the soccer field. These may include soccer-specific drills, dribbling drills, and light plyometric activities. Typically, these should be initiated in a single plane and at a submaximal (50%) speed. As she demonstrates success with these maneuvers, the intensity of the drills can be increased by adding multiplanar movements, focusing more on single-limb activities, and increasing the speed to 75% and eventually to 100%. If she is able to successfully execute these drills, a final progression to "live-game" activity should be executed during a simulated game or during a scrimmage situation. If she successfully completes this phase of rehabilitation without episodes of giving-way, consideration can be made to return to sport. Objective criteria to evaluate readiness to return to sport may include patient-reported outcomes such as the International Knee Documentation Committee (IKDC) self-report measure,[22] single-limb hop testing,[21] and functional movement tools such as a drop vertical jump maneuver.[38]

Evidence-Based Clinical Recommendations

SORT: Strength of Recommendation Taxonomy
A: Consistent, good-quality patient-oriented evidence
B: Inconsistent or limited-quality patient-oriented evidence
C: Consensus, disease-oriented evidence, usual practice, expert opinion, or case series

1. An objective algorithmic assessment can be used to identify "copers"—those ACL-deficient individuals who may be able to return to high-level functional activity without surgical ACL reconstruction and without repeated giving-way episodes. **Grade A**

2. Participation in interventions that incorporate neuromuscular re-education and improve lower extremity strength, balance, and proprioception increases the likelihood that ACL-deficient individuals can successfully return to pivoting and cutting activity without undergoing ACL reconstruction. **Grade B**

3. ACL-deficient individuals who choose nonoperative management should participate in a structured, functional reintegration program before returning to sport. **Grade C**

COMPREHENSION QUESTIONS

26.1 Which of the following is *not* a criterion for a patient with an anterior cruciate ligament tear to be classified as a potential "coper"?

A. 80% limb symmetry score or greater on all single-limb hop testing

B. Knee Outcome Survey of ADLs of 80% or greater

C. Reports of no more than one episode of giving way since injury

D. No asymmetries with movement patterns on a drop vertical jump assessment

26.2 Open kinetic chain (OKC) knee extension exercises should be performed in which of the following ranges of motion to minimize anterior shear forces within the ACL-deficient knee joint?

A. 90° flexion to full extension

B. 90° flexion to 10° flexion

C. 90° flexion to 45° flexion

D. 90° flexion to 60° flexion

ANSWERS

26.1 **D.** The drop vertical jump assessment is not a criterion to be considered a coper. All other answers were included in the algorithm defined by Fitzgerald et al.[2,7]

26.2 **C.** 90° to 45° is a safe range to perform OKC knee extension with ACL deficiency because it minimizes the anterior shear forces at the tibiofemoral joint.

REFERENCES

1. Hurd WJ, Axe MJ, Snyder-Mackler L. A 10-year prospective trial of a patient management algorithm and screening examination for highly active individuals with anterior cruciate ligament injury: part 1, outcomes. *Am J Sports Med.* 2008;36:40-47.

2. Fitzgerald GK, Axe MJ, Snyder-Mackler L. Proposed practice guidelines for nonoperative anterior cruciate ligament rehabilitation of physically active individuals. *J Orthop Sports Phys Ther.* 2000;30:194-203.

3. Duthon VB, Barea C, Abrassart S, Fasel JH, Fritschy D, Menetrey J. Anatomy of the anterior cruciate ligament. *Knee Surg Sports Traumatol Arthrosc.* 2006;14:204-213.

4. Butler DL, Noyes FR, Grood ES. Ligamentous restraints to anterior-posterior drawer in the human knee. A biomechanical study. *J Bone Joint Surg Am.* 1980;62:259-270.

5. Linko E, Harilainen A, Malmivaara A, Seitsalo S. Surgical versus conservative interventions for anterior cruciate ligament ruptures in adults. *Cochrane Database Syst Rev.* 2005(2):CD001356.

6. Noyes FR, Matthews DS, Mooar PA, Grood ES. The symptomatic anterior cruciate-deficient knee. Part II: the results of rehabilitation, activity modification, and counseling on functional disability. *J Bone Joint Surg Am.* 1983;65:163-174.

7. Fitzgerald GK, Axe MJ, Snyder-Mackler L. A decision-making scheme for returning patients to high-level activity with nonoperative treatment after anterior cruciate ligament rupture. *Knee Surg Sports Traumatol Arthrosc.* 2000;8:76-82.

8. Levy AS, Wetzler MJ, Lewars M, Laughlin W. Knee injuries in women collegiate rugby players. Am J Sports Med. 1997;25:360-362.

9. Beynnon BD, Johnson RJ, Abate JA, Fleming BC, Nichols CE. Treatment of anterior cruciate ligament injuries, part I. Am J Sports Med. 2005;33:1579-1602.

10. Lohmander LS, Ostenberg A, Englund M, Roos H. High prevalence of knee osteoarthritis, pain, and functional limitations in female soccer players twelve years after anterior cruciate ligament injury. Arthritis Rheum. 2004;50:3145-3152.

11. von Porat A, Roos EM, Roos H. High prevalence of osteoarthritis 14 years after an anterior cruciate ligament tear in male soccer players: a study of radiographic and patient relevant outcomes. Ann Rheum Dis. 2004;63:269-273.

12. Spindler KP, Wright RW. Clinical practice. Anterior cruciate ligament tear. N Engl J Med. 2008;359:2135-2142.

13. Daniel DM, Stone ML, Dobson BE, Fithian DC, Rossman DJ, Kaufman KR. Fate of the ACL-injured patient. A prospective outcome study. Am J Sports Med. 1994;22:632-644.

14. Kennedy JC, Alexander IJ, Hayes KC. Nerve supply of the human knee and its functional importance. Am J Sports Med. 1982;10:329-335.

15. McHugh MP, Tyler TF, Gleim GW, Nicholas SJ. Preoperative indicators of motion loss and weakness following anterior cruciate ligament reconstruction. J Orthop Sports Phys Ther. 1998;27:407-411.

16. Ageberg E, Pettersson A, Friden T. 15-year follow-up of neuromuscular function in patients with unilateral nonreconstructed anterior cruciate ligament injury initially treated with rehabilitation and activity modification: a longitudinal prospective study. Am J Sports Med. 2007;35:2109-2117.

17. Berchuck M, Andriacchi TP, Bach BR, Reider B. Gait adaptations by patients who have a deficient anterior cruciate ligament. J Bone Joint Surg Am. 1990;72:871-877.

18. Friden T, Roberts D, Zatterstrom R, Lindstrand A, Moritz U. Proprioceptive defects after an anterior cruciate ligament rupture—the relation to associated anatomical lesions and subjective knee function. Knee Surg Sports Traumatol Arthrosc. 1999;7:226-231.

19. Haus J, Halata Z. Innervation of the anterior cruciate ligament. Int Orthop. 1990;14:293-296.

20. Hurd WJ, Axe MJ, Snyder-Mackler L. A 10-year prospective trial of a patient management algorithm and screening examination for highly active individuals with anterior cruciate ligament injury: part 2, determinants of dynamic knee stability. Am J Sports Med. 2008;36:48-56.

21. Noyes FR, Barber SD, Mangine RE. Abnormal lower limb symmetry determined by function hop tests after anterior cruciate ligament rupture. Am J Sports Med. 1991;19:513-518.

22. Irrgang JJ, Snyder-Mackler L, Wainner RS, Fu FH, Harner CD. Development of a patient-reported measure of function of the knee. J Bone Joint Surg Am. 1998;80:1132-1145.

23. Logerstedt DS, Snyder-Mackler L, Ritter RC, Axe MJ, Godges JJ. Orthopaedic Section of the American Physical Therapy Association. Knee stability and movement coordination impairments: knee ligament sprain. J Orthop Sports Phys Ther. 2010;40:A1-A37.

24. Chmielewski TL, Hurd WJ, Rudolph KS, Axe MJ, Snyder-Mackler L. Perturbation training improves knee kinematics and reduces muscle co-contraction after complete unilateral anterior cruciate ligament rupture. Phys Ther. 2005;85:740-749.

25. Chmielewski TL, Rudolph KS, Snyder-Mackler L. Development of dynamic knee stability after acute ACL injury. J Electromyogr Kinesiol. 2002;12:267-274.

26. Snyder-Mackler L, Delitto A, Bailey SL, Stralka SW. Strength of the quadriceps femoris muscle and functional recovery after reconstruction of the anterior cruciate ligament. A prospective, randomized clinical trial of electrical stimulation. J Bone Joint Surg Am. 1995;77:1166-1173.

27. Beynnon BD, Johnson RJ, Fleming BC. The science of anterior cruciate ligament rehabilitation. Clin Orthop Relat Res. 2002(402):9-20.

28. Beynnon BD, Fleming BC, Johnson RJ, Nichols CE, Renstrom PA, Pope MH. Anterior cruciate ligament strain behavior during rehabilitation exercises in vivo. Am J Sports Med. 1995;23:24-34.

29. Hewett TE, Paterno MV, Myer GD. Strategies for enhancing proprioception and neuromuscular control of the knee. *Clin Orthop Relat Res.* 2002(402):76-94.

30. Paterno MV, Hewett TE, Noyes FR. The return of neuromuscular coordination after anterior cruciate ligament reconstruction. *J Orthop Sports Phys Ther.* 1998;27:94.

31. Paterno MV, Hewett TE, Noyes FR. Gender differences in neuromuscular coordination of controls, ACL-deficient knees and ACL-reconstructed knees. *J Orthop Sports Phys Ther.* 1999;29:A-45.

32. Friden T, Roberts D, Ageberg E, Walden M, Zatterstrom R. Review of knee proprioception and the relation to extremity function after an anterior cruciate ligament rupture. *J Orthop Sports Phys Ther.* 2001;31:567-576.

33. Gokeler A, Benjaminse A, Hewett TE, et al. Proprioceptive deficits after ACL injury: are they clinically relevant? *Br J Sports Med.* 2012;46:180-192.

34. Irrgang JJ, Neri R. The rationale for open and closed kinetic chain activities for restoration of proprioception and neuromuscular control following injury? In Lephart SM, Fu FH, eds. *Proprioception and Neuromuscular Control in Joint Stability.* Champaign, IL: Human Kinetics; 2000.

35. Schmitt L, Byrnes R, Cherny C, et al. Cincinnati Children's Hospital Medical Center: Evidence-based clinical care guideline for return to activity after lower extremity injury. Available at: http://www.cincinnatichildrens.org/svc/alpha/h/health-policy/otpt.htm, Guideline 38, pages 1-13, May 24, 2010. Accessed January 16, 2012.

36. Chmielewski TL, Hurd WJ, Snyder-Mackler L. Elucidation of a potentially destabilizing control strategy in ACL deficient non-copers. *J Electromyogr Kinesiol.* 2005;15:83-92.

37. Myer GD, Paterno MV, Ford KR, Quatman CE, Hewett TE. Rehabilitation after anterior cruciate ligament reconstruction: criteria based progression through the return to sport phase. *J Orthop Sports Phys Ther.* 2006;36:385-402.

38. Paterno MV, Schmitt LC, Ford KR, et al. Biomechanical measures during landing and postural stability predict second anterior cruciate ligament injury after anterior cruciate ligament reconstruction and return to sport. *Am J Sports Med.* 2010;38:1968-1978.

Knee Medial Collateral Ligament (MCL) Sprain

Janice K. Loudon

CASE 27

A 16-year-old high school football player was injured when he was hit on the lateral side of the right knee while running with the football. He immediately fell to the turf and was unable to bear weight on his right leg. He did not return to play. After a sideline examination, the team doctor diagnosed him with a grade II medial collateral ligament sprain. The football player's goal is to return to play as soon as possible.

▶ What examination signs may be associated with this diagnosis?
▶ What are the most appropriate examination tests?
▶ Based on his diagnosis, what do you anticipate will be the contributors to activity limitations?
▶ What are the most appropriate physical therapy interventions?
▶ What are the most appropriate physical therapy outcome measures for return to sport?
▶ What is his rehabilitation prognosis?

KEY DEFINITIONS

GRADE II LIGAMENT SPRAIN: Ligament injury that involves tearing of 25% to 75% of the ligament; signs and symptoms include pain, swelling, loss of motion, and possible joint instability

MEDIAL COLLATERAL LIGAMENT (MCL): Major ligament of the knee that maintains medial stability

VALGUS STRESS: Force applied to the lateral side of a joint that creates tensile stress to the medial joint

Objectives

1. Describe the anatomy of the medial collateral ligament of the knee.
2. Identify the most accurate clinical tests for assessing an MCL sprain.
3. Differentiate between the different grades of MCL sprains.
4. Prescribe appropriate therapeutic exercises for an individual with a grade II MCL sprain.
5. Describe the functional tests needed for return to sport after an MCL sprain.

Physical Therapy Considerations

PT considerations during management of the individual with a diagnosis of a grade II medial collateral ligament sprain:

▶ **General physical therapy plan of care/goals:** Decrease pain; increase joint range of motion; increase lower quadrant strength; prevent or minimize loss of aerobic fitness capacity

▶ **Physical therapy interventions:** Patient education regarding functional anatomy and injury pathomechanics; modalities and manual therapy to decrease pain; muscular flexibility exercises; resistance exercises to increase muscular endurance capacity of the core and to increase strength of lower extremity muscles; aerobic exercise program; knee brace

▶ **Precautions during physical therapy:** Monitor vital signs; address precautions or contraindications for exercise, based on the stages of healing

▶ **Complications interfering with physical therapy:** Excessive swelling; excessive scarring that limits normal knee range of motion

Understanding the Health Condition

Knee injuries are common in sporting activities. According to the American Association of Orthopaedic Surgeons (AAOS), in 2003 approximately 19.4 million individuals sought medical treatment for knee injuries and one of the most commonly

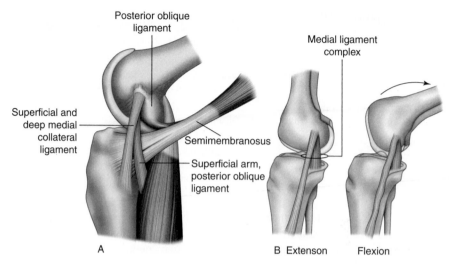

Posterior oblique
ligament

Medial ligament
complex

Superficial and
deep medial
collateral
ligament

Semimembranosus

Superficial arm,
posterior oblique
ligament

A

B Extenson   Flexion

Figure 27-1. A. Medial side of the knee, showing the superficial and deep portions of the medial collateral ligament. **B.** In knee extension, posterior fibers of the MCL are relatively tight. In knee flexion, tension in the posterior fibers decreases. (Reproduced with permission from Cole BJ, Sekiya JK. *Surgical Techniques of the Shoulder, Elbow, and Knee in Sports Medicine.* Philadelphia: Saunders; 2008. Figure 4-55.)

injured ligaments is the medial collateral ligament (MCL).[1,2] Anatomically, the MCL complex contains three components: the superficial MCL (sMCL), the deep MCL (dMCL), and the posterior oblique ligament (POL). These three components blend and exist as a continuous band of tissue (Fig. 27-1). The sMCL is a flat band that originates on the femur, proximal and posterior to the medial epicondyle and distal to the adductor tubercle.[3] It courses distally to attach to the medial tibia, eventually blending with the periosteum.[4] These fibers attach just posterior to the distal attachment of the closely aligned tendon of the sartorius and gracilis muscles. The length of the sMCL ranges from 6 to 12 cm depending on the size of the individual.[5] The sMCL is extracapsular and is separated from the dMCL by a bursa. The dMCL is also termed the medial capsular ligament and can be further divided into the meniscofemoral and meniscotibial portions. The deep fibers of the MCL originate slightly anterior and distal to the femoral attachment of the sMCL. The dMCL is composed of short vertically oriented bands that directly attach to the medial meniscus and the knee capsule. This anatomical relationship accounts for the high association of medial meniscal tears with MCL sprains. The third component of the MCL complex is a fibrous bundle that is located posterior to the sMCL and is termed the posterior oblique ligament (POL).[6] The POL blends with the posterior medial joint capsule, medial meniscus, and semimembranosus tendon sheath. Some authors refer to this anatomical area as the posteromedial corner.[5,7] The detailed anatomy of the MCL complex is described in Table 27-1.

The MCL complex is the primary stabilizer of the medial knee to direct valgus stress.[8] Grood et al.[9] determined that the MCL is the primary restraint for valgus at 5° of knee flexion (57% of anatomical restraint) and 25° (78% of anatomical restraint) of knee flexion. Portions of the MCL complex are taut throughout knee range of

Table 27-1 ANATOMY OF THE MCL COMPLEX	
Structure	**Anatomical Attachments**
Superficial MCL	Originates on the distal femur, proximal and posterior to the medial epicondyle and distal to the adductor tubercle Courses distally attaching to medial tibia, eventually blending with the periosteum
Deep MCL	Broader, shorter, and deeper to the superficial MCL Attaches to the joint capsule and medial meniscus
Posterior oblique ligament	Originates posterior to the sMCL Blends with posterior medial joint capsule, medial meniscus, and semimembranosus tendon sheath

motion (ROM; Fig. 27-1B). The anterior fibers of the sMCL are taut in flexion and the posterior fibers are taut in extension. The MCL is dynamically reinforced by the pes anserine and semimembranosus muscles when the knee is extended.[10] The meniscofemoral ligament of the dMCL is a secondary stabilizer to valgus stress at all angles of knee motion.[8] In addition to protecting against valgus stress, the MCL complex contributes to restraining rotatory motion (tibial external rotation) and anterior-posterior translation.[11]

Modes for which the MCL is injured include contact and noncontact incidents in which valgus stress is directed at a flexed knee. An isolated injury to the MCL often occurs from a direct blow to the lateral aspect of the thigh while the foot is planted, which produces a direct valgus moment. This type of injury is common in football and rugby. The dMCL fibers are shorter and experience a greater percentage of stretch when subject to valgus strain.[8] Therefore, the dMCL is ruptured more frequently than the superficial MCL. In addition, most MCL injuries occur at the femoral origin or in the mid-substance directly over the joint line.

A second mechanism of injury to the MCL is a valgus stress coupled with tibial external rotation. This pivoting maneuver occurs commonly in sports such as skiing, basketball, and soccer. With this type of injury, the POL is injured first followed by the deep and superficial fibers of the MCL.[6] Other injured structures may include the cruciate ligaments or medial meniscus.

Ligament sprains are commonly graded based on signs and symptoms from the clinical examination. The physical therapist needs to be cognizant of the fact that an individual may have laxity at the knee joint, but present functionally and without instability. The grade of ligament injury is based on the amount of laxity (in millimeters) as compared to the stable extremity. A grade I sprain involves microscopic tears of the superficial and deep MCL with no resultant instability or laxity detected with an applied valgus stress. A grade II MCL sprain is an incomplete tear with microscopic and gross disruption of fibers of the superficial and deep MCL. There are 5° to 15° of valgus instability at 30° of knee flexion with a definite end point. At full knee extension, there is no straight plane valgus or rotational instability. A grade III MCL sprain is a complete tear of the MCL complex with more than 15 mm of instability to valgus stress at 30° knee flexion and possibly at full knee extension. Rotational instability is often present. Table 27-2 outlines the grades of MCL ligament sprains.[10]

Table 27-2	GRADES OF MEDIAL COLLATERAL LIGAMENT SPRAIN		
Grade	Damage	Clinical Exam	Laxity (mm)
I	Microscopic tear of superficial and deep MCL	No increase in medial joint line opening at 30° knee flexion Tenderness with palpation over ligament Stiffness	0-5
II	Microscopic and gross disruption of superficial and deep fibers of MCL	Increased laxity at 30° knee flexion, but firm end feel Swelling Pain with palpation Limited knee ROM, especially extension Antalgic gait	5-10
III	Complete tear of MCL complex	Instability at 30° knee flexion and full extension Empty end feel Loss of full knee ROM Pain and swelling Limited weightbearing tolerance	>10

Physical Therapy Patient/Client Management

Most MCL sprains can be managed nonoperatively. Ruptured MCLs (grades I and II) can generally heal spontaneously and sufficiently such that nonsurgical management has become the treatment of choice.[12] However, remodeling of the collagen fibers takes years and the mechanical properties of the healed MCL remain inferior to those of the normal MCL.[13,14] The intact, normal MCL has strain rates that are 30 times higher along its longitudinal direction compared to its transverse direction.[15] Physical therapy interventions include therapeutic exercise and may include ultrasound.[16] The primary goal for most injured athletes/individuals is to return to pain-free sport or activity as quickly and as safely as possible in a manner that does not overload the healing tissues.

Examination, Evaluation, and Diagnosis

A comprehensive musculoskeletal examination should be conducted to rule out other potential sources of knee pain including: injuries to the anterior cruciate ligament or meniscus, adolescent epiphyseal fracture, or patellofemoral pain. During the subjective examination, the physical therapist identifies the mechanism of injury, location of pain, if tearing or popping occurred on the medial side of the knee, and the athlete's functional limitations.

The objective examination includes assessment of ROM, swelling, muscle strength, palpation, and special tests. In the acute phase after injury, knee ROM is usually limited in flexion and extension primarily due to swelling. Swelling localized to the medial aspect of the knee is consistent with isolated MCL complex injury because the MCL is extra-articular and rarely results in intra-articular swelling. Significant traumatic effusion is a sign of anterior cruciate ligament rupture.[11] Muscle strength, especially the quadriceps, may be deficient due to pain and swelling. Palpation should include the entire course of the MCL complex. Tenderness may be noted over the adductor tubercle, medial epicondyle, joint line, and/or proximal tibia.

Special tests for the MCL complex include the two-part **valgus stress test** and the Swain test (Table 27-3). The valgus stress test is performed with the knee at 30° of flexion (Fig. 27-2) and with the knee in full extension (Fig. 27-3). At 30° of knee flexion, medial laxity of 0 to 5 mm compared to the uninvolved limb indicates tearing of the superficial MCL (grade I sprain).[17] Greater than 5 mm of laxity is a grade II sprain and suggests further injury to the deep MCL, POL, and posteromedial corner.[18] With the knee in full extension, a valgus stress test will be negative for an isolated superficial MCL injury (grade I and II sprains).[18] If this test is positive at full knee extension, then the entire MCL complex and cruciate ligaments are compromised. The sensitivity of the valgus stress test at 30° flexion is excellent (91%).[19,20]

Table 27-3   SPECIAL TESTS ASSOCIATED WITH THE MEDIAL COLLATERAL LIGAMENT COMPLEX

Tests	Patient Position	Findings	Sensitivity	Specificity
Valgus stress test with knee at 30° flexion (Fig. 27-2)	Patient is supine with the test leg slightly over the side of the table. The therapist lifts the test leg using the table to support the femur. The therapist bends the knee to 30°. The therapist then applies a valgus stress to the limb at the knee.	Increased laxity as compared to the uninvolved side.	91%[20]	49%[20]
Valgus stress test with knee in full extension (Fig. 27-3)	Patient is supine with the test leg slightly over the side of the table. The therapist lifts the test leg using the table to support the femur. The therapist keeps the knee in full extension and then applies a valgus stress to the limb at the knee.	Increased laxity as compared to the uninvolved side.	NA	NA
Swain test (Fig. 27-4)	The patient is sitting on the side of the table. Therapist passively rotates the tibia into external rotation.	Pain along the medial side of joint indicates injury to MCL complex.	NA	NA

Abbreviation: NA, not available.

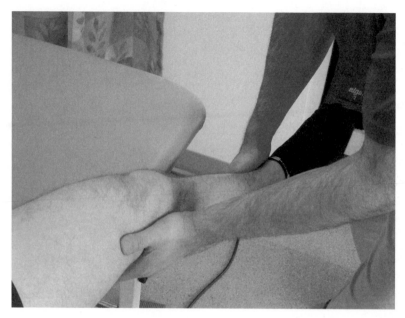

Figure 27-2. Valgus stress test at 30° knee flexion.

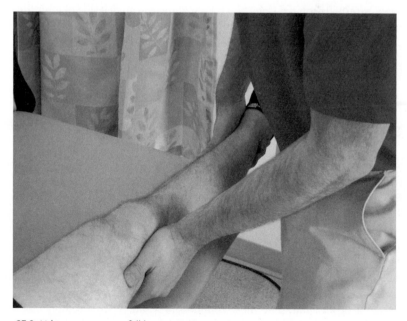

Figure 27-3. Valgus stress test at full knee extension.

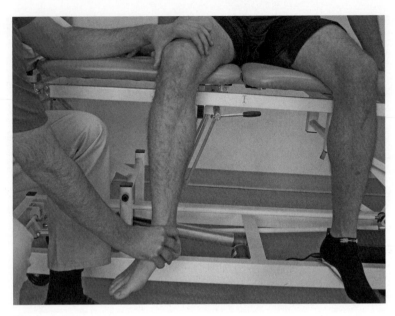

Figure 27-4. Swain test.

The Swain test is an examination for testing chronic MCL injury and rotatory instability.[21] This test is performed with the knee flexed to 90° and the tibia is passively externally rotated (Fig. 27-4). Pain along the medial side of joint indicates injury to MCL complex.

To exclude a physeal injury in adolescents, a stress radiograph should be performed. Magnetic resonance imaging (MRI) is usually not indicated for an isolated MCL injury.

Plan of Care and Interventions

Treatment of grade I and grade II MCL sprains is similar, with the exception that grade I injuries are progressed at a faster rate with regards to weightbearing, ROM, and strengthening. Grade III sprains are initially treated conservatively, but if instability and loss of function persists, then surgery is warranted.[22] Indications for operative treatment of an MCL injury include: a large bony avulsion; concomitant tibial plateau fracture; and/or associated cruciate ligament injury. Approximately 80% of grade III MCL injuries have associated anterior cruciate ligament or meniscal damage, so surgery for this grade is not uncommon.[23] Surgical fixation can be achieved by the orthopaedist performing a primary repair or a reconstruction with an autograft or allograft. The most common procedures are a semimembranosus tendon reconstruction (Slocum procedure) or advancing the tibial MCL (Mauck procedure). **Prognosis for nonoperative isolated grade III MCL sprains is good.**[6]

Table 27-4 REHABILITATION FOR MCL SPRAIN[26,28]	
Phase I (1 wk)	Rehabilitation brace (limited motion) Partial weightbearing with crutches Low intensity ultrasound over MCL Exercise in brace (3 times per day) • Straight leg raise (limit hip adduction) • Active ankle ROM • Active knee flexion to 90° • Active hip flexion and extension • Upper extremity active exercise • Ice, compression on knee Stationary cycling without resistance
Phase II (2 wk)	Progress to full weightbearing Aerobic exercise Knee ROM without pain Ultrasound over MCL Partial squats Step-up and step-down exercises Stationary cycling
Phase III (3 wk)	Closed-chain exercises with good form (no valgus loading) Progress knee flexion and extension (pain-free) If no effusion and full motion, • Functional exercises including straight ahead level running • Balance exercises
Phase IV (after 3 wk)	Agility exercises

The rehabilitation program following an MCL sprain can be divided into four phases (Table 27-4). The phase time is dependent on the grade of injury. For example, an individual with a grade I MCL sprain may be able to return to sport in 10 days, whereas an individual with a grade II sprain can be expected to be going through rehabilitation for up to 6 weeks.[24]

Phase I begins postinjury and lasts up to 1 week. MCL injuries are best treated with early mobilization and strengthening. Active motion significantly reduces laxity and increases the tensile strength of the healing superficial MCL compared to immobilization of the limb.[25] That being said, there may be a brief period of knee immobilization and symptomatic management with ice, elevation, and compression. A grade II/III sprain requires a longer immobilization period with limited ROM. In these circumstances, a long-legged rehabilitation brace is worn that limits knee ROM in the extremes of extension and flexion. During phase I, **low-intensity ultrasound** may be beneficial in improving synthesis of type I collagen.[16] The athlete may need crutches and be allowed to bear weight as tolerated. For more severe sprains, crutches may be needed for longer (up to 3 months for grade III).[26] Active knee flexion should begin during this phase, but needs to be pain-free and limited to 90° of knee flexion. Basic straight leg raises should also be prescribed limiting hip adduction initially. Stationary cycling can be performed pain-free and resistance-free.

Phase II begins at approximately 2 weeks postinjury. Individuals with grade II or III injuries start later. During this phase, the athlete is progressed to full weight-bearing. Range of motion should be advanced working toward full motion. Lower extremity strengthening is continued and weightbearing exercises are introduced. Examples of these exercises are partial motion squats and step-up and step-down exercises. Aerobic cross training should be emphasized and may include cycling, upper extremity ergometer, or swimming.

Phase III is characterized by functional training and begins around 3 weeks. Closed-chain exercises are continued with an emphasis on controlling valgus loading. An anteromedial lunge may be used for this purpose (Fig. 27-5). The athlete must be able to lunge without allowing the knee to collapse toward the midline. Balance training is also included. A running program can be initiated when the athlete has good leg control, full ROM, and no knee effusion.

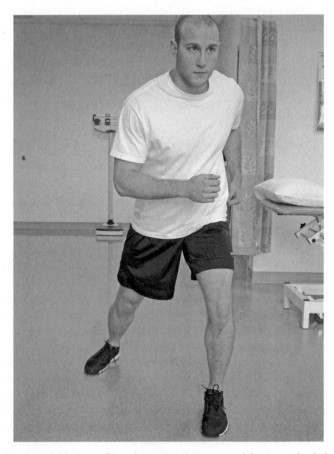

Figure 27-5. Anteromedial lunge performed to assess the patient's ability to avoid right knee valgus.

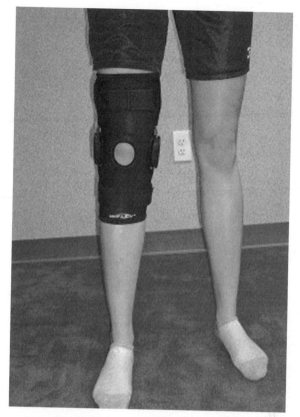

Figure 27-6. Functional brace. (Reproduced with permission from De Carlo M, Armstrong B. Rehabilitation of the knee following sports injury. *Clin Sports Med.* 2010 Jan;29(1):81-106.)

Phase IV is the phase in which the athlete is working to return to sport. Agility exercises and sport-specific skills are emphasized. A functional brace is worn for return to sport especially with contact sports (Fig. 27-6). The brace may be worn up to 6 months. The brace should be a lightweight hinged knee brace with medial and lateral upright supports to control frontal plane stresses.[27] Most athletes with MCL sprains can **return to sport** within 8 weeks. The return to sport criteria are listed in Table 27-5.

Table 27-5   FULL RETURN-TO-SPORT CRITERIA[26]
No swelling
Minimal to no pain that is localized over the superficial MCL
Full knee ROM
Knee stable when tested in full extension
Minimal valgus opening at 30° knee flexion with definite end point
Strength of quadriceps and hamstrings equal to 90% of that of the contralateral limb
Good movement performance with functional tests (*e.g.*, no valgus knee moment with cutting, landing from jump)

Evidence-Based Clinical Recommendations

SORT: Strength of Recommendation Taxonomy

A: Consistent, good-quality patient-oriented evidence
B: Inconsistent or limited-quality patient-oriented evidence
C: Consensus, disease-oriented evidence, usual practice, expert opinion, or case series

1. Valgus stress testing is sensitive for diagnosing a medial collateral ligament (MCL) sprain. **Grade A**

2. The functional outcome for an individual with an isolated nonoperative grade III MCL injury is good. **Grade B**

3. Low-intensity ultrasound improves collagen synthesis and strength of the injured MCL. **Grade B**

4. Most athletes are able to return to sport 8 weeks following MCL sprain. **Grade C**

COMPREHENSION QUESTIONS

27.1 Valgus stress to the knee in weightbearing is the most common mechanism of injury to a medial collateral ligament. The second most common mechanism of injury is

  A. Tibial external rotation

  B. Tibial internal rotation

  C. Knee hyperextension

  D. Deceleration

27.2 The medial collateral ligament complex comprise three components that include the superficial band, deep band, and the _____.

  A. Medial meniscus

  B. Posterior cruciate ligament

  C. Posterior oblique ligament

  D. Meniscofemoral ligament

ANSWERS

27.1 **A.** Based on the origin and insertion of the MCL, tibial external rotation will cause the MCL to become taut, putting it at higher risk of injury.

27.2 **C.** The fibrous bundle that is located posterior to the sMCL is termed the posterior oblique ligament (POL).[6] The POL blends with the posterior medial joint capsule, medial meniscus, and semimembranosus tendon sheath. Some authors refer to this anatomical area as the posteromedial corner.[5,7]

REFERENCES

1. American Academy of Orthopaedic Surgeons. Common knee injuries. 2007. Available at: http://orthoinfo.aaos.org/topic.cfm?topic=a00325. Accessed November 10, 2011.

2. Phisitkul P, James SL, Wolf BR, Amendola A. MCL injuries of the knee: current concepts review. *Iowa Orthop J.* 2006;26:77-90.

3. LaPrade RF, Engebretsen AH, Ly TV, Johansen S, Wentorf FA, Engebretsen L. The anatomy of the medial part of the knee. *J Bone Joint Surg Am.* 2007;89:2000-2010.

4. Warren LF, Marshall JL. The supporting structures and layers on the medial side of the knee: an anatomical analysis. *J Bone Joint Surg Am.* 1979;61:56-62.

5. Robinson JR, Sanchez-Ballester J, Bull AM, Thomas Rde W, Amis AA. The posteromedial corner revisited. An anatomical description of the passive restraining structures of the medial aspect of the human knee. *J Bone Joint Surg Br.* 2004;86:674-681.

6. Marchant MH Jr, Tibor LM, Sekiya JK, Hardaker WT Jr, Garrett WE Jr, Taylor DC. Management of medial-sided knee injuries, part 1: medial collateral ligament. *Am J Sports Med.* 2011;39:1102-1113.

7. Sims WF, Jacobson KE. The posteromedial corner of the knee: medial-sided injury patterns revisited. *Am J Sports Med.* 2004;32:337-345.

8. Robinson JR, Bull AM, Thomas RR, Amis AA. The role of the medical collateral ligament and posteromedial capsule in controlling knee laxity. *Am J Sports Med.* 2006;34:1815-1823.

9. Grood ES, Noyes FR, Butler DL, Suntay WJ. Ligamentous and capsular restraint preventing medial and lateral laxity in intact human cadaver knees. *J Bone Joint Surg Am.* 1981;63:1257-1269.

10. Hughston JC, Andrews JR, Cross MJ, Moschi A. Classification of knee ligament instabilities. Part 1. The medial compartment and cruciate ligament. *J Bone Joint Surg Am.* 1976;58:159-172.

11. Griffith CJ, LaPrade RF, Johansen S, Armitage B, Wijdicks C, Engebretsen L. Medial knee injury: part 1, static function of the individual components of the main medial knee structures. *Am J Sports Med.* 2009;37:1762-1770.

12. Frank C, Woo SL, Amiel D, Harwood F, Gomez M, Akeson W. Medial collateral ligament healing. A multidisciplinary assessment in rabbits. *Am J Sports Med.* 1983;11:379-389.

13. Scheffler SU, Clineff TD, Papageorgiou CD, Debski RE, Ma CB, Woo SL. Structure and function of the healing medial collateral ligament in a goat model. *Ann Biomed Eng.* 2001;29:173-180.

14. Woo SL, Gomez MA, Inoue M, Akeson WH. New experimental procedures to evaluate the biomechanical properties of healing canine medial collateral ligaments. *J Orthop Res.* 1987;5:425-432.

15. Quapp KM, Weiss JA. Material characterization of human medial collateral ligament. *J Biomech Eng.* 1998;120:757-763.

16. Sparrow KJ, Finucane SD, Owen JR, Wayne JS. The effects of low-intensity ultrasound on medial collateral ligament healing in the rabbit model. *Am J Sports Med.* 2005;33:1048-1056.

17. Grood ES, Noyes FR, Butler DL, Suntay WJ. Ligamentous and capsular restraints preventing medial and lateral laxity in intact human cadaver knees. *J Bone Joint Surg Am.* 1981;63:1257-1269.

18. Haimes JL, Wroble RR, Grood ES, Noyes FR. Role of the medial structures in the intact and anterior cruciate ligament-deficient knee. Limits of motion in the human knee. *Am J Sports Med.* 1994;22:402-409.

19. Kastelein M, Wagemakers HP, Luijsterburg PA, Verhaar JA, Koes BW, Bierma-Zeinstra SW. Assessing medial collateral ligament knee lesions in general practice. *Am J Med.* 2008;121:982-988.

20. Simonsen O, Jensen J, Mouritsen P, Lauritzen J. The accuracy of clinical examination of injury of the knee joint. *Injury.* 1984;16:96-101.

21. Lonergan KT, Taylor DC. Medial collateral ligament injuries of the knee: an evolution of surgical reconstruction. *Tech Knee Surg.* 2002;1:137-145.

22. Indelicato PA. Isolated medial collateral ligament injuries in the knee. *J Am Acad Orthop Surg.* 1995;3:9-14.

23. Hastings DE. The non-operative management of collateral injuries to the knee joint. *Clin Orthop Relat Res.* 1980;147:22-28.

24. Holden DL, Eggert AW, Butler JE. The nonoperative treatment of grade I and II medial collateral ligament injuries to the knee. *Am J Med.* 1983;11:340-344.

25. Hart DP, Dahners LE. Healing of the medial collateral ligaments in rats. The effects of repair, motion, and secondary stabilizing ligaments. *J Bone Joint Surg Am.* 1987;69:1194-1199.

26. Brotzman SB. *Handbook of Orthopaedic Rehabilitation.* St. Louis, MO: Mosby; 1996.

27. Reider B. Medial collateral ligament injuries in athletes. *Sports Med.* 1996;21:147-156.

28. Czerniecki JM, Lippert R, Olerud JE. A biomechanical evaluation of tibiofemoral rotation in anterior cruciate deficient knees during walking and running. *Am J Sports Med.* 1988;16:327-331.

Knee Posterior Collateral Ligament (PCL) Sprain

Matt Mymern
Laurie Griffin

A 24-year-old male is referred to a physical therapy clinic after sustaining a right knee injury playing soccer 6 days ago. The patient reports that the injury occurred when another player tackled him. He describes the impact as a posterior and laterally directed force to the medial tibia. Since the incident, he reports pain with prolonged walking and difficulty descending stairs. The patient reports minimal to no knee instability. Anti-inflammatory medication decreases the pain and allows him to descend stairs without difficulty. The patient reports a history of right patellar tendinitis. The patient's medical history is unremarkable.

► What examination signs may be associated with this suspected diagnosis?
► What are the most appropriate examination tests?
► What are the most appropriate physical therapy interventions?

KEY DEFINITIONS

POSTERIOR CRUCIATE LIGAMENT (PCL): Intracapsular ligament of the knee that extends from the posterior intercondylar region of the tibia to the medial femoral condyle; the PCL limits posterior translation of the tibia

POSTEROLATERAL CORNER (PLC): Region of the knee composed of the popliteofibular ligament, fibular collateral ligament, and the popliteus muscle

VARUS FORCE: Force applied to a limb that results in the distal aspect of the limb moving toward the midline of the body

Objectives

1. Describe pathomechanics for a posterior cruciate ligament injury.
2. Identify appropriate clinical special tests to evaluate a patient with potential injury to the posterior cruciate ligament.
3. Implement evidence-based rehabilitation treatments for posterior cruciate ligament injuries.

Physical Therapy Considerations

PT considerations during management of the individual with a diagnosis of PCL injury:

▶ **General physical therapy plan of care/goals:** Decrease pain and swelling, prevent muscular inhibition, normalize gait abnormalities, restore range of motion (ROM), maintain cardiovascular fitness

▶ **Physical therapy interventions:** Patient education; home exercise program (HEP); modalities; manual therapy to decrease pain, swelling, and increase ROM; patellar mobilization; gait training

▶ **Precautions during physical therapy:** Assess vital signs, monitor neurovascular status (*e.g.*, distal pulses, sensory and motor function); decrease posterior tibial shear forces

▶ **Complications interfering with physical therapy:** Fibular nerve dysfunction with possible progression into foot drop, which may require the need for ankle-foot orthosis

Understanding the Health Condition

The PCL is approximately twice as thick and strong as the anterior cruciate ligament (ACL).[1,2] The PCL is 13 millimeters (mm) wide and 38 mm long.[1,2] It originates from the anterolateral aspect of the medial femoral condyle near the intercondylar notch.[1–3] The PCL inserts on the posterior tibial plateau, approximately one centimeter distal to the joint line. The PCL is intracapsular; however, it is isolated with the ACL from the synovial cavity. The PCL can be further divided into an anterolateral bundle and posteromedial bundle. The anterolateral bundle is larger and represents 65% of the substance.[1-3] In knee flexion, the anterolateral bundle is taut and the posteromedial bundle is lax. The posteromedial bundle, comprising the remaining 35% of the PCL substance, is taut in knee extension, while the antero-medial bundle is lax.[1-3]

Several PCL injury mechanisms have been described in the literature. A common mechanism is a posteriorly directed force to the tibia, which creates a supraphysi-ologic load to the PCL. The classic example is a football player's shoulder pad or hel-met coming into direct contact with a player's tibia during a tackle. Another example is the enormous posteriorly directed force that occurs during a motor vehicle accident when the passenger's tibia strikes the dashboard. Traumatic hyperextension of the knee may also cause a PCL injury (e.g., slide tackle in soccer when the player's foot is securely planted on the turf). If the mechanism of injury also involves forceful twist-ing, other structures may be compromised, resulting in a multiligamentous injury.[3-5]

PCL injuries are categorized by the extent of the damage into three grades.[5] In grade I injuries, the ligament is stretched and only mildly damaged (up to 25% of the ligament substance is torn). Posterior translation of the tibia on the femur may be up to 5 mm greater than the uninvolved side. In a grade II injury, the ligament is considered moderately damaged (25%-50% of the ligament substance is torn). A posterior translation difference of 6 to 10 mm compared to the uninvolved side is expected. A grade III injury is a completely torn ligament; the tear may occur at any part of the PCL. Translation difference of >10 mm is expected in the grade III tear.[6] PCL injuries may occur in isolation or in combination with other soft tissue damage. An isolated PCL injury means that only the PCL is damaged. Combined ligament injuries of the PCL may involve several structures, most often the posterolateral structures of the knee[3-5] including the popliteofibular ligament, fibular collateral ligament, and popliteus muscle.[7]

Physical Therapy Patient/Client Management

Many approaches can be utilized in the management of both nonoperative and surgically indicated knee injuries. There is limited research to determine the **most effective rehabilitative program during the acute stage** (approximately the first 6 weeks after injury). During this time, treatment includes edema management, soft tissue massage, range of motion, patellofemoral mobilization, gait training, and isometric muscle activation.[7-9] For chronic management of a PCL injury (greater than 6 weeks after initial injury), a trial of bracing may be appropriate. It may also be recommended to have serial radiographs to identify any arthritic changes or con-comitant meniscal involvement in the chronic injured knee.[10]

Plans of care and treatments are individualized and depend on the mechanism of injury to the PCL and any associated ligamentous damage. Medial knee injuries may heal with appropriate conservative care; however, damage to the lateral and posterolat-eral structures (e.g., PCL injury) may be more successfully managed with surgical inter-vention.[11] A surgical consultation should always be considered for patients who are unable to fulfill their daily, occupational, or athletic demands. The plan of care should address options to prevent posterior tibial translation due to a lax PCL. The goal is to maintain anatomical positioning as best as possible to prevent progressive disability.

Examination, Evaluation, and Diagnosis

Isolated injury to the PCL or combined ligamentous injury occurs less frequently than injuries to other areas of the knee. Hence, less research has been directed to the posterolateral aspect of the knee. Posterior cruciate ligament injuries have been reported in 1% to 40% of acute injuries[12,13] and up to 40% of knee injuries in the traumatic setting.[11] Acute injuries to the PCL are the noncontact type (e.g., work-related injuries, sports injuries, and low energy or low velocity falls). The most common cause of traumatic PCL injury is motor vehicle collision, followed by high energy or high velocity sporting injuries.[14] Due to the lack of research into long-term outcomes following PCL injuries, it is difficult to predict whether patients with PCL injury will be able to return to their premorbid level of activity or if they will have persistent chronic symptoms.[15]

To enable a comprehensive examination, both lower extremities should be exposed to compare overall alignment of the limbs, joint effusion, and previous scars. Gait should be specifically examined for a varus thrust mechanism or hyperextension thrust pattern, both of which indicate chronic injury of the PCL and posterolateral corner.[10,16,17] A varus thrust gait, which is common in patients with chronic posterolateral deficiency, indicates lateral compartment opening as the knee shifts into varus upon foot strike.[16] An abnormal gait pattern secondary to chronic posterolateral deficiency of the knee may result in degenerative changes if not addressed with treatment.

A neurovascular screen should be performed to determine if any involvement to the common fibular nerve has occurred. This is not uncommon because of the location of the fibular nerve and popliteal artery in relation to the lateral compartment and the varus stress that occurs with PCL injuries. Sensation or strength changes reflective of the function of the common fibular nerve and its branches should be assessed. Damage should be suspected if the patient presents with numbness or altered sensation on the dorsum of the foot (excluding the first dorsal web space) or weakness in ankle dorsiflexion or eversion, or great toe extension.[17] Injury to the popliteal artery can be evaluated by the Ankle-Brachial Index (ABI). An ABI < 0.9 has been reported to be 95% to 100% sensitive and 80% to 100% specific in detecting arterial injuries that require surgical intervention.[18]

Palpation and special tests provide additional objective data to further refine or refute a hypothesis during the examination process. The anterior joint line can be palpated with the patient supine, knees flexed to 90°, and feet flat on the table. Normally, the anterior border of the medial tibial plateau should be approximately 1 cm anterior to the medial femoral condyle.[17] An injury to the PCL can be suspected by the degree of posterior subluxation of the tibial plateau in comparison to the femoral condyle.[17] Table 28-1 describes special tests that can be performed to further rule in or rule out injury to the PCL and/or associated ligamentous injury.

Table 28-1   SPECIAL TESTS TO RULE IN OR RULE OUT PCL AND/OR CONCOMITANT LIGAMENTOUS INJURY

Special Test	Positioning	Findings
Godfrey test 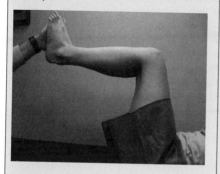	Patient is supine with hips and knees flexed to 90°. Therapist views patient's knees from the side.	Using the tibial tuberosity as a landmark, the therapist observes the patient's knees from the lateral aspect. If the PCL is lax (or torn), gravity allows the tibia to rest in a posteriorly subluxed position, which can be seen as a posterior sag.[10]
Active quads test 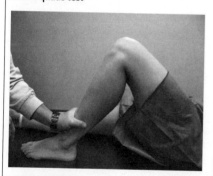	Patient is supine with involved hip and knee flexed to 90°. Therapist stabilizes foot and asks patient to contract quadriceps.	As quadriceps contract, therapist observes for reduction of the posteriorly subluxed tibia.[17] (55% sensitivity, 97% specificity[15])
Posterior drawer test 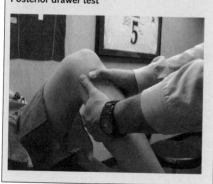	Patient is supine with hips flexed to 45° and involved knee flexed to 90°. Therapist pushes proximal tibia posteriorly.	Therapist feels the movement to assess posterior tibial plateau translation. Grade I injury = 0-5 mm translation Grade II injury = 6-10 mm translation Grade III injury = 11 mm or more[6]

(Continued)

Table 28-1 SPECIAL TESTS TO RULE IN OR RULE OUT PCL AND/OR CONCOMITANT LIGAMENTOUS INJURY (*CONTINUED*)

Special Test	Positioning	Findings
Reverse pivot shift 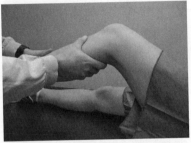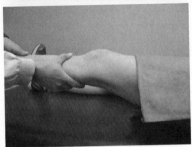	Patient is supine with hip flexed 90°, tibia externally rotated at the foot, knee is flexed to 70°-80°. Therapist applies valgus stress to the knee while extending the knee.	The patient and therapist perceive an audible "clunk" when the posteriorly subluxed tibia suddenly reduces as the knee approaches full extension.[13,19,20] For posterolateral corner injuries[16]: positive predictive value 68%; negative predictive value 89%
External rotation recurvatum 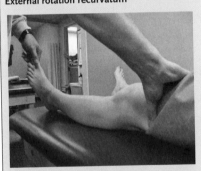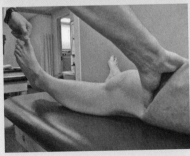	Patient is supine with legs extended. Therapist lifts the patient's great toe off the plinth and compares bilaterally.	A positive test is defined as an increase in knee recurvatum, varus, or external rotation of the tibia, likely due to posterolateral opening of the joint.[10] Positive test may detect both an ACL and PCL injury has occurred.[7]

(Continued)

Table 28-1 SPECIAL TESTS TO RULE IN OR RULE OUT PCL AND/OR CONCOMITANT LIGAMENTOUS INJURY (*CONTINUED*)		
Special Test	Positioning	Findings
Dial test 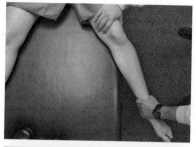 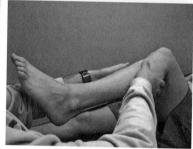	Patient is supine or prone. Therapist externally rotates the tibia at the foot and examines for differences in external rotation with the knee flexed at 30° and 90°. Therapist compares the difference of tibial external rotation bilaterally at 30° and 90° of knee flexion.	If a difference of 10°-15° is noted between the injured and contralateral leg, injury of the PCL and posterolateral corner may be suspected. If a difference is noted at only 30° of knee flexion, injury to the posterolateral corner may be likely.[16] If tibial external rotation is increased at 30° and 90° compared to the uninvolved side, both posterolateral corner and the PCL may be involved.[21–23]

Imaging is generally performed to determine the integrity or the extent of damage to the PCL after an injury has occurred. This is usually performed before a patient is referred for physical therapy. If available, the physical therapist should thoroughly review the radiographs. Anteroposterior, lateral, and oblique images can determine the presence of a fracture to the tibial plateau, femoral condyles, or patella.[10] A lateral view may identify significant posterior tibial subluxation if gross instability is present.[16] Differentiation between a complete and partial PCL tear has not yet been determined to be reliable with stress radiographs. For a stress radiograph, the therapist applies a varus stress to the knee that is flexed 20° to identify if any lateral joint opening occurs. Grade III injury to the posterolateral corner should be considered if lateral opening of approximately 4.0 mm occurs.[7] Standing weightbearing anteroposterior and sunrise views may show joint space narrowing in individuals with chronic PCL injury.[9] The sunrise view is a tangential view of the patella taken with the patient prone and knee flexed to 115°. The beam is directed on the patella with a 15° angulation. Magnetic resonance imaging (MRI) has become the gold standard to examine PCL integrity.[24] An MRI scan may be performed to further examine a knee when the diagnosis is uncertain or when complex injury to the knee has occurred because it allows for examination of intra-articular structures and any concurrent osteochondral injury.

Plan of Care and Interventions

To formulate a treatment plan, the physical therapist must take into consideration the patient's primary complaints, activity level, occupational demands, any comorbidities and whether the PCL injury is acute or chronic.

For the acute PCL injury like the one sustained by this patient, conservative management has not been well studied. Grade I or II isolated PCL injuries may be managed without operative treatment. One of the main goals is to maintain the knee in the best possible anatomical position. Cosgarea and Jay[19] and LaPrade[17] recommend immobilizing the patient's knee in extension by a knee immobilizer brace for 2 to 4 weeks to limit gravitational pull on the anterolateral bundle of the PCL. The authors also recommend decreasing inflammation, maintaining knee range of motion (ROM) through passive ROM and **avoiding hamstring over-activation** (i.e., isolated resistive hamstring exercises) too early in the rehabilitation.[17,19,25] Knee passive ROM in the prone position, patellar mobilization, **quadriceps muscle activation (i.e., quad sets)** and ice are also recommended. Table 28-2 provides a description of the exercises that should be the primary focus from onset of injury to approximately 6 weeks. Bracing a PCL-injured knee may assist in maintaining the posteriorly subluxed tibia in a more neutral position which may reduce stress on the healing structures, allowing for healing in a more anatomical position. However, evidence to support the effectiveness of PCL-specific bracing to improve long-term stability is lacking.

Operative management is considered for individuals with grade III PCL injuries, as well as for those who have failed conservative treatment with grade II PCL injuries. A multitude of techniques are available to perform a PCL reconstruction; however, the newer methods that reconstruct both bundles with allograft should, in theory, result in improved stability.[3,26] However, the evidence is inconclusive regarding which surgical technique results in the best outcomes.

One of the concerns after surgical intervention is how to maintain proper positioning of the PCL to avoid stretching of the graft over time due to the posterior tibial sag from the effects of gravity. **Different bracing protocols** are described in the literature with some authors recommending a knee immobilizer in full extension at all times for 3 to 6 weeks postoperatively.[27-29] Spiridonov et al.[27] recommend the use of a Jack PCL brace (Cascade Orthopedic Supply, Inc.) that applies an anteriorly directed force on the tibia starting postoperative day 3.

In a review article, Edson et al.[28] reported that completely avoiding knee ROM for the first 5 weeks after surgical intervention allows patients to maintain static stability of the PCL graft. Fanelli et al.[29] recommended a period of only 3 weeks of knee immobilization. However, several investigators have allowed for early limited PROM immediately postoperative day 1.[17,19,31] Other immediate postoperative interventions include patellar mobilizations, quadriceps re-education activities, ankle pumps, and ice.[27,29]

After 5 weeks postoperatively, knee ROM and partial weightbearing can be initiated with a continued avoidance of isolated hamstring contractions.[13,17,28,30] Overly aggressive flexion ROM should be avoided to prevent undue stress on the healing graft. Only a small number of patients have been found to require a manipulation under anesthesia or debridement due to loss of knee flexion ROM.[17]

Table 28-2   KNEE EXERCISES TO MAINTAIN ROM AND DECREASE INFLAMMATION IN ACUTE PHASE AFTER PCL INJURY

Therapeutic Exercise	Starting Position	Exercise Technique
Prone passive ROM 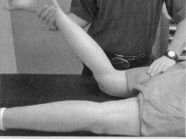 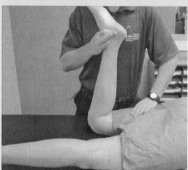	Patient prone on table. Therapist or caregiver flexes patient's knee to end range, as tolerated by the patient.	Instruct patient to avoid hamstring activation and to remain passive during ROM. Prone positioning decreases the force of gravity and posterior tibial positioning.
Patellar mobilizations 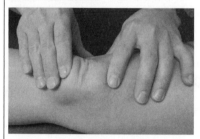 Superior-inferior 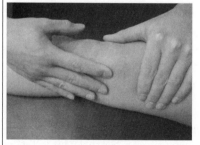 Medial-lateral	Patient supine with legs extended and quadriceps relaxed.	Instruct patient to mobilize the patella in superior-inferior and medial-lateral directions.

(Continued)

Table 28-2 KNEE EXERCISES TO MAINTAIN ROM AND DECREASE INFLAMMATION IN ACUTE PHASE AFTER PCL INJURY (*CONTINUED*)

Therapeutic Exercise	Starting Position	Exercise Technique
Quadriceps muscle sets	Patient supine or in long sitting.	Instruct patient to actively draw the patella superiorly while contracting the quadriceps. Hold 5 s, repeat 20 times.

At 10 weeks postoperatively, Edson et al.[28] advise that passive ROM remains the focus of the rehabilitative program, as well as initiation of gait training and proprioceptive training. Patients may still be weaning off of their crutches until the tenth week after surgery.[11] A goal for the end of the third postoperative month is to have approximately of 100° to 110° of passive knee flexion. Fanelli et al.[29,30] recommend an eventual transition at postoperative week 11 to a PCL functional brace.

Quelard et al.[31] recommend a **postoperative rehabilitation program** allowing for progressive weightbearing at the tenth week after surgery, avoiding open kinetic chain hamstring exercise for 5 months with a plan to return to training at 8 months. With the described protocol by Quelard et al.,[31] significant improvement in differential laxity, International Knee Documentation Committee (IKDC) scores and Tegner Lysholm Knee Scale scores were found after an average of 5 years follow-up. The majority of patients can expect to return to sports and heavy labor 9 months after surgical repair of the PCL.[11,26,28]

Evidence-Based Clinical Recommendations

SORT: Strength of Recommendation Taxonomy

A: Consistent, good-quality patient-oriented evidence
B: Inconsistent or limited-quality patient-oriented evidence
C: Consensus, disease-oriented evidence, usual practice, expert opinion, or case series

1. Current evidence guides acute rehabilitative protocols for conservative or surgically managed knees with PCL injury. **Grade C**

2. Limiting isolated hamstring strengthening and promoting strengthening of the quadriceps improve stability and decrease tibial sag of the knee with a PCL injury. **Grade B**

3. Bracing that prevents further posterior tibial sag (*e.g.*, knee extension immobilizer, brace providing anteriorly directed force on tibia) is beneficial for individuals with PCL-deficient knees. **Grade C**

4. Individuals with surgical repair of the PCL and postoperative rehabilitation have demonstrated statistically significant improvements in differential laxity, IKDC scores, and Tegner and Lysholm scores at 5 years follow-up. **Grade B**

COMPREHENSION QUESTIONS

28.1 A patient is referred to a physical therapy clinic with a diagnosis of a PCL tear. He expresses concern about surgical repair and states that he would rather conservatively rehabilitate his knee. Which of the following sets of interventions would be the *most* appropriate plan to assist the patient in the acute stage of rehabilitation?

A. Supine ROM, towel under the knee with quad sets, patellar mobilization, ice

B. Prone passive knee ROM, towel under proximal tibia during gastrocnemius-soleus towel stretching in long sitting position, quad sets, patellar mobilization, ice

C. Prone active knee ROM, hamstring sets, patellar mobilization, ice

D. Supine passive ROM, hamstring sets, patellar mobilization, ice

28.2 A patient complains of knee instability. In the physical therapy examination, he has positive posterior drawer and quadriceps active tests. Which additional special test should the physical therapist perform to help *rule in* a posterior lateral corner injury versus an isolated PCL tear?

A. Godfrey

B. Anterior drawer

C. Dial

D. External rotation recurvatum

28.3 With respect to the anatomy of the PCL, which of the following is a true statement?

A. The anteromedial bundle is larger of the two bundles and is taut in extension.

B. The anteromedial bundle is smaller of the two bundles and is lax in flexion.

C. The posteromedial bundle is larger of the two bundles and is taut in extension.

D. The posteromedial bundle is smaller of the two bundles and is lax in flexion.

ANSWERS

28.1 **B.** Prone ROM decreases the effect of gravity and any posterior tibial translation with ROM. Support under the proximal tibia also assists in preventing posterior tibial sag and reduces hamstring involvement with gastrocnemius-soleus stretching in the long sitting position. Hamstring activation will be limited because this position promotes further posterior tibial translation, decreasing stress to the healing posterolateral structures.[8,11,25,29,30]

28.2 **C.** If a difference is noted from the contralateral side of 10° to 15° on the dial test, injury of the PCL and posterolateral corner may be suspected. If a difference is noted at only 30° of flexion, injury to the posterolateral corner may be likely.[9] If tibial external rotation is increased at 30° and 90° compared to the contralateral side, both posterolateral corner and the PCL may be involved.[16,21,23] The posterior tibial sag noted on the Godfrey test indicates that the PCL is lax (option A). The anterior drawer test is commonly used to assess for anterior cruciate ligament laxity, not PCL laxity (option B). A positive external rotation recurvatum test may detect both an ACL and PCL injury. (option D).

28.3 **D.**

REFERENCES

1. Lopes OV Jr, Ferretti M, Shen W, Ekdahl M, Smolinski P, Fu FH. Topography of the femoral attachment of the posterior cruciate ligament. *J Bone Joint Surg Am*. 2008;90:249-255.

2. Tajima G, Nozaki M, Iriuchishima T, et al. Morphology of the tibial insertion of the posterior cruciate ligament. *J Bone Joint Surg Am*. 2009;91:859-866.

3. Moorman CT III, Murphy Zane MS, Bansai S, et al. Tibial insertion of the posterior cruciate ligament: a sagittal plane analysis using gross, histologic, and radiographic methods. *Arthroscopy*. 2008;24:269-275.

4. Matava MJ, Ellis E, Gruber B. Surgical treatment of posterior cruciate ligament tears: an evolving technique. *J Am Acad Orthop Surg*. 2009;17:435-446.

5. Wind WM Jr, Bergfeld JA, Parker RD. Evaluation and treatment of posterior cruciate ligament injuries: revisited. *Am J Sports Med*. 2004;32:1765-1775.

6. American Medical Association. Committee on the medical aspects of sports. *Standard Nomenclature of Athletic Injuries*. Chicago, IL: American Medical Association;1968:92-101.

7. Lunden JB, Bzdusek PJ, Monson JK, Malcomson KW, LaPrade RF. Current concepts in the recognition and treatment of posterolateral corner injuries of the knee. *J Orthop Sports Phys Ther*. 2010;40:502-516.

8. Feagin JA, Steadman JR. *The Crucial Principles in Care of the Knee*. Philadelphia, PA: Wolters Kluwer/Lippincott Williams & Wilkins; 2008:203-219.

9. Rigby JM, Porter KM. Posterior cruciate ligament injuries. *Trauma*. 2010;12:175-181.

10. Lopez-Vidriero E, Simon DA, Johnson DH. Initial evaluation of posterior cruciate ligament injuries: history, physical examination, imaging studies, surgical and nonsurgical indications. *Sports Med Arthrosc*. 2010;18:230-237.

11. Fanelli GC, Edson CJ. Posterior cruciate ligament injuries in trauma patients: Part II. *Arthroscopy*. 1995;11:526-529.

12. Gray H. *Anatomy of the Human Body*. 20th ed. Philadelphia, PA: Lea and Febiger; 1918.

13. LaPrade RF, Terry GC. Injuries to the posterolateral aspect of the knee. Association of anatomic injury patterns with clinical instability. *Am J Sports Med*. 1997;25:433-438.

14. Schulz MS, Russe K, Weiler A, Eichhorn HJ, Strobel MJ. Epidemiology of posterior cruciate ligament injuries. *Arch Orthop Trauma Surg*. 2003;123:186-191.

15. McAllister DR, Petrigliano FA. Diagnosis and treatment of posterior cruciate ligament injuries. *Curr Sports Med Rep*. 2007;6:293-299.

16. Miller MD, Cooper DE, Fanelli GC, Harner CD, LaPrade RF. Posterior cruciate ligament: current concepts. *Instr Course Lect*. 2002;51:347-351.

17. LaPrade RF. *Posterolateral Knee Injuries: Anatomy, Evaluation, and Treatment*. New York: Thieme; 2006.

18. Johnson ME, Foster L, DeLee JC. Neurologic and vascular injuries associated with knee ligament injuries. *Am J Sports Med*. 2008;36:2448-2462.

19. Cosgarea AJ, Jay PR. Posterior cruciate ligament injuries: evaluation and management. *J Am Acad Orthop Surg*. 2001;9:297-307.

20. Covey CD, Sapega AA. Injuries of the posterior cruciate ligament. *J Bone Joint Surg Am*. 1993;75:1376-1386.

21. Levy BA, Stuart MJ, Whelan DB. Posterolateral instability of the knee: evaluation, treatment, results. *Sports Med Arthrosc*. 2010;18:254-262.

22. Parolie JM, Bergfeld JA. Long-term results of nonoperative treatment of isolated posterior cruciate ligament injuries in the athlete. *Am J Sports Med*. 1986;14:35-38.

23. Veltri DM, Deng XH, Torzilli PA, Warren RF, Maynard MJ. The role of the cruciate and posterolateral ligaments in stability of the knee. A biomechanical study. *Am J Sports Med*. 1995;23:436-443.

24. Feltham GT, Albright JP. The diagnosis of PCL injury: literature review and introduction of two novel tests. *Iowa Orthop J*. 2001;21:36-42.

25. Fanelli GC, Edson CJ. Combined posterior cruciate ligament-posterolateral reconstructions with Achilles tendon allograft and biceps femoris tendon tenodesis: 2- to 10-year follow-up. *Arthroscopy*. 2004;20:339-345.

26. Harner CD, Janaushek MA, Kanamori A, Yagi M, Vogrin TM, Woo SL. Biomechanical analysis of a double-bundle posterior cruciate ligament reconstruction. *Am J Sports Med*. 2000;28:144-151.

27. Spiridonov SI, Slinkard NJ, LaPrade RF. Isolated and combined grade-III posterior cruciate ligament tears treated with double-bundle reconstruction using an endoscopically placed femoral tunnels and grafts: operative technique and clinical outcomes. *J Bone J Surg Am*. 2011;93:1773-1780.

28. Edson CJ, Fanelli GC, Beck JD. Postoperative rehabilitation of the posterior cruciate ligament. *Sports Med Arthrosc*. 2010;18:275-279.

29. Fanelli GC. Posterior cruciate ligament rehabilitation: how slow should we go? *Arthroscopy*. 2008;24:234-235.

30. Fanelli GC, Beck JD, Edson CJ. Double bundle posterior cruciate ligament reconstruction: surgical technique and results. *Sports Med Arthrosc*. 2010;18:242-248.

31. Quelard B, Sonnery-Cottet B, Zayni R, et al. Isolated posterior cruciate ligament reconstruction: is non-aggressive rehabilitation the right protocol? *Orthop Traumatol Surg Res*. 2010;96:256-262.

Knee Meniscus Sprain

Jason Brumitt

CASE 29

A 24-year-old female injured her right knee 2 days ago during a city-league basketball game. She was unable to continue playing after the injury and required "a little" assistance from a teammate to get to her car. She was evaluated by her primary care provider (PCP) the next day. The PCP recommended the use of over-the-counter nonsteroidal anti-inflammatory medication, and referred the patient to physical therapy. Five days postinjury, the patient reports to the physical therapist that the injury occurred when she planted her right leg and rotated to the right to evade a defender. She denies hearing a pop; however, she reports that the immediate pain was severe (8 out of 10 on a visual analog scale). Her current pain level is 5 out of 10. The patient's pain and mechanism of injury are consistent with a meniscus injury.

▶ What examination signs may be associated with this suspected diagnosis?
▶ What are the most appropriate examination tests?

Table 29-1	2 × 2 TABLE FOR DIAGNOSTIC TESTS	
	Disease/Health Condition Present	Disease/Health Condition Absent
Test positive	True positive (A)	False positive (B)
Test negative	False negative (C)	True negative (D)

Sensitivity = A/(A + C); specificity = D/(B + D)

KEY DEFINITIONS

SENSITIVITY: Ability of a diagnostic test to correctly identify individuals who have the target disease or health condition in a patient population (Table 29-1)

SPECIFICITY: Ability of a diagnostic test to correctly identify individuals who do not have the target disease or health condition (Table 29-1)

SnNout: Mnemonic for a highly sensitive test (high <u>s</u>e<u>n</u>sitivity, <u>n</u>egative, rules <u>out</u>)[1]

SpPin: Mnemonic for a highly specific test (high <u>sp</u>ecificity, <u>p</u>ositive, rules <u>in</u>)[1]

Objectives

1. Describe the anatomy and function of the menisci.
2. Describe the pathomechanics associated with a meniscal injury.
3. Recognize symptoms associated with a meniscal injury.
4. Describe appropriate clinical examination tests that may help rule in a diagnosis of a meniscus sprain.

Physical Therapy Considerations

PT considerations during management of the individual with a suspected meniscus sprain:

▶ **General physical therapy plan of care/goals:** Rule out other knee injuries; decrease pain; increase muscular flexibility; increase or prevent loss of knee range of motion; increase lower quadrant strength; prevent or minimize loss of aerobic fitness capacity

▶ **Physical therapy interventions:** Modalities to reduce pain; interventions to restore range of motion deficits; therapeutic exercises to restore muscular strength and aerobic fitness

▶ **Precautions during physical therapy:** Monitor vital signs; avoid exercises that place a rotatory force on the knee during acute and subacute phases of healing

▶ **Complications interfering with physical therapy:** Damage to additional knee structures such as anterior cruciate or medial collateral ligaments; articular cartilage pathology; osteochondritis dissecans, fracture, tumor,[2] cysts[3]

Understanding the Health Condition

The menisci are wedge-shaped fibrocartilage structures located on the proximal (articular) portion of the tibia. Each knee has a lateral and medial meniscus: the lateral meniscus (circular shaped) is smaller than the medial meniscus (C-shaped; Fig. 29-1). The menisci have several attachments on the tibia: the anterior and posterior horns via insertional ligaments, the joint capsule, the anterior intermeniscal ligament, and the coronary ligaments. The lateral meniscus has additional attachments to the meniscofemoral ligaments and a portion of the popliteal tendon.[4,5] The medial meniscus attaches to the deep portion of the medial collateral ligament of the knee.[5]

The menisci provide several functions at the knee. Their primary function is to protect the joint by serving as shock absorbers to transmit loads across the joint.[4] The menisci also help improve joint congruence and overall stability.[4] Additional roles include lubricating the joint and aiding nutrition to the cartilage.[6]

Meniscus injuries are typically the result of a violent twisting motion. An example of a meniscal injury mechanism is a basketball player attempting to evade a defender by planting the leg then quickly rotating the body to move in another direction. The rotation stress that is created through the loaded knee may sprain or tear a portion of the meniscus. The meniscus is also at risk for injury during valgus forces at the knee. It is common for the meniscus to be sprained in conjunction with either an anterior cruciate ligament (ACL) or medial collateral ligament (MCL) sprain. Eighty-two to ninety-six percent of knees with an ACL sprain have an associated meniscal injury.[7] Isolated sprains of the meniscus are also common. In some orthopaedic surgery practice settings, upward of 20% of all surgical procedures for the knee are for the meniscus.[6]

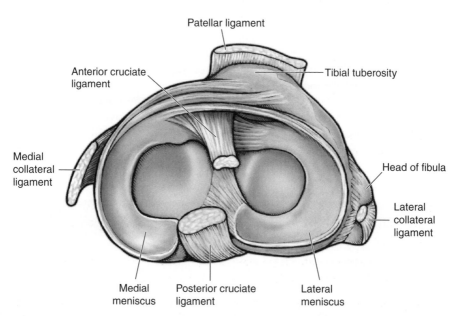

Figure 29-1. The menisci of the right knee. (Reproduced with permission from Morton DA, Foreman KB, Albertine KH, eds. *The Big Picture: Gross Anatomy.* New York: McGraw-Hill; 2011. Figure 36-5C.)

Examination, Evaluation, and Diagnosis

Diagnosis is based on patient history and a clinical examination. Table 29-2 presents key questions that should be asked during the subjective (patient history) portion of the examination. A patient may describe that the injury occurred when rotating or twisting. The date of injury provides information regarding the stage of healing and may aid prognosis. An audible popping sound is frequently associated with a ligament tear (*e.g.*, ACL). However, a "pop" is *not* usually associated with an isolated meniscus injury. Swelling is common and may impair range of motion and/or contribute to pain (secondary to stimulation of mechanoreceptors). A patient with a meniscal injury may report pain "in the knee" and/or pain along the joint line. The patient may also describe that her knee "catches" or "locks."

Table 29-3 presents a sample physical examination for a patient with suspected knee pathology. The information obtained during the subjective portion of the examination helps to guide decision making as to which tests to administer. Special tests for meniscal pathology may be performed in standing, supine, and prone positions (Table 29-4).

The patient's gait and/or ability to bear weight through the involved extremity may contraindicate performing a test in standing (*i.e.*, Thessaly test). However, if the patient is able to ambulate with assistance, the Thessaly test may be performed at this time. Other special tests are performed in supine (McMurray's test, joint line tenderness) or in prone positions (Apley's compression test).

In addition to the tests presented in Table 29-4, there are other tests (*e.g.*, Ege's test) that are reported to assess the integrity of the meniscus.[8-11] In general, the diagnostic utility of all special tests reported to identify a meniscus injury is questionable.[12-14] In 2007, Hegedus et al.[12] performed a meta-analysis of common special tests for the meniscus. They found that there was no single test that was able to help the physical therapist identify a knee with a meniscal injury. Since that report, additional studies have presented diagnostic accuracy statistics for the joint line tenderness test, the Thessaly test, and the joint fullness test in detecting meniscal injury.[8-10,15] In some cases, higher sensitivity and specificity values were reported, especially in situations where the diagnostic utility of performing two tests was assessed.[10,15] Additional studies are warranted to support the values reported in recent investigations.

Table 29-5 presents **sensitivity and specificity for some special tests** that are reported to identify meniscal pathology.[8-10,15,16] The **gold standard** for determining

Table 29-2 INTERVIEW QUESTIONS THAT SHOULD BE ASKED IF A MENISCAL INJURY IS SUSPECTED
When and how did you injure your knee? (*i.e.*, mechanism of injury)
How long have you been experiencing this pain?
Did you hear a "pop"?
Was there any swelling (immediately postinjury or residual)?
Where is your pain located?
Does the knee "lock" or does it "catch"?

Table 29-3   PHYSICAL EXAMINATION FOR INDIVIDUALS WITH SUSPECTED KNEE PATHOLOGY

Standing
- General observation (view patient anteriorly, posteriorly, and laterally in static and dynamic postures)
- Gait
- Special and functional tests (Table 29-4)

Sitting
- Active and passive range of motion (goniometry)
- Muscular flexibility testing
- Resisted testing (*i.e.*, manual muscle testing)
- Neurovascular testing

Supine
- Observation
- Active and passive range of motion (goniometry)
- Muscular flexibility testing
- Resisted testing (*i.e.*, manual muscle testing)
- Special tests (Table 29-4)
- Joint play
- Palpation

Sidelying
- Resisted testing
- Special tests (Table 29-4)

Prone
- Muscular flexibility testing
- Resisted testing
- Special tests (Table 29-4)

Table 29-4   SPECIAL TESTS REPORTED TO IDENTIFY MENISCAL INJURY

Test	Patient Position	Test Performance	Positive Findings
McMurray's test (Fig. 29-2)	Supine on table	Therapist grasps the foot at the heel with one hand and the knee with the other hand. Palpate the tibiofemoral joint line with one finger and the thumb. Passively fully flex the knee and then either rotate the leg internally or externally. Passively extend the knee. Repeat again, extending the knee from the flexed position and with the leg rotated the opposite direction.	Audible or palpable click
Thessaly test[8,9]	Standing in single limb stance on involved leg, placing hands on therapist's hands to assist balance	Patient flexes involved leg to either 5° (Fig. 29-3) or 20° (Fig. 29-4). Patient is instructed to rotate her body to the left then rotate body to the right while maintaining the desired degree of knee flexion. This movement is repeated three times.	Reproduction of symptoms/pain

(Continued)

Table 29-4   SPECIAL TESTS REPORTED TO IDENTIFY MENISCAL INJURY (CONTINUED)

Test	Patient Position	Test Performance	Positive Findings
Bounce home test (Fig. 29-5)	Supine on table	Therapist supports the involved lower extremity with one hand at the posterior side of the knee and the other hand supports the foot. The hip is passively flexed to approximately 45° and the knee passively flexed to approximately 25°-30°. Without informing the patient, the therapist quickly removes his hand from the knee, allowing the knee to passively extend.	Reproduction of pain Inability to achieve full extension
Joint line tenderness (Fig. 29-6)	Supine on table, hips flexed to 45° and knees to approximately 90°	Therapist palpates the tibiofemoral joint line on each side.	Reproduction of pain
Joint line fullness (Fig. 29-6)	Supine on table, hips flexed to 45° and involved knee flexed 70°-90° to assess medial compartment and 30°-45° to assess lateral compartment	Therapist palpates the tibiofemoral joint line for "palpable fullness."	Fullness that limits/prevents "normal joint compression"
Apley's compression test (Fig. 29-7)	Prone on table with involved knee flexed to 90°	Therapist grasps the foot and ankle of involved lower extremity with both hands. The therapist's leg is used to apply gentle pressure to the patient's posterior thigh to stabilize it. A compressive force is applied through the foot directed toward the knee. Maintain compression while internally and externally rotating the leg.	Reproduction of symptoms/pain

the presence or absence of a meniscus injury is arthroscopy.[17] Some tests have a wide range of sensitivity and specificity scores. The higher the sensitivity and specificity, the greater the confidence one has in the results from a test. For example, a positive Thessaly test at 20° of knee flexion (sensitivity: 89%-92%, specificity: 96%-97%) may help rule *in* a meniscal injury because of its high specificity (SpPin), whereas a negative Thessaly test may help rule *out* a

Table 29-5   SENSITIVITY AND SPECIFICITY ASSOCIATED WITH SELECTED SPECIAL TESTS FOR MENISCAL PATHOLOGY

Author (Year)	Population	Test	Sensitivity (%)	Specificity (%)
Kocher et al.[16] (2001)	113 patients (49 boys, 64 girls; mean age 11.9 y)	1. Clinical exam 2. MRI	1. 62.1,[a] 50.0[b] 2. 79.3,[a] 66.7[b]	1. 80.7,[a] 89.2[b] 2. 92.0,[a] 82.8[b]
Karachalios et al.[9] (2005)	213 patients (56 females; mean age 29.4 y) and 197 volunteers (53 females; mean age 31.1 y)	1. McMurray's test 2. Apley's compression test 3. Joint line tenderness 4. Thessaly test at 5° 5. Thessaly test at 20°	1. 48,[a] 65[b] 2. 41,[a] 41[b] 3. 71,[a] 78[b] 4. 66,[a] 81[b] 5. 89,[a] 92[b]	1. 94,[a] 86[b] 2. 93,[a] 86[b] 3. 87,[a] 90[b] 4. 96,[a] 91[b] 5. 97,[a] 96[b]
Harrison et al.[8] (2009)	116 patients (57 females) with suspected meniscal injury	1. Thessaly test	1. 90.3	1. 97.7
Konan et al.[10] (2009)	109 patients (29 females; mean age 39 y)	1. McMurray's test 2. Joint line tenderness 3. Thessaly test at 20° 4. McMurray's test and joint line tenderness 5. Thessaly test at 20° and joint line tenderness	1. 50,[a] 21[b] 2. 83,[a] 68[b] 3. 59,[a] 31[b] 4. 91,[a] 75[b] 5. 93,[a] 78[b]	1. 77,[a] 94[b] 2. 76,[a] 97[b] 3. 67,[a] 95[b] 4. 91,[a] 99[b] 5. 92,[a] 98[b]
Couture et al.[15] (2011)	100 patients (43 females; mean age 46.1 y) to have knee arthroscopic surgery	1. Joint line tenderness 2. McMurray's test 3. Joint line fullness	1. 90,[a] 87[c] 2. 28,[a] 32[c] 3. 73,[a] 70[c]	1. 0,[a] 30[c] 2. 87,[a] 78[c] 3. 73,[a] 82[c]

[a] Right meniscus
[b] Left meniscus
[c] Combined results for right and left meniscus

meniscal injury because of its high sensitivity (SnNout).[1,9] Since the ability of one test to accurately diagnose a meniscus injury may not be strong, some authors have reported that one's "diagnostic certainty" may be increased by performing several tests.[10,15] Konan et al.[10] found that combining the results from the Thessaly test performed at 20° of knee flexion and the joint line tenderness test had greater sensitivity and specificity values than when either of the test results were analyzed individually.

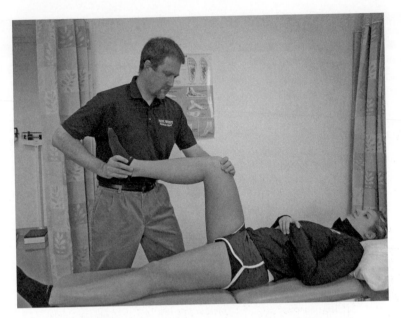

Figure 29-2. McMurray's test.

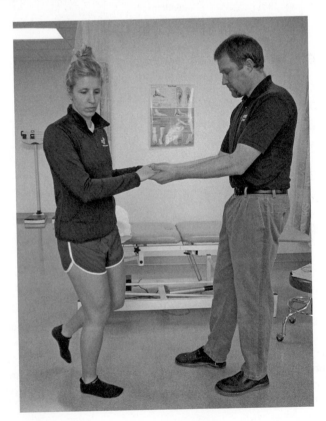

Figure 29-3. Thessaly test at 5°.

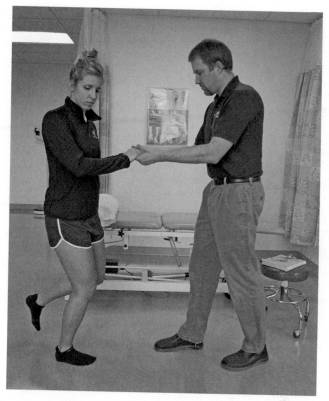

Figure 29-4. Thessaly test at 20°.

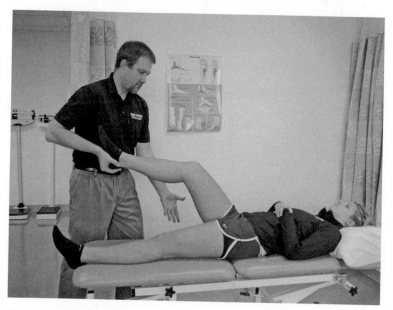

Figure 29-5. Bounce home test.

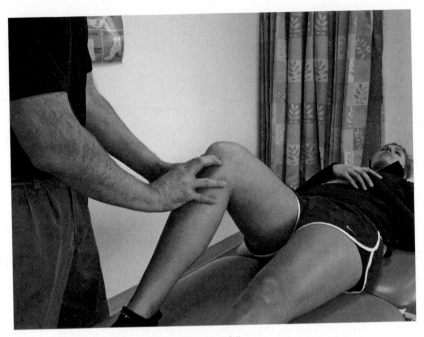

Figure 29-6. Test for joint line tenderness or joint line fullness.

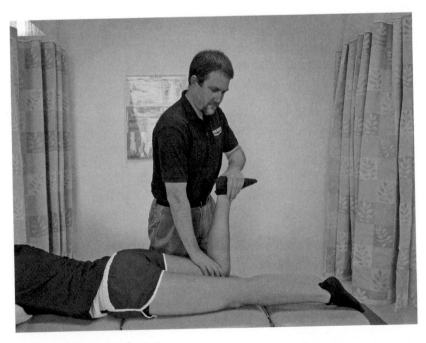

Figure 29-7. Apley's compression test.

Plan of Care and Interventions

The physical therapy plan of care is dependent on the severity of the meniscal sprain and the patient's point of entry into the healthcare system. Physical therapy treatment may include modalities to reduce pain (*e.g.*, whirlpool, electrical stimulation, cryotherapy), interventions to restore range of motion deficits (therapeutic exercise progression, joint mobilization/manual therapy), and therapeutic exercises to restore muscular strength and aerobic fitness.[18] The ability to progress the patient may be limited by the location of the tear (less vascular inner 2/3 versus the outer 1/3 of the meniscus), the extent (size) of the tear, and/or the presence of comorbid conditions. If a patient has been referred by a PCP or self-referred, the physical therapist may initiate treatment for a patient with a suspected meniscal sprain. However, if the patient fails to improve with treatment, referral to an orthopaedic surgeon is necessary. Arthroscopy, the gold standard test for meniscal pathology, confirms the presence of a meniscus injury in individuals who have elected to treat knee pain with surgery.

Evidence-Based Clinical Recommendations

SORT: Strength of Recommendation Taxonomy
A: Consistent, good-quality patient-oriented evidence
B: Inconsistent or limited-quality patient-oriented evidence
C: Consensus, disease-oriented evidence, usual practice, expert opinion, or case series

1. Special tests that can be performed by the physical therapist to identify meniscal pathology have moderate to high sensitivity and specificity. **Grade B**

2. The gold standard test to confirm or rule out a meniscus injury is arthroscopy. **Grade A**

COMPREHENSION QUESTIONS

29.1 The Thessaly test is performed with the patient's knee in ___ and ___ degrees of knee flexion.

    A. 5, 10

    B. 10, 20

    C. 5, 20

    D. 20, 30

29.2 According to Couture et al.,[15] the McMurray's test has poor sensitivity (28%) for detecting medial meniscus pathology; however, the test is associated with a high specificity (87%). If a patient with a suspected meniscus injury has a positive McMurray's test, which of the following is true?

A. The patient does not have a medial meniscus injury.

B. A positive McMurray's test will help to rule in a meniscal injury.

C. A positive McMurray's test will help to rule out a meniscal injury.

D. The patient has a medial meniscus injury.

ANSWERS

29.1 **C.**

29.2 **B.** If a positive test is found with a test that has a high specificity, then the test may help to rule in the target disorder (SpPin). In this case, the McMurray's test was associated with a high specificity (87%). Option D is incorrect because, although one might suspect that there is a meniscus injury based on the high specificity, it would be incorrect to state that the patient *does* have an injury. It is accurate to state that the post-test *probability* of a meniscal tear is higher in the presence of a positive test with high specificity. However, arthroscopy is the gold standard test to confirm the presence or absence of a meniscus injury.

REFERENCES

1. Sackett DL. *Evidence-Based Medicine: How to Practice and Teach EBM*. Edinburgh: Churchill Livingstone; 2000.

2. Muscolo DL, Ayerza MA, Makino A, Costa-Paz M, Aponte-Tinao LA. Tumors about the knee misdiagnosed as athletic injuries. *J Bone Joint Surg Am.* 2003;85A:1209-1214.

3. Pinar H, Boya H, Satoglu IS, Oztekin HH. A contribution to Pisani's sign for diagnosing lateral meniscal cysts: a technical report. *Knee Surg Sports Traumatol Arthrosc.* 2009;17:402-404.

4. Masouros SD, McDermott ID, Amis AA, Bull AM. Biomechanics of the meniscus-meniscal ligament construct of the knee. *Knee Surg Sports Traumatol Arthrosc.* 2008;16:1121-1132.

5. Kohn D, Moreno B. Meniscus insertion anatomy as a basis for meniscus replacement: a morphologic cadaveric study. *Arthroscopy.* 1995;11:96-103.

6. Renstrom P, Johnson RJ. Anatomy and biomechanics of the menisci. *Clin Sports Med.* 1990;9: 523-538.

7. Bellabarba C, Bush-Joseph CA, Bach BR Jr. Patterns of meniscal injury in the anterior-cruciate deficient knee: a review of the literature. *Am J Orthop.* 1997;26:18-23.

8. Harrison BK, Abell BE, Gibson TW. The Thessaly test for detection of meniscal tears: validation of a new physical examination technique for primary care medicine. *Clin J Sport Med.* 2009;19:9-12.

9. Karachalios T, Hantes M, Zibis AH, Zachos V, Karantanas AH, Malizos KN. Diagnostic accuracy of a new clinical test (the Thessaly test) for early detection of meniscal tears. *J Bone Joint Surg Am.* 2005;87:955-962.

10. Konan S, Rayan F, Haddad FS. Do physical diagnostic tests accurately detect meniscal tears? *Knee Surg Sports Traumatol Arthrosc.* 2009;17:806-811.

11. Solomon DH, Simel DL, Bates DW, Katz JN, Schaffer JL. The rational clinical examination. Does this patient have a torn meniscus or ligament of the knee? Value of the physical examination. *JAMA.* 2001;286:1610-1620.

12. Hegedus EJ, Cook C, Hasselblad V, Goode A, McCrory DC. Physical examination tests for assessing a torn meniscus in the knee: a systematic review with meta-analysis. *J Orthop Sports Phys Ther.* 2007;37:541-550.

13. Malanga GA, Andrus S, Nadler SF, McLean J. Physical examination of the knee: a review of the original test description and scientific validity of common orthopedic tests. *Arch Phys Med Rehabil.* 2003;84:592-603.

14. Stratford PW, Binkley J. A review of the McMurray test: definition, interpretation, and clinical usefulness. *J Orthop Sports Phys Ther.* 1995;22:116-120.

15. Couture JF, Al-Juhani W, Forsythe ME, Lenczner E, Marien R, Burman M. Joint line fullness and meniscal pathology. *Sports Health.* 2012;4:47-50.

16. Kocher MS, DiCanzio J, Zurakowski D, Micheli LJ. Diagnostic performance of clinical examination and selective magnetic resonance imaging in the evaluation of intraarticular knee disorders in children and adolescents. *Am J Sports Med.* 2001;29:292-296.

17. Jackson JL, O'Malley PG, Kroenke K. Evaluation of acute knee pain in primary care. *Ann Intern Med.* 2003;139:575-588.

18. Lim HC, Bae JH, Wang JH, Seok CW, Kim MK. Non-operative treatment of degenerative posterior root tear of the medial meniscus. *Knee Surg Sports Traumatol Arthrosc.* 2010;18:535-539.

Tibial Stress Fracture

Michael D. Rosenthal
Shane A. Vath

A local fireman who has no significant prior running experience plans to enter a marathon in 7 months. He has 28 weeks to train so he begins running 1 mile every other day. He adds an additional mile weekly to ensure he will be able to successfully progress his running distance to 26 miles in time for the race. After 3 weeks of running, he noted medial shin pain that occurred near the end of his runs or during his cool-down walking period. The leg pain dissipated after sitting and resting for a few hours and was not present upon awakening or through-out the next day. He continued his training, which resulted in a gradual increase and earlier onset of pain. He experienced leg pain at the beginning of runs that would ease with continued running. He ignored the pain and continued his running program. After 6 weeks of training, his leg pain occurred at the beginning of runs and no longer resolved with cessation of running. The pain intensity increased and he could not continue running. He began taking nonsteroidal anti-inflammatory drugs (NSAIDs), which allowed him to complete one more week of painful training. However, the pain increased with continued running despite use of NSAIDs. The patient now had shin pain at rest that increased with stand-ing and walking activities. He also experienced pain while resting in bed. He had mild to moderate discomfort when awakening and the symptoms continued with increasing intensity during and following prolonged standing and walking activi-ties. After prolonged sitting, symptoms eased but remained present. The patient was frustrated and concerned about his ability to run the local marathon so he self-referred to an outpatient physical therapy clinic for evaluation and treatment. At the time of evaluation, the patient had not run for 2 days. As he stood in the waiting area and walked through the therapy office, his gait was notably antalgic, with an exaggerated lean over the more involved side. Strength testing, range of motion (ROM), and visual inspection were all normal. Diffuse medial shin pain was reproduced with ROM and strength testing. The most significant finding on examination was localized tenderness to palpation about 2 cm in length along the medial tibia (right side greater than left). The tenderness was at the junction of the mid- to distal one-third of the tibias. There was also mild bilateral tenderness over the central third of the medial tibias. Other than his recent increase in training, the patient's past medical history was unremarkable. Signs, symptoms, and history are consistent with tibial stress fractures. The fireman's main goal is to return to his training program and run pain-free as soon as possible to meet his goal of completing the local marathon.

▶ Based on the patient's suspected diagnosis, what do you anticipate may be the contributing factors to the condition?
▶ What physical examination signs may be associated with this diagnosis?
▶ What ancillary tests are most sensitive and specific for diagnosing a tibial stress fracture?

KEY DEFINITIONS

EXTRINSIC RISK FACTORS: Characteristics of an individual's training or competition schedule that may influence the likelihood of sustaining a stress fracture (*e.g.*, training regimen, shoe selection, training surface or terrain, type of sport)

INTRINSIC RISK FACTORS: Characteristics of the individual that may influence the likelihood of sustaining a stress fracture (*e.g.*, sex, knee alignment, leg length discrepancy, nutritional factors, hormonal factors)

OSTEOBLASTS: Cells that produce bone matrix, ultimately resulting in increased bone strength and healing of a (stress) fracture

OSTEOCLASTS: Cells that resorb bone, which can ultimately produce a resorption cavity and decrease in bone strength

TIBIAL STRESS FRACTURE: Overuse injury that primarily occurs due to a significant increase in training volume (usually running); marked by localized tenderness of 2 to 3 cm along the medial tibia; pain at rest and at night are common

Objectives

1. Describe tibial stress fracture symptoms and potential intrinsic and extrinsic risk factors associated with this diagnosis.

2. Identify rationale for referral for further evaluation and imaging.

3. Identify commonly used clinical tests for diagnosing tibial stress fractures.

Physical Therapy Considerations

PT considerations during management of the individual with a suspected diagnosis of medial tibial stress fracture:

▶ **General physical therapy plan of care/goals:** Differential diagnosis; consultation with an orthopaedic provider; decrease pain; protect from further injury with immobilization and/or appropriate assistive devices to normalize gait and reduce tibial load; provide education regarding diagnosis and prognosis; minimize lower extremity deconditioning (strength and endurance) without interrupting healing; aid in managing progression back to running by educating patient on training variables (frequency, intensity, type, duration) and recommended progression each week to reduce likelihood of further injury

▶ **Physical therapy interventions:** Patient education regarding functional anatomy and injury pathomechanics; modalities; muscular flexibility and joint mobility exercises; resistance exercises to promote maintenance and recovery of muscular endurance and strength; alternate low impact aerobic conditioning to allow fitness training; gradual progression of impact loading exercises; orthotic fabrication; continue discussion with patient to minimize likelihood that frustration with injury will alter mood

▶ **Precautions during physical therapy:** Avoid stress to the lower extremity that may result in fracture completion; monitor response of shin pain to prescribed exercise program and reduce tissue loads if patient experiences increased symptoms; address precautions or contraindications for exercise based on patient's pre-existing condition(s); monitor response to reduced activity and impact on individual's career, sport, or leisure activities

▶ **Complications interfering with physical therapy:** Patient/client who is unwilling or unable to alter training regimen; work schedule; comorbidities (*e.g.*, hormonal status, nutritional status, overall health status)

Understanding the Health Condition

The tibia is the major weightbearing bone in the leg. Ninety percent of the lower extremity load is carried by the tibia with the fibula taking the remaining 10%.[1] The tibia is prismoid in shape, having a broadened flat plateau proximally which articulates with the femoral condyles. Below the knee, the diameter lessens to its smallest size in the area between the middle third and distal third of the length of the bone. Near the ankle, the tibia expands again to form the tibial plafond, a concave dense region that articulates with the talar dome. The shaft of the tibia is made up of three surfaces: the anterior border or crest, the medial border, and the lateral border. There are multiple intrinsic and extrinsic muscles that attach to the tibia. These muscles are contained within four compartments: anterior, lateral, superficial posterior, and deep posterior. The borders of each compartment are defined by varying proportions of tough fascia, soft tissue, and bone. Variability in borders makes some compartments more or less compliant and able to tolerate increases in size (whether due to muscle hypertrophy or edema), which may result in increased intra-compartmental pressures. The fascia of the anterior compartment attaches to the medial border of the tibia. The fibula attaches to the tibia by a tough interosseous membrane, proximal and distal bony articulations, and associated ligaments. The tibia undergoes varied loading throughout the gait cycle and is somewhat impacted by bony anatomy and running style. With running, the tibia is cyclically loaded with vertical forces measuring 2.5 to 2.8 times body weight.[2]

Medial tibial pain accounts for 13% to 17% of all running injuries.[3] Stress fractures are typically one of the top five most common running injuries and account for 5% to 50% of all musculoskeletal running injuries.[4,5] The tibia is the most common location of stress fracture,[6-8] accounting for 33% to 55% of all stress fractures.[9-11] The majority of tibial stress fractures occur over the posteromedial aspect at the junction of the mid- to distal third of its length (Fig. 30-1). Tibial stress fractures can also occur in the region of the medial tibial plateau (Fig. 30-2) and the anterior cortex of the tibia. For patients with anterior tibial cortex stress fractures, poor blood supply to the area and tension, vice compression, and forces to the region of injury have been associated with delayed and problematic return to sports.[12]

Stress fractures are an overuse injury experienced primarily by individuals who undergo a rapid increase in running or other high impact activities. Stress fractures often occur during the second and third weeks following an increase in training

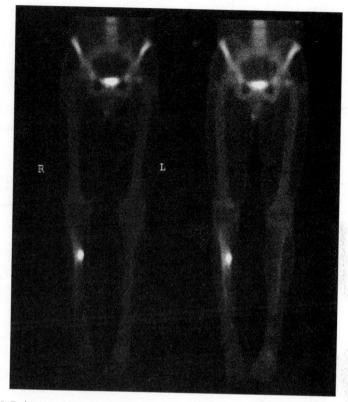

Figure 30–1. Technetium bone scan image of a patient with a right mid-tibia stress fracture. The brighter regions, where more of the radioactive technetium is taken up by osteoblast cells, indicate an increased rate of bone turnover.

volume, but have also been reported at later stages of training.[13] Development of a stress fracture is the result of an accumulation of microtrauma from repetitive loading, continuation of loading, and loss of bone homeostasis due to inadequate rest and repair.[14] Responses to bone loading occur along a continuum—beginning with normal remodeling and then advancing to accelerated remodeling, stress reaction, stress injury, stress fracture, and complete fracture when excessive loading without adequate rest is continued.[12] Effective training programs that include well-planned loading and rest periods promote bony adaptation and subsequent increases in bone mass (strength). Bone is a dynamic tissue that undergoes an ongoing remodeling process with both osteoclast and osteoblast activity. Osteoclastic activity creates tunnels within the bone that weaken the bone and result in pain with repeated loading. If loading is continued and the healing process interrupted, osteoclastic activity outpaces osteoblastic activity and microfracture lines can propagate across the bone, resulting in a stress fracture. Regardless of the etiology of stress fracture, relative rest allows the body to restore balance and heal appropriately. However, continued training, cyclic impact loading, and inadequate recovery periods will increase shin pain and may allow a stress fracture to progress to a complete fracture.

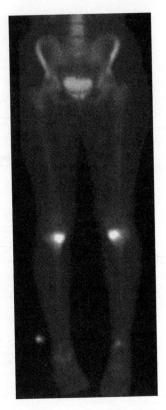

Figure 30-2. Technetium bone scan image of patient with bilateral medial tibial plateau stress fractures.

Muscular strength and performance are thought to mitigate ground reaction forces and protect against the development of stress fractures.[12] As muscle fatigue develops, muscular shock absorption decreases and the bone experiences a significantly greater load, with reports indicating ground reaction and shear strain forces increasing by 25% to 35%.[15]

Stress fractures may be the result of extrinsic, intrinsic, and/or a combination of these factors. **Extrinsic factors** that have been proposed to contribute to the onset of stress fracture include rapid increase in training (intensity, frequency, and duration), suboptimal or inappropriate footwear, and training surface. Proposed **intrinsic risk factors** include: sex (more common in women), race (more common in white and Asian women than African American women), biomechanical factors (*e.g.*, bone geometry, kinetic chain strength and stability, pes cavus, pes planus, etc.), anatomic factors (*e.g.*, foot shape, leg length discrepancy, knee alignment), hormonal factors, and nutritional factors.[12,16–18] The components of the female athlete triad greatly increase the risk of stress fracture.[12] These include decreased bone mineral density (osteopenia or osteoporosis), altered nutritional status (disordered eating) and hormonal factors (menstrual cycle irregularity). In contrast, having a higher level of physical fitness and a history of previous impact loading sports activity seem to be protective of overuse injuries.[19] Untrained individuals are 10 times more likely to develop overuse injuries when compared to individuals who have a higher level of physical fitness.[20]

Examination, Evaluation, and Diagnosis

A thorough patient history often helps the physical therapist to develop a reasonable differential diagnosis prior to initiating the physical examination. The therapist should gather information regarding: past medical history, history of similar symptoms, previous medical attention sought for the condition and type of medical providers seen, whether a diagnosis had been established, past imaging studies and results, easing and aggravating factors, and current status of symptoms (improving, worsening, or static). In addition, the physical therapist should inquire about the patient's specific training routine, including: frequency, intensity, type of training (sprints, hills, etc.), distance, types of running surfaces on which the individual trains, and which positions or activities reproduce symptoms during daily activity. The therapist should also explore what is motivating the individual to perform his current exercise program (e.g., job qualification or training, sport, leisure, health).

Patients presenting with suspicion of tibial stress fracture are most likely to report a recent history of increased running volume. However, given the spectrum of bone stress injury, it may be difficult to base the diagnosis purely on a clinical examination. Furthermore, the physical therapist must remember that it is possible to have a concomitant condition (e.g., periostitis). Early symptoms of a tibial stress fracture may be similar to those of medial tibial stress syndrome (MTSS). Differential diagnoses for tibial stress fracture include: MTSS, chronic periostalgia secondary to tension between fascial attachments to the periosteum, exercise-induced compartment syndrome, tendinitis, periostitis, muscle hernia, intermittent claudication, venous insufficiency, and osteoid osteoma.

The primary symptoms associated with tibial stress fracture are local tenderness and swelling. Initial symptoms are typically mild and resolve with prolonged sitting or sleep. If the aggravating activity is continued, the symptoms tend to worsen and pain limits the patient's ability to perform the desired activity. If the individual is not involved in an organized sport or lacks a specific training goal, he will typically refrain from further training due to pain and the symptoms will resolve over time. With continued training, the condition typically worsens. Symptoms become more frequent, have an earlier onset, interrupt the ability to train, and are present for longer durations after cessation of activity. In many cases, patients experience pain at rest that increases after prolonged standing and eases somewhat after prolonged sitting. Pain at rest, especially at night, is also common with stress fractures.

A key physical examination finding is localized tenderness within a 2- to 3-cm region, often accompanied by swelling. This contrasts from the diffuse pain over an area greater than 5 cm, which is more indicative of MTSS.[21] Numerous **special tests** have been reported in the literature to assist in the clinical diagnosis of tibial stress fracture (Table 30-1). None of the special tests has been consistently shown to demonstrate high diagnostic value.

Radiographic examination is often conducted to aid in diagnosing tibial stress fracture. However, changes on plain radiographs are usually not present for at least 2 to 3 weeks after onset of symptoms, are often normal for up to 3 months, and in some cases remain normal.[22,23] Abnormal findings on radiographs indicating stress fracture may include periosteal thickening and subtle or distinct lucency.[23]

Table 30-1	SPECIAL TESTS ASSOCIATED WITH TIBIAL STRESS FRACTURES	
Test	Patient Position	Findings
Fulcrum test	Patient sits at edge of treatment table. Therapist grasps ankle with one hand and provides a medial/lateral stress to the tibia in the symptomatic region.	Increased pain or reproduction of the patient's pain is a positive sign for potential tibial stress fracture.
Percussion test	Patient lies supine on treatment table. The therapist passively elevates the straight leg off the examination table and provides a rapid percussive force through the heel along the long axis of the leg/tibia.	Increased pain or reproduction of the patient's pain is a positive sign for potential tibial stress fracture.
Tuning fork test[27]	Patient lies supine on treatment table. The knee is flexed to approximately 90° to relax the posterior leg musculature. The therapist strikes a 128 Hz tuning fork and applies it to the tibia at the region of tenderness. The tuning fork may be held stationary or slowly moved across the region of tenderness.	Increased pain or reproduction of the patient's pain is a positive sign for potential tibial stress fracture.
Ultrasound test[28]	Patient lies supine on treatment table. The knee is flexed to approximately 90° to relax the posterior leg musculature. Continuous therapeutic ultrasound of 1 MHz for 3-5 min is applied to the region of greatest tenderness to palpation. The ultrasound head is moved over an area equal to approximately three times the size of the sound head at an intensity of 0.5-3.0 W/cm^2.	Increased pain or reproduction of the patient's pain is a positive sign for potential tibial stress fracture.
Single-leg hop	Patient stands on one leg and performs a vertical jump. This more provocative test should only be performed if previous tests do not reproduce symptoms, or to aid in determining ability to return to impact activities.	Reproduction of the patient's pain is a positive sign for potential tibial stress fracture.

Periosteal thickening, the most common finding, is a non-sensitive finding that is often present in individuals with an extensive physical training background. As a result, technetium bone scan, computed tomography, and magnetic resonance imaging are utilized to improve sensitivity and specificity in diagnosing tibial pain.[24,25] The current criterion standard ("gold standard") for diagnosis of tibial stress fractures is **magnetic resonance imaging,**[25,26] but the results of any and all imaging studies should be supported by the comprehensive patient history and physical examination.

Plan of Care and Interventions

Physical therapy interventions should address findings from the history and musculoskeletal examination. If the physical therapist suspects a stress fracture, the individual should be advised to maintain a decreased weightbearing status on the involved extremity(ies) using crutches and referred to an orthopaedic specialist for further evaluation and management. If diagnosis of a tibial stress fracture is confirmed via imaging, the therapist can be involved in developing a comprehensive rehabilitation program to minimize deconditioning, optimize return to preinjury activity levels, and address intrinsic and extrinsic factors to mitigate the potential for reinjury.

Evidence-Based Clinical Recommendations

SORT: Strength of Recommendation Taxonomy

A: Consistent, good-quality patient-oriented evidence
B: Inconsistent or limited-quality patient-oriented evidence
C: Consensus, disease-oriented evidence, usual practice, expert opinion, or case series

1. Extrinsic risk factors are associated with development of tibial stress fractures. **Grade A**

2. Intrinsic risk factors are associated with development of tibial stress fractures. **Grade B**

3. Special clinical tests can assist in the diagnosis of tibial stress fractures. **Grade B**

4. Magnetic resonance imaging is the most specific and sensitive tool for diagnosis of tibial stress fractures. **Grade A**

COMPREHENSION QUESTIONS

30.1 What is the *most* common cause of tibial stress fracture?

   A. Training errors (extrinsic risk factor)

   B. Pes planus (intrinsic risk factor)

   C. Incorrect shoe selection (extrinsic risk factor)

   D. High body mass index (intrinsic risk factor)

30.2 What is the *most* sensitive and specific imaging modality for diagnosis of tibial stress fracture?

   A. Bone densitometry

   B. Magnetic resonance imaging

   C. Technetium bone scan

   D. Standard (plain) radiographs

ANSWERS

30.1 **A.** The most prevalent cause of tibial stress fracture is training errors.[14]

30.2 **B.** MRI is considered the gold standard for diagnosing tibial stress fractures. It provides the most sensitive and specific information when evaluating bone stress injuries.[25,26] While the technetium bone scan provides a high level of sensitivity, the specificity is not as high as MRI.

REFERENCES

1. Takebe K, Nakagawa A, Minami H, Kanazawa H, Hirohata K. Role of the fibula in weight-bearing. *Clin Orthop Relat Res*. 1984;184:289-292.

2. Miller DI. Ground reaction forces in distance running. In: Cavanagh PR, ed. *The Biomechanics of Distance Running*. Champaign, IL: Human Kinetics; 1990:203-224.

3. Taunton JE, Clement DB, Webber D. Lower extremity stress fractures in athletes. *Phys Sportsmed*. 1981;9:77-86.

4. Bennell KL, Malcolm SA, Brukner PD, et al. A 12-month prospective study of the relationship between stress fractures and bone turnover in athletes. *Calcif Tissue Int*. 1998;63:80-85.

5. Losito JM, Laird RC, Alexis MR, Mora J. Tibial and proximal fibular stress fracture in a rower. *J Am Pod Med Assoc*. 2003;9:340-343.

6. James SL, Bates BT, Osternig LR. Injuries to runners. *Am J Sports Med*. 1978;6:40-50.

7. Kowal DM. Nature and causes of injuries in women resulting from an endurance training program. *Am J Sports Med*. 1980;8:265-269.

8. McBryde AM Jr. Stress fractures in runners. *Clin Sports Med*. 1985;4:737-752.

9. Brukner P, Bradshaw C, Khan KM, White S, Crossley K. Stress fractures: a review of 180 cases. *Clin J Sport Med*. 1996;6:85-89.

10. Giladi M, Milgrom C, Simkin A. Stress fractures and tibial bone width: a risk factor. *J Bone Joint Surg*. 1987;69:326-329.

11. Matheson GO, Clement DB, McKenzie DC, Taunton JE, Lloyd-Smith DR. Macintyre JG. Stress fractures in athletes. A study of 320 cases. *Am J Sports Med*. 1987;15:46-58.

12. Brukner P, Bennell K, Matheson G. *Stress Fractures*. Victoria, Australia: Human Kinetics; 1999.

13. Burr DB. Bone, exercise, and stress fractures. *Exerc Sport Sci Rev*. 1997;25:171-194.

14. Pepper M, Akuthota V, McCarty EC. The pathophysiology of stress fractures. *Clin Sports Med*. 2006;25:1-16.

15. Beck BR. Tibial stress injuries. An aetiological review for the purposes of guiding management. *Sports Med*. 1998;26:265-79.

16. Pester S, Smith PC. Stress fractures in the lower extremities of soldiers in basic training. *Orthop Rev*. 1992;21:297-303.

17. Arendt E, Agel J, Heikes C, Griffiths H. Stress injuries to bone in college athletes: a retrospective review of experience at a single institution. *Am J Sports Med*. 2003;31:959-968.

18. Armstrong DW III, Rue JP, Wilckens JH, Frassica FJ. Stress fracture injury in young military men and women. *Bone*. 2004;35:806-816.

19. Milgrom C, Simkin A, Eldad A, Nyska M, Finestone A. Using bone's adaptation ability to lower the incidence of stress fractures. *Am J Sports Med*. 2000;28:245-251.

20. Rosendal L, Langberg H, Skov-Jensen A, Kjaer M. Incidence of injury and physical performance adaptations during military training. *Clin J Sport Med*. 2003;13:157-163.

21. Batt ME, Ugalde V, Anderson MW, Shelton DK. A prospective controlled study of diagnostic imaging for acute shin splints. *Med Sci Sports Exerc.* 1998;20:1564-1571.

22. Savoca CJ. Stress fractures. A classification of the earliest radiographic signs. *Radiology* 1971;100: 519-524.

23. Deutsch AL, Coel MN, Mink JH. Imaging of stress injuries to bone. Radiography, scintigraphy and MR imaging. *Clin Sports Med.* 1997;16:275-290.

24. Gaeta M, Minutoli F, Vinci S, et al. High-resolution CT grading of tibial stress reactions in distance runners. *Am J Roentgenol.* 2006;187:789-793.

25. Fredericson M, Bergman AG, Hoffman KL, Dillingham MS. Tibial stress reaction in runners. Correlation of clinical symptoms and scintigraphy with a new magnetic resonance imaging grading system. *Am J Sports Med.* 1995;23:472-481.

26. Young AJ, McAllister DR. Evaluation and treatment of tibial stress fractures. *Clin Sports Med.* 2006;25:117-128.

27. Lesho EP. Can tuning forks replace bone scans for identification of tibial stress fractures? *Mil Med.* 1997;162:802-803.

28. Romani WA, Perrin DH, Dussault RG, Ball DW, Kahler DM. Identification of tibial stress fractures using therapeutic continuous ultrasound. *J Orthop Sports Phys Ther.* 2000;30:444-452.

DISCLAIMER

The views expressed in this article are those of the authors and do not necessarily reflect the official policy or position of the Department of the Navy, Department of Defense, or the U.S. Government.

Medial Tibial Stress Syndrome

Michael D. Rosenthal
Shane A. Vath

A 25-year-old businessman initiated a running program with a goal to get into shape and lose weight. The program consisted of running 2 miles 4 to 5 times per week and he continued this regimen for 4 weeks. He initially noted medial shin pain after 2 weeks of running that occurred near the end of his runs or with cool-down walking. When the pain started to interfere with his desired exercise program, he self-referred to an outpatient physical therapy clinic for evaluation and treatment. Signs, symptoms, and history are consistent with medial tibial stress syndrome (MTSS). The individual's main goal is to return to pain-free running and improve his fitness.

► Based on the patient's suspected diagnosis, what do you anticipate may be the contributing factors to the condition?
► What examination signs may be associated with this diagnosis?
► What are the most appropriate physical therapy interventions?
► What are possible complications that may limit the effectiveness of physical therapy?

KEY DEFINITIONS

EXTRINSIC RISK FACTORS: Characteristics of an individual's training or competition schedule that may influence the likelihood of developing MTSS (e.g., training regimen, shoe selection, training surface or terrain, type of sport)

INTRINSIC RISK FACTORS: Characteristics of the individual that may influence the likelihood of developing MTSS (e.g., sex, lower extremity strength, hip ROM, body mass index, navicular drop)

MEDIAL TIBIAL STRESS SYNDROME: Overuse injury that primarily occurs with a rapid increase in frequency, intensity, and duration of impact activities (usually running); marked by diffuse tenderness >5 cm in length along the posteromedial border of the tibia of one or both legs, and most commonly affects the middle to distal thirds of the tibia

Objectives

1. Describe medial tibial stress syndrome and identify potential risk factors that may result in this condition.
2. Provide appropriate patient education regarding MTSS.
3. Design and prescribe appropriate resistance exercises to treat MTSS.
4. Prescribe alternate aerobic activities aimed to improve fitness that minimize lower extremity loads and risk for further injury.
5. Discuss an appropriate plan for increasing activity and returning to impact activities while preventing a recurrence of the condition.

Physical Therapy Considerations

PT considerations during management of the individual with a diagnosis of medial tibial stress syndrome:

▶ **General physical therapy plan of care/goals:** Differential diagnosis; decrease pain; protect from further progression of the injury; provide education regarding diagnosis and prognosis; increase muscular flexibility and lower extremity strength; minimize lower extremity deconditioning (strength and endurance) without interrupting healing; encourage low-impact aerobic conditioning to maintain or increase aerobic fitness; aid in managing progression back to running by educating patient on training variables (frequency, intensity, type, duration) and recommended progression each week to reduce likelihood of further injury

▶ **Physical therapy interventions:** Patient education regarding functional anatomy and injury pathomechanics; modalities and manual therapy to decrease pain; muscular flexibility exercises; lower extremity resistance exercises to increase strength and muscular endurance; low-impact aerobic exercise program; trial use of foot orthoses

▶ **Precautions during physical therapy:** Monitor response of shin pain to pre-scribed exercise program and reduce tissue loads if patient experiences increased pain; address precautions or contraindications for exercise based on patient's pre-existing condition(s); monitor response to reduced activity and impact on individual's career, sport, or leisure activities; continue open line of discussion with patient during period of care to ensure frustration with injury does not lead to altered mood and/or depression

▶ **Complications interfering with physical therapy:** Patient/client who is unwill-ing or unable to alter their training regimen; work schedule; comorbidities (*e.g.*, connective tissue disorders, nutritional status, overall health status)

Understanding the Health Condition

Medial tibial pain accounts for 13% to 17% of all running injuries[1-3] and stress injuries account for 15% to 20% of all musculoskeletal running injuries.[4,5] Medial tibial stress syndrome (MTSS) is a painful overuse injury experienced primar-ily by individuals who undergo a rapid increase in running or other high-impact activities. The term "shin splints" is often used in the literature and by patients and medical professionals to describe exercise-related leg pain. While used to describe a multitude of leg conditions, and frequently used in reference to MTSS, shin splints is not a specific diagnosis. It is important that physical therapists realize shin splints is a nonspecific term. Therapists should utilize more appropriate terminology in the differential diagnosis of patients with leg pain. MTSS has been reported to occur in conjunction with posterior exertional compartment syndrome in 15% of cases. In 25% of cases, MTSS coexists with other conditions such as periostitis, sequelae from prior tibial fracture, and muscle herniation through fascial defect.[6,7] Differential diagnoses for medial tibial pain includes: tibial bone stress injury (including tibial stress fracture, covered in Case 30), chronic periostalgia secondary to tension between fascia attachments to the periosteum, exertional compartment syndrome, tendinopathy, periostitis, muscle hernia, intermittent claudication, venous insufficiency, chronic deep posterior compartment syndrome, infection, peripheral neuropathy, lumbosacral radicu-lopathy, and neoplasm.[8-10]

The pertinent anatomy associated with MTSS includes the muscles within the leg that are contained within four compartments (Fig. 31-1): anterior (tibialis anterior, extensor digitorum longus, extensor hallucis longus, fibularis tertius), lateral (fibu-laris longus, fibularis brevis), superficial posterior (gastrocnemius, soleus, plantaris), and deep posterior (popliteus, tibialis posterior, flexor digitorum longus, flexor hallucis longus). The borders of each compartment are defined by varying pro-portions of fascia, soft tissue, and bone. Variability in borders makes some com-partments more or less compliant and able to tolerate increase in size (whether due to muscle hypertrophy or edema), which may result in increased intra-compartmental pressures. The fascia of the anterior compartment attaches to the medial border of the tibia.

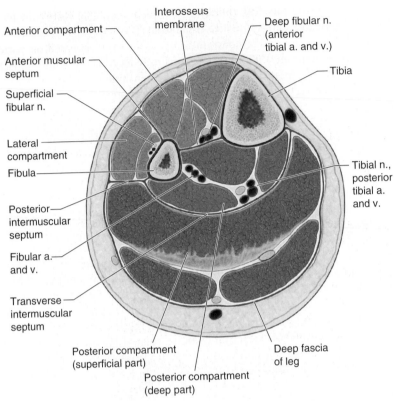

Figure 31-1. Cross-section of the right leg. (Reproduced with permission from Morton DA, Foreman KB, Albertine KH, eds. *The Big Picture: Gross Anatomy*. New York: McGraw-Hill; 2011. Figure 37-1A.)

Only recently, it has been agreed that MTSS is the result of a bone stress injury and not the result of an inflammatory process of the periosteum.[11-13] MTSS represents the early stages of the continuum of stress injury to bone.[14] Normally, when the tibia is exposed to higher loads, osteoclast activity (bone resorption) produces channeling within the tibia that can be more pronounced on the concave portion of the posteromedial aspect of the tibia. Next, osteoblast activity (bone formation) produces periosteal thickening, which results in stronger bone that is more able to tolerate the increased loads. However, if the activity of osteoclasts outpaces that of osteoblasts during the ongoing process of bone remodeling, tunnels will be produced within the bone, causing structural weakness that may result in pain with repeated loading. If repetitive high-impact loading is continued, the healing process is further interrupted and microfracture lines can propagate across the bone—resulting in a stress fracture. Bone biopsies have shown osseous metabolic changes with inflammatory changes at periosteal attachments (tendinous and deep crural fascia connections to the bone).[15] Plain radiographs of patients with nonacute MTSS may show thickening of the posteromedial tibial cortex in response to osteoblastic activity (Fig. 31-2) in contrast to the clear, consistent tibial cortical thickness in those without MTSS (Fig. 31-3).[16] A technetium bone scan in the patient with MTSS demonstrates diffuse

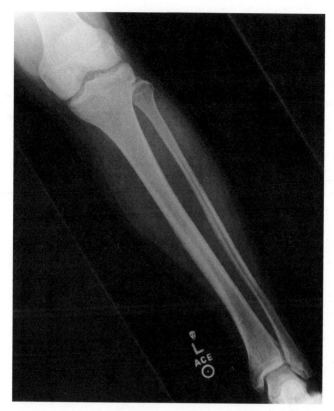

Figure 31-2. Anteroposterior plain radiograph of the leg of a patient with MTSS. Note region of periosteal thickening in the mid-distal third of the medial tibia.

uptake, oriented vertically, along the posteromedial tibia (Fig. 31-4). This pattern is distinctly different from the localized uptake in the patient with a tibial stress fracture (Case 30, Fig. 30-1). In 18 adult male athletes with longstanding cases of MTSS, Magnusson et al.[17] noted that the posteromedial tibial border was 15% more porous than control subjects and 23% more porous than athletic controls, indicating that, despite thickening of the cortex, MTSS is associated with areas of low bone mineral density.

While the pathoanatomy underlying MTSS has recently been agreed upon, the pathomechanics remain disputed. One plausible cause is tibial bending as a result of the recurrent impact loading. Another potential cause is traction produced by muscular and fascial insertions about the posteromedial tibia. Stickley et al.[18] suggest the potential for a traction-induced injury from the pull of the deep crural fascia, but not from the muscles of the deep and superficial posterior compartments. Bouche and Johnson[19] reported that the tension produced by the deep posterior compartment muscles upon the distal tibial fascia increased the tension on the medial tibia crest. Additional authors attribute MTSS symptoms to a short tibialis posterior tendon or traction from the soleus and/or flexor digitorum longus on the tibia, which corresponds to the typical area of tenderness.[20–22] Stress to the tibia may also increase

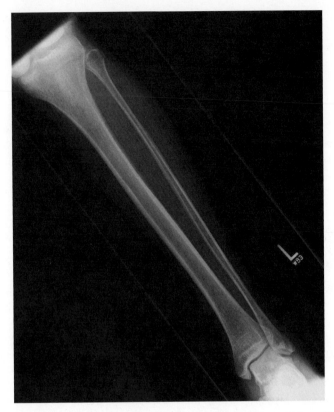

Figure 31-3. Anteroposterior plain radiograph of the leg of a patient without a history of MTSS. Note the clear, consistent periosteal thickness in the medial tibial metaphysis.

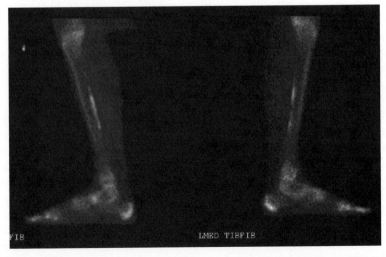

Figure 31-4. Bone scan showing vertically oriented, nonfocal, radioisotope uptake consistent with the diagnosis of MTSS.

due to muscular fatigue with running which reduces muscular shock absorption and shifts the load to the tibia.[17] Regardless of the cause or causes of MTSS, relative rest allows the body to restore balance and heal appropriately.

The primary symptom associated with MTSS is diffuse pain along the posteromedial border of the tibia, most commonly affecting the mid to distal thirds of the tibia.[23–25] Diffuse pain over an area greater than 5 cm is indicative of MTSS, while a smaller region of 2 to 3 cm of localized tenderness potentially accompanied by swelling is more indicative of tibial stress fractures.[25,26] Initial symptoms are typically mild and resolve with prolonged sitting or sleep. If the aggravating activity is continued, the symptoms tend to worsen and pain limits ability to perform the desired activity. If the individual is not involved in an organized sport or lacks a specific training goal, he will typically refrain from further training, which allows the pain to resolve over time. With continued training, the condition typically worsens with pain that becomes more frequent, with earlier onset, interrupts the ability to train, and presents for longer durations after cessation of activity. In many cases, patients experience pain with prolonged standing. Less commonly, pain occurs in prolonged non-weightbearing positions.

Numerous intrinsic and extrinsic risk factors have been proposed to contribute to the development of MTSS. The available research is neither extensive nor is there consensus for support of any single contributing factor. **Extrinsic factors** that have been reported to increase the likelihood of developing MTSS include: rapid increase in weekly training (increasing intensity appears more important than increasing frequency and distance), insufficient footwear, running history of less than 5 years, previous history of MTSS or stress fracture, and use of orthotics.[14,27,28] Further research is necessary to validate many of the reported extrinsic risk factors.[14] Proposed **intrinsic risk factors** include: overpronation, sex (greater risk in women), high body mass index, higher percentage of lower extremity body weight, increased tibial internal rotation during loading phase of running/walking, female athlete triad, and increased hip internal and external rotation.[14,23,25–29] MTSS is likely the result of a combination of these factors.

Physical Therapy Patient/Client Management

The physical therapist may be the first medical professional sought out by a patient for evaluation and treatment of exertional leg pain. Patients may also be referred by other healthcare professionals who commonly evaluate patients with musculoskeletal conditions. If referred to the physical therapist, it is not uncommon for the patient to present with a generalized diagnosis of "leg pain" or "shin splints." Patients may have had imaging studies (e.g., x-rays, bone scans, etc.) prior to referral, but therapists may not have available resources for reviewing the images or have access to the radiology report. When presenting to physical therapy, the athlete is often seeking relief of symptoms with the ability to continue high-impact activities. The physical therapist must perform a thorough subjective and objective evaluation. The training regimen should be explored to allow the therapist to provide appropriate education on training variables and progressive return to high-impact activities. The primary goal for most injured athletes, workers and individuals is to maintain the greatest level of fitness possible while returning to pain-free sport or activity as quickly and as safely as possible. A systematic loading program should be utilized to provide appropriate stress to tissues throughout the healing process.

Examination, Evaluation, and Diagnosis

Individuals presenting with symptoms consistent with MTSS are likely involved in high-impact activities and have had a rapid increase in training. Individuals frequently report diffuse posteromedial shin pain in one or both legs after performing high-impact activities. Typically, pain progresses in the following manner: pain after exercise that resolves with rest; pain during exercise that is reduced with continued training, but returns after activity and resolves slowly with rest; pain during activity that prohibits continued training and continues during and interrupts daily activities. During the history portion of the examination, the physical therapist should obtain information regarding the patient's past medical history. If the patient has experienced similar symptoms previously, it is imperative to learn whether he sought out medical attention, what type of medical providers were seen, whether there was an established diagnosis, and the results of any previous imaging studies. Patient questioning should include easing/aggravating factors and status of symptoms (improving, worsening, or static). In addition, the physical therapist should inquire about the patient's specific training routine, including: frequency, intensity, type of training (sprints, hills, etc.), distance, types of running surfaces on which the individual trains, and which positions or activities reproduce symptoms during daily activity. Females should be questioned regarding frequency of menstrual cycle and for presence or history of disordered eating. The therapist should explore what is motivating the individual to perform the exercise program (job qualification or training, sport, or leisure/health). A thorough history often enables the therapist to develop a reasonable differential diagnosis prior to initiating the physical examination.

Patients presenting with suspicion of MTSS are likely to report a recent history of increased running volume. However, given the spectrum of bone stress injury, it may be difficult to base the diagnosis purely on a clinical examination. Furthermore, the physical therapist must remember that it is possible to have a concomitant condition. Early symptoms of MTSS may be similar to that of tibial stress fracture. A key physical examination finding that helps distinguish MTSS from tibial stress fracture is diffuse tenderness of 5 cm or greater.[25] Numerous special tests have been reported in the literature to assist in the clinical diagnosis of MTSS and tibial stress fracture. These tests were discussed in Case 30. None of the special tests has been consistently shown to demonstrate high diagnostic value.

Radiographic examination should be considered if the individual is adherent to the conservative management program, but is not experiencing a reduction in tibial pain after 3 to 4 weeks. Radiographs should be considered earlier if there is an increase in pain despite treatment compliance. Plain radiographs are typically of minimal benefit and usually do not begin to demonstrate any abnormalities for 14 to 21 days and in some cases remain normal.[16,30] Abnormal findings on radiographs consistent with MTSS consist of periosteal thickening.[16] Although periosteal thickening is the most common finding, this is a nonsensitive finding that is often present in individuals with an extensive physical training background. As a result, technetium bone scan, computed tomography, and magnetic resonance imaging are widely utilized to improve sensitivity and specificity in diagnosing tibial pain.[31,32]

Plan of Care and Interventions

There is a **lack of intervention studies** to guide clinical interventions to accelerate recovery from MTSS. There have been only three randomized controlled trials (all conducted in military populations) on the treatment of MTSS.[13] Relative rest is agreed upon as equal to, if not better than, other treatment options. Physical therapy interventions should be directed at the etiology of the painful overuse syndrome, which most commonly involves an overly aggressive training progression. Relative rest to reduce cyclic loading of the tibias and soft tissues especially during weightbearing is the primary treatment for MTSS. Aquatic therapy, cycling, rowing, gravity-reduced walking/jogging (e.g., harness supported treadmill activity or AlterG anti-gravity treadmills), and elliptical trainers may be incorporated to promote physical conditioning during the period of relative rest as long as the patient adheres to pain-free activity levels. Before returning to running, the patient should have pain-free full weightbearing ambulation with daily activities. Occasionally, assistive devices (e.g., axillary crutches) may be required to reduce the load sufficiently to ensure ambulation is pain-free. Without appropriate rest, the condition typically progresses in severity.

Ice is helpful in reducing MTSS-related pain.[31,33] Nonsteroidal anti-inflammatory drugs (NSAIDs) may be utilized to provide pain relief.[34] However, utilizing NSAIDs to decrease pain and allow increased tolerance for exercise or excessive daily activity may result in progression of the injury and longer duration of symptoms. During the period of relative rest, the individual should experience a gradual reduction in pain in conjunction with some increase in functional ability. If pain continues despite relative rest (i.e., pain-free activity) for approximately 2 weeks, then weightbearing activity should be reduced (authors' clinical experience). If pain increases, function is reduced, or the patient experiences a lack of improvement, then daily activity should be assessed and adjusted appropriately. Although researchers have found an association between orthotics and an increased risk of MTSS, orthotics have been shown to help reduce symptoms associated with MTSS.[35-37] The response to orthotics is dependent on the individual patient, ranging from immediate relief to improvement over days to weeks. While shoe selection based upon foot type has been long advocated, current literature suggests no significant effect of shoe selection on preventing leg injuries in military populations.[38] Posterior leg stretching (e.g., gastrocnemius-soleus, posterior tibialis, etc.) has been advocated primarily on the basis of the muscular insertions at or about the region of MTSS.[18,19,22] A prospective study by Loudon and Dolphino[39] assessed calf stretching and off-the-shelf shoe inserts in 23 adults with symptoms of MTSS. The authors reported that 65% of the subjects had a 50% reduction in pain at the end of the 3-week intervention. While the results of this study may support calf stretching in the treatment of MTSS, the study did not isolate stretching as an independent intervention and did not include a comparison or control group. In addition, limited passive ankle dorsiflexion was not found to be a risk factor for MTSS by Moen et al.[28] Ultrasound, phonophoresis, cortisone injections, bone electrical stimulators, and acupuncture have not been shown to be beneficial in treating exercise-induced leg pain, including MTSS.[30,31,40–42]

If the condition fails to improve after 4 weeks of physical therapy interventions, we recommend that the patient be referred to another healthcare provider (such as an orthopaedic surgeon) who specializes in musculoskeletal injuries for additional evaluation, work-up, and to ensure that no other condition is responsible for symptoms. In recalcitrant cases of MTSS, fasciotomy of the superficial and deep posterior compartments has been performed with reports of up to 72% to 78% improvement following fasciotomy.[43–45] Surgery involving cauterizing the periosteum of the tibia had a 90% success rate at 6-month follow-up.[8] Surgical intervention may act to denervate the periosteum.[46] Although significant improvement in pain has been reported following surgery, the rate of return to presymptomatic levels of activity has been reported at less than 50%.[45]

Evidence-Based Clinical Recommendations

SORT: Strength of Recommendation Taxonomy

A: Consistent, good-quality patient-oriented evidence
B: Inconsistent or limited-quality patient-oriented evidence
C: Consensus, disease-oriented evidence, usual practice, expert opinion, or case series

1. Extrinsic risk factors are associated with development of MTSS. **Grade C**

2. Intrinsic risk factors are associated with development of MTSS. **Grade B**

3. Interventions such as ice and stretching are associated with better patient outcomes than relative rest in the management of MTSS. **Grade C**

COMPREHENSION QUESTIONS

31.1 What intrinsic risk factor for MTSS is *most* consistently supported in the literature?

A. Higher BMI

B. Limited hip range of motion

C. Limited ankle range of motion

D. Overpronation

31.2 What treatment approach has been demonstrated to be *most* effective in the management of MTSS?

A. Acupuncture

B. Laser treatment

C. Relative rest

D. Phonophoresis

ANSWERS

31.1 **D.** Overpronation is the most widely reported and agreed upon intrinsic risk factor for the development of MTSS.[15]

31.2 **C.** There is a lack of intervention studies to guide the management of MTSS. There have been only three randomized controlled trials (all conducted in military populations) on the treatment of MTSS. Relative rest is agreed upon as equal to, if not better than, other treatment options.

REFERENCES

1. Taunton JE, Clement DB, Webber D. Lower extremity stress fractures in athletes. *Phys Sportsmed.* 1981;9:77-86.

2. Clement DB, Taunton JE, Smart GW, McNicol KL. Survey of overuse running injuries. *Phys Sportsmed.* 1981;9:47-58.

3. Epperly T, Fields K. Epidemiology of running injuries. In: O'Conner FG, Wilder R, Nirschl R, eds. *Textbook of Running Medicine.* New York, NY: McGraw-Hill; 2001:1-11.

4. Bennell KL, Malcolm SA, Thomas SA, Wark JD, Brukner PD. The incidence and distribution of stress fractures in competitive track and field athletes. A twelve-month prospective study. *Am J Sports Med.* 1996;24:211-217.

5. Brubaker CE, James SL. Injuries to runners. *J Sports Med.* 1974;2:189-198.

6. Styf J. Diagnosis of exercise-induced pain in the anterior aspect of the lower leg. *Am J Sports Med.* 1988;16:165-169.

7. Styf JR, Korner LM. Diagnosis of chronic anterior compartment syndrome in the lower leg. *Acta Orthop Scand.* 1987;58:139-144.

8. Detmer DE. Chronic shin splints: classification and management of medial tibial stress syndrome. *Sports Med.* 1986;3:436-446.

9. Chambers HG. Medial tibial stress syndrome: evaluation and management. *Oper Techniq Sports Med.* 1995;3:274-277.

10. Edwards PH Jr, Wright ML, Hartman JF. A practical approach for the differential diagnosis of chronic leg pain in the athlete. *Am J Sports Med.* 2005;33:1241-1249.

11. Tweed JL, Avil SJ, Campbell JA, Barnes MR. Etiologic factors in the development of medial tibial stress syndrome: a review of the literature. *J Am Podiatr Med Assoc.* 2008;98:107-111.

12. Craig DI. Current developments concerning medial tibial stress syndrome. *Phys Sportsmed.* 2009;37:39-44.

13. Moen MH, Tol JL, Weir A, Steuenebrink M, De Winter TC. Medial tibial stress syndrome: a critical review. *Sports Med.* 2009;39:523-546.

14. Brukner P, Bennell K, Matheson G. *Stress Fractures.* Victoria, Australia: Blackwell Science Asia; 1999.

15. Johnell O, Rausing A, Wendeberg M, Westlin N. Morphological bone changes in shin splints. *Clin Orthop Relat Res.* 1982;167:180-184.

16. Deutsch AL, Coel MN, Mink JH. Imaging of stress injuries to bone. Radiography, scintigraphy and MR imaging. *Clin Sports Med.* 1997;16:275-290.

17. Magnusson HI, Westlin NE, Nyqvist F, Gardsell P, Seeman E, Karlsson MK. Abnormally decreased regional bone density in athletes with medial tibial stress syndrome. *Am J Sports Med.* 2001;29:712-715.

18. Stickley CD, Hetzler RK, Kimura IF, Lozanoff S. Crural fascia and muscle origins related to medial tibial stress syndrome symptom location. *Med Sci Sports Exec.* 2009;41:1991-1996.

19. Bouche RT, Johnson CH. Medial tibial stress syndrome (tibial fasciitis): a proposed pathomechanical model involving fascial traction. *J Am Podiatr Med Assoc.* 2007;97:31-36.

20. Saxena A, O'Brien T, Bunce D. Anatomic dissection of the tibialis posterior muscle and its correlation to medial tibial stress syndrome. *J Foot Surg.*1990;29:105-108.

21. Michael RH, Holder LE. The soleus syndrome. A cause of medial tibial stress (shin splints). *Am J Sports Med.*1985;13:87-94.

22. Beck BR, Osternig LR. Medial tibial stress syndrome. The location of muscles in the leg and relation to symptoms. *J Bone Joint Surg Am.* 1994;76:1057-1061.

23. Yates B, White S. The incidence and risk factors in the development of medial tibial stress syndrome among naval recruits. *Am J Sports Med.* 2004;32:772-780.

24. Bennett JE, Reinking MF, Pluemer B, Pentel A, Seaton M, Killian C. Factors contributing to the development of medial tibial stress syndrome in high school runners. *J Orthop Sports Phys Ther.* 2001;31:504-510.

25. Batt ME, Ugalde V, Anderson MW, Shelton DK . A prospective controlled study of diagnostic imaging for acute shin splints. *Med Sci Sports Exerc.* 1998;30:1564-1571.

26. Anderson MW, Ugalde V, Batt M, Gacayan J. Shin splints: MR appearance in a preliminary study. *Radiology.* 1997:204:177-180.

27. Burne SG, Khan KM, Boudville PB, et al. Risk factors associated with exertional medial tibial pain: a 12-month prospective clinical study. *Br J Sports Med.* 2004;38:441-445.

28. Moen MH. Bongers T, Bakker EW, et al. Risk factors and prognostic indicators for medial tibial stress syndrome. *Scan J Med Sci Sports.* 2012;22:34-39.

29. Lauder TD, Williams MV, Campbell CS, Davis G, Sherman R, Pulos E. The female athlete triad: prevalance in military women. *Mil Med.* 1999;164:630-635.

30. Savoca CJ. Stress fractures. A classification of the earliest radiographic signs. *Radiology.* 1971;100: 519-524.

31. Fredericson M, Bergman AG, Hoffman KL, Dillingham MS. Tibial stress reactions in runners. Correlation of clinical symptoms and scintigraphy with a new magnetic resonance imaging grading system. *Am J Sports Med.* 1995;23:472-481.

32. Gaeta M, Minutoli F, Vinci S, et al. High-resolution CT grading of tibial stress reactions in distance runners. *AJR Am J Roentgenol.* 2006;187:789-793.

33. Andrish JT, Bergfeld JA, Walheim J. A prospective study of the management of shin splints. *J Bone Joint Surg Am.* 1974;56:1697-1700.

34. Couture CJ, Karlson KA. Tibial stress injuries; decisive diagnosis and treatment of 'shin splints.' *Phys Sportsmed.* 2002;30:29-36.

35. Schwellnus MP, Jordaan G, Noakes TD. Prevention of common overuse injuries by the use of shock absorbing insoles. A prospective study. *Am J Sports Med.* 1990;18:636-641.

36. Hubbard TJ, Carpenter EM, Cordova ML. Contributing factors to medial tibial stress syndrome: a prospective investigation. *Med Sci Sports Exerc.* 2009;41:490-496.

37. Eickhoff CA, Hossain SA, Slawski DP. From the field. Effects of prescribed foot orthoses on medial tibial stress syndrome in collegiate cross-country runners. *Clin Kinesiol.* 2000;54:76-80.

38. Knapik JJ, Trone DW, Swedler DI, et al. Injury reduction effectiveness of assigning running shoes based on plantar shape in marine corps basic training. *Am J Sports Med.* 2010;38:1759-1767.

39. Loudon JK. Dolphino MR. Use of foot orthoses and calf stretching for individuals with medial tibial stress syndrome. *Foot Ankle Spec.* 2010;3:15-20.

40. Beck BR. Tibial stress injuries. An aetiological review for the purposes of guiding management. *Sports Med.* 1998;26:265-279.

41. Morris RH. Medial tibial syndrome: a treatment protocol using electric current. *Chiropractic Sports Med.* 1991;5:5-8.

42. Schulman RA. Tibial shin splints treated with a single acupuncture session: case report and review of the literature. *J Am Med Acupuncture*. 2002;13:7-9.

43. Clanton TO, Solcher BW. Chronic leg pain in the athlete. *Clin Sports Med*. 1994;13:743-759.

44. Holen KJ, Engebretsen L, Grontvedt T, Rossvoll I, Hammer S, Stoltz V. Surgical treatment of medial tibial stress syndrome (shin splint) by fasciotomy of the superficial posterior compartment of the leg. *Scand J Med Sci Sports*. 1995;5:40-43.

45. Yates B, Allen MJ, Barnes MR. Outcome of surgical treatment of medial tibial stress syndrome. *J Bone Joint Surg Am*. 2003;85-A:1974-1980.

46. Wallensten R. Results of fasciotomy in patients with medial tibial syndrome or chronic anterior-compartment syndrome. *J Bone Joint Surg Am*. 1983;65:1252-1255.

DISCLAIMER:

The views expressed in this chapter are those of the authors and do not necessarily reflect the official policy or position of the Department of the Navy, Department of Defense, or the U.S. Government.

Achilles Tendinosis

Jason Brumitt

A 35-year-old male was referred by his orthopaedic physician to an outpatient physical therapy clinic with a diagnosis of Achilles tendinosis on his right side. He has experienced a gradual increase in pain for 2 years. His worsening symptoms have limited his ability to run or play basketball. Previous therapies (nonsteroidal anti-inflammatories, ultrasound, manual therapy, custom orthotics) have failed to improve symptoms. His orthopaedist has recommended surgery. However, the patient would like to try physical therapy again.

▶ Based on the patient's diagnosis, what do you anticipate may be the contributing factors to his condition?
▶ What are the most appropriate physical therapy interventions?

KEY DEFINITIONS

ECCENTRIC EXERCISE: Form of exercise in which the muscle(s) are allowed to lengthen gradually in the presence of an applied load

MICRODIALYSIS: Laboratory technique in which a catheter is inserted into a tendon at the site of suspected degenerative changes in order to study metabolism within the tendon

NEOVASCULARIZATION: Growth of new blood vessels

TENDINOPATHY: General term for a diseased state of a tendon; tendinosis may be referred to as a chronic tendinopathy

TENDINOSIS: Chronic, painful degenerative condition of a tendon marked by *absence* of inflammation, a loss of function, and the presence of a thickened region (*i.e.*, a painful nodule)

Objectives

1. Describe the differences between tendinitis and tendinosis.
2. Describe the pathophysiology associated with Achilles tendinosis.
3. Prescribe an evidence-based resistance training program for an individual with Achilles tendinosis.

Physical Therapy Considerations

PT considerations during management of the individual with a diagnosis of Achilles tendinosis:

▶ **General physical therapy plan of care/goals:** Decrease pain; increase muscular flexibility; increase active and/or passive range of motion; increase lower quadrant strength; prevent or minimize loss of aerobic fitness capacity

▶ **Physical therapy interventions:** Patient education regarding functional anatomy and injury pathomechanics; muscular flexibility exercises; resistance exercises to increase muscular strength of the gastrocnemius and soleus; aerobic exercise program

▶ **Precautions during physical therapy:** Monitor vital signs

▶ **Complications interfering with physical therapy:** Patient noncompliance with exercise program

Understanding the Health Condition

The Achilles tendon is the strongest tendon in the human body; however, it is at risk for acute injury (tendinitis), degeneration (tendinosis), and/or rupture.[1-3] The tendon is the distal extension of the gastrocnemius and soleus muscles and inserts into the calcaneus. A region of decreased blood supply is frequently found at the midportion of the tendon (2-6 cm proximal to its insertion site)—a location associated with Achilles tendon injuries.

Tendinosis is a chronic, painful state marked by a different pathophysiology than that associated with an acute tendon injury (tendinitis).[4] Tendinosis is thought to be the result of overuse and age-related changes with a failure of proper tissue healing.[2] In a study of ten adults undergoing surgery for Achilles tendinopathy, de Mos et al.[5] found increased water content, matrix degeneration, increased collagen turnover rate, a high amount of denatured or damaged collagen, and increased enzymatic activity. Athletic individuals (males > females) between the ages of 35 to 50 years have an increased risk of injury to the Achilles tendon. Achilles tendinosis has been most frequently reported in runners, basketball players, and soccer players.[3,6,7] Degenerative tendon conditions have also been identified in nonactive individuals.[8] Left untreated, pain will persist and the condition may lead to rupture of the Achilles tendon.

Tendinosis is distinct from acute tendinitis because it is *not* associated with local chemically mediated inflammation.[9-10] Intratendinous microdialysis studies have investigated the metabolism within the tendonitic Achilles. Prostaglandins associated with chemical inflammation are *absent*, suggesting that if any swelling is present it may be the result of neurogenic inflammation.[9-10] In fact, neuropeptides (substance P and calcitonin gene-related peptide) that may contribute to neurogenic inflammation have been identified in individuals with Achilles tendinosis.[10-12] Microdialysis techniques have also identified glutamate (an excitatory neurotransmitter) and lactate in the midportion of the tendonitic Achilles.[7,13] Alfredson et al.[13] have suggested that the fourfold increase in glutamate observed in subjects with Achilles tendinosis may serve as a mediator of pain in this chronic condition. It had been theorized that exercise may decrease glutamate concentration within the tendon; however, glutamate levels in the Achilles of patients with tendinosis were unchanged after completion of a 12-week treatment program of an eccentric exercise program.[13] Alfredson et al.[7] have also suggested that the presence of lactate in the tendonitic Achilles indicates an anaerobic state; however, it has yet to be determined whether ischemia is a precursor to tendinosis or the result of tendonitic changes.

In patients with Achilles tendinosis, neovascularization has been visualized (utilizing grey-scale ultrasonography and color Doppler techniques) primarily on the ventral side of the Achilles at the tendon's midportion (the region of the thickened painful nodule). These blood vessels are not present in individuals without Achilles tendinosis.[14,15] The neovascularization in the region of the Achilles may occur in response to a hypoxic environment and/or increased glutamate concentrations.[15] Accompanying the neovascularization are sensory and sympathetic nerves.[15-17]

Physical Therapy Patient/Client Management

The primary physical therapy interventions for a patient with Achilles tendinosis should be therapeutic exercise (specifically eccentric exercises).[4,10] Additional treatments including modalities, soft tissue mobilization, footwear evaluation, and/or orthotics have been suggested as potentially useful adjuncts.[4,10] Patients who fail to benefit from physical therapy interventions may benefit from a topical glyceryl trinitrate patch, glucocorticoid injection, or extracorporeal shock wave therapy.[4,10] Sclerosing injections or surgery are invasive treatments performed by orthopaedic physicians for patients who fail to improve with the aforementioned treatments.[4,10]

Examination, Evaluation, and Diagnosis

A diagnosis of tendinosis is based on clinical examination findings and may be confirmed with imaging studies.[4] Diagnostic imaging techniques (ultrasonography, magnetic resonance imaging) or biopsy are used by physicians to confirm the diagnosis.[4] The patient with suspected or confirmed Achilles tendinosis typically reports a history of pain, an inability to participate in sports without pain, and/ or a loss of function. The patient may present with a lack of strength and/or pain during manual muscle testing. In some individuals, a functional movement (*e.g.*, a heel raise on the involved side) must be performed to reproduce the pain. An elite athlete may need to perform a single-legged vertical jump or hop to reproduce his symptoms. The patient may present with asymmetrical or deficient range of motion patterns including a lack of dorsiflexion.[18] Palpation of the tendon may reveal tenderness and a nodule usually at the mid-portion of the tendon (2-6 cm proximal to the insertion site). To help rule out an Achilles tendon rupture, the physical therapist should confirm that the patient has a negative Thompson test (*i.e.*, with an intact Achilles tendon, the non-weightbearing, involved ankle should passively plantarflex when the therapist squeezes the calf).

Plan of Care and Interventions

Therapeutic exercise, modalities, orthotics, and manual therapy techniques have been suggested as potential interventions for patients with a diagnosis of Achilles tendinosis. There is a growing body of evidence that suggests eccentric exercises should be a prescribed as a primary intervention in a conservative treatment program.

Alfredson et al.[19] found that a 12-week **eccentric exercise program** for the gastrocnemius and the soleus helped to significantly decrease pain and increase calf strength in recreational adult runners with Achilles tendinosis. Thirty recreational athletes who had failed to improve with prior bouts of physical therapy and other conservative treatments were either in the experimental group (n = 15; mean age 44.3 ± 7.0 years) or the control group (n = 15; mean age 39.6 ± 7.9 years). At the end of the 12-week training period, all individuals in the experimental group were able to return to preinjury training levels, whereas those in the control group (who did not receive any treatment) elected to have surgery. There were only

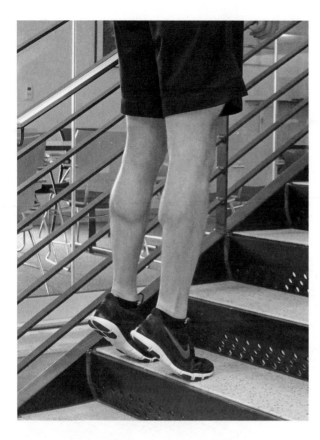

Figure 32-1. Patient elevates body by plantarflexing uninvolved left ankle. At the top of the motion (full plantarflexion), the patient stands with both ankles in plantarflexion and then shifts all of his weight to the involved right leg.

two exercises prescribed for the experimental group; each exercise was performed twice daily with 3 sets of 15 repetitions. To perform each exercise, the patient first assumes an upright posture with his forefeet supported on a step or stair. Next, the patient elevates his body by plantarflexing his *uninvolved* ankle. Then the patient shifts his weight to load the injured lower extremity (Fig. 32-1). Finally, the patient performs the eccentric component of the exercise by lowering the heel of his *symptomatic* limb below the plane of the step. Figures 32-2 and 32-3 demonstrate this eccentric component with emphasis on the gastrocnemius and soleus, respectively. Subjects in the experimental group were instructed to complete all repetitions even in the presence of pain. Once each subject was able to perform the exercises without pain, he/she was instructed to perform the exercises with weight in a backpack or to perform the exercises with a standing calf machine. Both groups realized significant improvements in pain (measured by a visual analog scale) from baseline. However, all 15 subjects in the experimental group were able to return to running (preinjury level) at the completion of the 12-week rehabilitation program, whereas it took an average of 24 weeks for subjects in the control group to return to running after surgery.[19]

Follow-up studies have investigated the mechanisms by which the eccentric training program has been successful in patients with Achilles tendinosis. It has

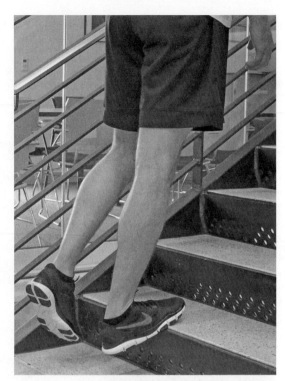

Figure 32-2. Eccentric component with emphasis on the gastrocnemius. After shifting weight to the involved right lower extremity, the patient lowers his body by allowing dorsiflexion at the ankle, keeping the right knee in full extension.

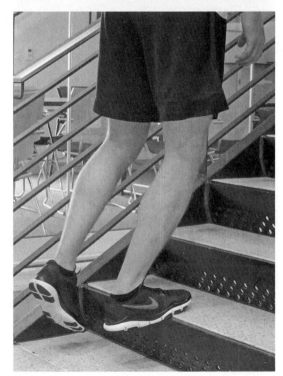

Figure 32-3. Eccentric component with emphasis on the soleus. After shifting weight to the involved right lower extremity, the patient lowers his body by allowing dorsiflexion at the ankle, keeping the right knee slightly flexed.

been shown that the eccentric training program increased the collagen synthesis rate in injured male soccer players, but not in healthy controls.[6] The training program also appeared to help decrease (i.e., normalize) tendon size.[20,21] The observed destruction of the new blood vessels and associated nerves after an eccentric program may account for the decrease in pain experienced by patients. It is thought that the forces generated during the eccentric exercises[19] destroy those structures.[5,22]

Combining eccentric exercise with laser therapy may also facilitate healing of Achilles tendinosis. Stergioulas et al.[23] compared outcomes between two groups that received either an eccentric training program with **low-level laser therapy** (LLLT) or the eccentric training program with a placebo laser treatment over an 8-week treatment period. Subjects in the experimental group received the LLLT treatment in six spots on the affected Achilles tendon (wavelength 820 nm; optical output 30 mW; irradiation area 0.5 cm^2; energy per session 0.9 J). At the final assessment point (4 weeks after completion of the study), those receiving the LLLT treatment reported significantly reduced pain, improved active dorsiflexion, decreased morning stiffness, and decreased tenderness to palpation compared to those receiving the placebo laser treatment.[21] The prescribed eccentric training program differed from Alfredson et al.[19] Instead of having the subjects perform 3 sets of 15 repetitions twice per day for 12 weeks, Stergioulas et al.[23] prescribed one set of 5 repetitions on day one with progression to 12 sets of 12 repetitions (with a 1-minute rest between sets) by week 4. This program was performed only 4 days per week for 2 months. Patients were instructed that mild pain (defined as < 50 mm on a 100-mm visual analog scale) was allowed during the performance of the exercise. They were instructed not to exercise if their postexercise pain was "disabling" or if it continued into the next day. Once the subject was able to meet this goal without pain, a 4-kg weight was added to the subject's backpack. Subjects were also instructed to perform 5 repetitions of both gastrocnemius and soleus stretches (15-second holds per repetition) at the start and end of each treatment session. Other investigations that combined eccentric exercise with either the use of night splints or an AirHeel brace were not associated with superior outcomes when compared to eccentric exercise alone.[24,25]

A majority of the research literature has assessed the positive outcomes associated with eccentric exercise for midportion Achilles tendinosis. A **modified eccentric training program appears to also help some patients with insertional Achilles tendinosis.**[26] Jonsson et al.[26] prescribed the same eccentric training protocol described by Alfredson et al.[19] (3 sets of 15 repetitions, twice per day for 12 weeks), except that the ankle was not allowed to load into dorsiflexion. In other words, eccentric loading was performed on a flat surface instead of over a stair (Figs. 32-4 and 32-5). Dorsiflexion was prohibited in order to avoid the mechanical impingement that occurs between the calcaneus, Achilles tendon, and the bursa, which results in increased compressive forces. Over two-thirds of patients with insertional Achilles tendinosis reported satisfaction and a return to preinjury activity with this modified eccentric training protocol.

An alternate exercise program for patients with Achilles tendinosis has been reported by Silbernagel et al.[27] Their four-phase exercise program starts with concentric heel raises (single- and double-legged standing and sitting toe raises) and

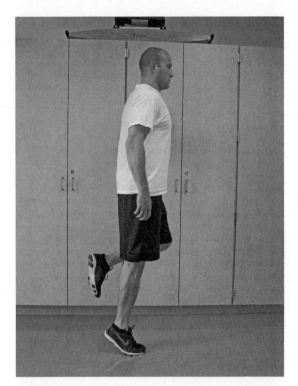

Figure 32-4. First, patient stands on uninvolved left leg and plantarflexes to elevate the body in order to avoid concentric plantarflexion on involved right leg. Next, he shifts his weight to the involved right leg to begin eccentric lowering of the body.

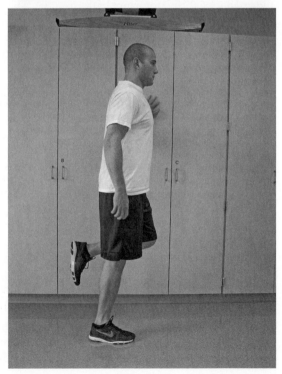

Figure 32-5. Patient eccentrically lowers the body to the floor (end position).

standing eccentric toe raises (eccentric loading of the involved ankle; similar to that described by Alfredson et al.[19]). Later stages included eccentric calf muscle training (with added weight) as described by Alfredson et al.,[19] double- and single-legged heel raises at the edge of a stair, quick-rebounding toe raises, and plyometrics.[27] Subjects experienced significant improvements in measures of pain, power, and muscular endurance compared to baseline measures. At the 5-year follow-up, a majority of subjects had made a full recovery.[28] Future investigations are warranted to determine which of the aforementioned programs lead to the best patient outcomes.

Alfredson et al.[10] have also recommended a treatment algorithm for patients who have failed to improve with an eccentric training program. First, after the initial exercise training period, a topical glyceryl nitrate patch (GNP) is applied to the tendon (up to 24 weeks) and the exercise program is continued. It has been proposed that GNP may release nitric oxide which may facilitate collagen synthesis, but there is disagreement in the literature regarding this proposed mechanism.[29,30] During this time, the authors recommended the addition of massage and electrotherapy to the involved tendon; however, there has been no evidence to support the effectiveness of these adjuncts. If the patient still has pain after 24 weeks of patch use and continued therapy, glucocorticoid injections and extracorporeal shock wave therapy may be initiated.[10,31] Sclerosing injections to the ventral portion of the tendon have been performed in order to destroy neovascularization.[10,32,33] Finally, if the aforementioned procedures fail, a surgical procedure (*e.g.*, debridement, reconstruction) should be considered.[10,34,35]

Evidence-Based Clinical Recommendations

SORT: Strength of Recommendation Taxonomy

A: Consistent, good-quality patient oriented evidence
B: Inconsistent or limited-quality patient-oriented evidence
C: Consensus, disease-oriented evidence, usual practice, expert opinion, or case series

1. An exercise program consisting of eccentric exercises for the gastrocnemius and soleus muscles helps reduce pain and restore function in patients with *midportion* Achilles tendinosis. **Grade A**

2. Low-level laser therapy added to an eccentric exercise program may provide superior pain reduction and increased ankle range of motion compared to the eccentric exercise program alone. **Grade B**

3. An exercise program consisting of modified eccentric exercises for the gastrocnemius and soleus may help reduce pain and restore function in patients with *insertional* Achilles tendinosis. **Grade B**

COMPREHENSION QUESTIONS

32.1 The reduction of pain experienced by patients after completing a 12-week eccentric exercise program for midportion Achilles tendinosis is thought to be due to destruction of which of the following structures?

A. New blood vessels and associated nerves

B. Tendon sheath

C. Collagen fibers

D. Scar tissue

32.2 Which of the following statements is accurate when performing an eccentric exercise intervention for midportion Achilles tendinosis (as described by Alfredson et al.[19])?

A. The ankle should be allowed to dorsiflex to 10°.

B. The patient should not experience pain during exercise.

C. The patient should not concentrically plantarflex the involved ankle.

D. The patient should eccentrically plantarflex the uninvolved ankle.

ANSWERS

32.1 **A.** Imaging studies performed after the completion of a training program have revealed a normalized tendon structure with a decrease in new blood vessels and associated nerves.

32.2 **C.** Alfredson et al.[19] described an eccentric exercise protocol that requires the patient to concentrically plantarflex the uninvolved ankle followed by eccentrically lowering of the body, allowing the involved ankle to dorsiflex as much as possible (the heel is lowered below top of the step/stair). Pain is allowed during the performance of these exercises.

REFERENCES

1. Mann RA, Chou L. Effective intervention for Achilles tendinitis and tendinosis: toe rise helps differentiate tendinitis from tendinosis. *J Musculoskeletal Med.* 1998;15:57-62.

2. Heckman DS, Gluck GS, Parekh SG. Tendon disorders of the foot and ankle, part 2: Achilles tendon disorders. *Am J Sports Med.* 2009; 37:1223-1234.

3. Schepsis AA, Jones H, Haas AL. Achilles tendon disorders in athletes. *Am J Sports Med.* 2002; 30:287-305.

4. Alfredson H. The chronic painful Achilles and patellar tendon: research on basic biology and treatment. *Scand J Med Sci Sports.* 2005;15:252-259.

5. de Mos M, van El B, DeGroot J, et al. Achilles tendinosis: changes in biochemical composition and collagen turnover rate. *Am J Sports Med.* 2007;35:1549-1556.

6. Langberg H, Ellingsgaard H, Madsen T, et al. Eccentric rehabilitation exercise increases peritendinous type I collagen synthesis in humans with Achilles tendinosis. *Scand J Med Sci Sports.* 2007;17:61-66.

7. Alfredson H, Bjur D, Thorsen K, Lorentzon R, Sandstrom P. High intratendinous lactate levels in painful chronic Achilles tendinosis. An investigation using microdialysis technique. *J Orthop Res.* 2002;20:934-938.

8. Astrom M. Partial rupture in chronic Achilles tendinopathy. A retrospective analysis of 342 cases. *Acta Orthop Scand.* 1998; 69:404-407.

9. Alfredson H, Lorentzon M, Backman S, Backman A, Lerner UH. cDNA-arrays and real-time quantitative PCR techniques in the investigation of chronic Achilles tendinosis. *J Orthop Res.* 2003;21:970-975.

10. Alfredson H, Cook J. A treatment algorithm for managing Achilles tendinopathy: new treatment options. *Br J Sports Med.* 2007;41:211-216.

11. Scott A, Khan KM, Roberts CR, Cook JL, Duronio V. What do we mean by the term "inflammation"? A contemporary basic science update for sports medicine. *Br J Sports Med.* 2004;38:372-380.

12. Andersson G, Danielson P, Alfredson H, Forsgren S. Presence of substance P and the neurokinin-1 receptor in tenocytes of the human Achilles tendon. *Regul Pept.* 2008;150:81-87.

13. Alfredson H, Lorentzon R. Intratendinous glutamate levels and eccentric training in chronic Achilles tendinosis: a prospective study using microdialysis technique. *Knee Surg Sports Traumatol Arthrosc.* 2003;11:196-199.

14. Ohberg L, Lorentzon R, Alfredson H. Neovascularization in Achilles tendons with painful tendinosis but not in normal tendons: an ultrasonographic investigation. *Knee Surg Sports Traumatol Arthrosc.* 2001;9:233-238.

15. Alfredson H, Ohberg L, Forsgren S. Is vasculo-neural ingrowth the cause of pain in chronic Achilles tendinosis? An investigation using ultrasonography and colour Doppler, immunohistochemistry, and diagnostic injections. *Knee Surg Sports Traumatol Arthrosc.* 2003;11:334-338.

16. Andersson G, Danielson P, Alfredson H, Forsgren S. Nerve-related characteristics of ventral paratendinous tissue in chronic Achilles tendinosis. *Knee Surg Sports Traumatol Arthrosc.* 2007;15: 1272-1279.

17. Bjur D, Alfredson H, Forsgren S. The innervation pattern of the human Achilles tendon: studies of the normal and tendinosis tendon with markers for general and sensory innervation. *Cell Tissue Res.* 2005;320:201-206.

18. Kaufman KR, Brodine SK, Shaffer RA, Johnson CW, Cullison TR. The effect of foot structure and range of motion on musculoskeletal overuse injuries. *Am J Sports Med.* 1999;27:585-593.

19. Alfredson H, Pietila T, Jonsson P, Lorentzon R. Heavy-load eccentric calf muscle training for the treatment of chronic Achilles tendinosis. *Am J Sports Med.* 1998;26:360-366.

20. Gardin A, Movin T, Svensson L, Shalabi A. The long-term clinical and MRI results following eccentric calf muscle training in chronic Achilles tendinosis. *Skeletal Radiol.* 2010;39:435-442.

21. Shalabi A, Kristoffersen-Wilberg M, Svensson L, Aspelin P, Movin T. Eccentric training of the gastrocnemius-soleus complex in chronic Achilles tendinopathy results in decreased tendon volume and intratendinous signal as evaluated by MRI. *Am J Sports Med.* 2004;32:1286-1296.

22. Ohberg L, Alfredson H. Effects of neovascularization behind the good results with eccentric training in chronic mid-portion Achilles tendinosis? *Knee Surg Sports Traumatol Arthrosc.* 2004;12:465-470.

23. Stergioulas A, Stergioula M, Aarskog R, Lopes-Martins RA, Bjordal JM. Effects of lower-level laser therapy and eccentric exercises in the treatment of recreational athletes with chronic achilles tendinopathy. *Am J Sports Med.* 2008;36:881-887.

24. Petersen W, Welp R, Rosenbaum D. Chronic Achilles tendinopathy: a prospective randomized study comparing the therapeutic effect of eccentric training, the airheel brace, and a combination of both. *Am J Sports Med.* 2007;35:1659-1667.

25. de Jonge S, de Vos RJ, Van Schie HT, Verhaar JA, Weir A, Tol JL. One-year follow-up of a randomised controlled trial on added splinting to eccentric exercises in chronic midportion Achilles tendinopathy. *Br J Sports Med.* 2010;44:673-677.

26. Jonsson P, Alfredson H, Sunding K, Fahlstrom M, Cook J. New regimen for eccentric calf-muscle training in patients with chronic insertional Achilles tendinopathy: results of a pilot study. *Br J Sports Med.* 2008;42:746-749.

27. Silbernagel KG, Thomee R, Eriksson BI, Karlsson J. Continued sports activity, using a pain-monitoring model, during rehabilitation in patients with Achilles tendinopathy: a randomized controlled study. *Am J Sports Med.* 2007;35:897-906.

28. Silbernagel KG, Brorsson A, Lundberg M. The majority of patients with Achilles tendinopathy recover fully when treated with exercise alone: a 5-year follow-up. *Am J Sports Med.* 2011;39: 607-613.

29. Paoloni JA, Appleyard RC, Nelson J, Murrell GA. Topical glycerin trinitrate treatment of chronic noninsertational achilles tendinopathy. A randomized, double-blind, placebo-controlled trial. *J Bone Joint Surg Am.* 2004;86-A:916-922.

30. Kane TP, Ismail M, Calder JD. Topical glyceryl trinitrate and noninsertional Achilles tendinopathy: a clinical and cellular investigation. *Am J Sports Med.* 2008; 36:1160-1163.

31. Rompe JD, Furia J, Maffulli N. Eccentric loading versus eccentric loading plus shock-wave treatment for midportion achilles tendinopathy: a randomized controlled trial. *Am J Sports Med.* 2009;37: 463-470.

32. Willberg L, Sunding K, Ohberg L, Forssblad M, Fahlstrom M, Alfredson H. Sclerosing injections to treat midportion Achilles tendinosis: a randomised controlled study evaluating two different concentrations of polidocanol. *Knee Surg Sports Traumatol Arthrosc.* 2008;16:859-864.

33. Lind B, Ohberg L, Alfredson H. Sclerosing polidocanol injections in mid-portion Achilles tendinosis: remaining good clinical results and decreased tendon thickness at 2-year follow-up. *Knee Surg Sports Traumatol Arthrosc.* 2006;14:1327-1332.

34. Maffulli N, Longo UG, Loppini M, Spiezia F, Denaro V. New options in the management of tendinopathy. *Open Access Journal of Sports Medicine.* 2010:1;29-37.

35. Alfredson H. Ultrasound and Doppler-guided mini-surgery to treat midportion Achilles tendinosis: results of a large material and randomised study comparing two scraping techniques. *Br J Sports Med.* 2011;45:407-410.

Plantar Fasciitis

Casey A. Unverzagt
Kyle Botten
Caryn Gehrke

CASE 33

A 45-year-old male self-referred to an outpatient physical therapy clinic with complaints of left heel pain for the past several months. He denies any specific trauma and also denies pain in the right heel or foot. He reports that ibuprofen helps his pain temporarily, but that overall the pain is getting worse. He reports that the pain is worse in the morning and evenings, and that he has had to terminate his walking program due to the pain. His goal is to eliminate his pain and return to walking 1 to 2 miles per day, 4 to 5 times per week.

► Based on the patient's subjective report, and likely diagnosis of plantar fasciitis, what do you anticipate may be the contributing factors to his condition?
► What examination signs may be associated with this diagnosis?
► What are the most appropriate physical therapy outcome measures to assess his functional capacity?
► What are the most appropriate physical therapy interventions?

KEY DEFINITIONS

PLANTAR FASCIITIS: Inflammatory condition affecting the plantar fascia and the perifascial structures of the foot

WINDLASS MECHANISM: Describes the manner by which the plantar fascia supports the foot during weightbearing; provides a model of the biomechanical stresses placed on the plantar fascia[1]

Objectives

1. Describe plantar fasciitis and identify potential risk factors associated with this diagnosis.

2. Describe appropriate joint range of motion and/or flexibility exercises for a person with plantar fasciitis.

3. Discuss current evidence supporting the use of appropriate modalities, taping, and orthotic fabrications for a person with plantar fasciitis.

Physical Therapy Considerations

PT considerations during management of the individual with a diagnosis of plantar fasciitis:

▶ **General physical therapy plan of care/goals:** Decrease pain; increase muscular flexibility; prevent or minimize loss of aerobic fitness capacity

▶ **Physical therapy interventions:** Patient education regarding functional anatomy and injury pathomechanics; modalities to decrease pain and inflammation; manual therapy to decrease pain and increase joint mobility; stretching exercises to address tight triceps surae and plantar fascia; orthotic fabrication

▶ **Precautions during physical therapy:** Address contraindications for exercise based on patient's pre-existing condition(s)

▶ **Complications interfering with physical therapy:** Lack of compliance with home exercise program

Understanding the Health Condition

The plantar fascia is a fascial layer investing the plantar aspect of the foot that originates from the calcaneus and, via a complex network, inserts on the plantar aspect of the forefoot.[2] Composed largely of collagen and elastic fibers, the plantar fascia's robust and fibrous structure serves to assist with weightbearing of the foot.[2] It is divided into two layers in the transverse plane: the superficial plantar fascia and the deep plantar fascia.[3] The deep plantar fascia is further divided into three layers in the coronal plane (central, lateral, and medial portions).[2] The superficial fascia

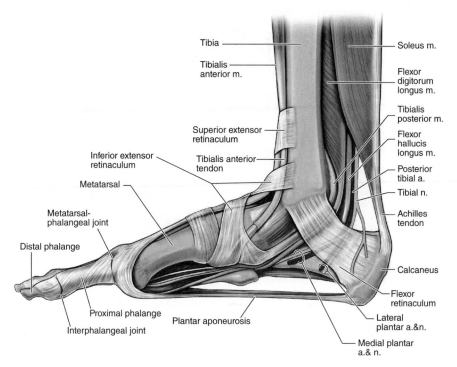

Figure 33-1. Lateral view of the plantar aponeurosis. (Reproduced with permission from Morton DA, Foreman KB, Albertine KH, eds. *The Big Picture: Gross Anatomy.* New York: McGraw-Hill; 2011. Figure 38-1.)

forms a tough and thick padding over the sole, and has strong *retinacula cutis* (skin ligaments) that tether the skin to the underlying plantar aponeurosis.[3] The deep fascia resembles that within the hand. There is a central plantar aponeurosis that extends forward and divides into digitations for the toes (Fig. 33-1).[3]

Plantar fasciitis is an inflammatory condition affecting the plantar fascia and the perifascial structures of the foot. Historically, therapists have attributed plantar fasciitis to faulty biomechanics such as excessive pronation.[1] However, a more recent review of the literature reveals that individuals with either a low-arched or higher-arched foot can experience plantar fasciitis.[1] It has been postulated that individuals with lower arches have conditions resulting from too much motion about the mid-foot and rearfoot, whereas individuals with high arches have conditions that result from too little motion.[1,4,5]

The "windlass mechanism" is a model used to provide an explanation of the bio-mechanical factors and stresses placed upon the foot and plantar fascia.[1] A windlass is a device used to move heavy weights, and it consists of a rope wound around a horizontal cylinder or barrel that is rotated by turning a crank or belt. The wind-lass effect of the plantar fascia can be illustrated when standing on the ball of the foot (*i.e.*, "tip toes"). The rope is analogous to the plantar fascia, and the cylinder is analogous to the metatarsophalangeal joints.[3] During the push-off phase of gait, dorsiflexion causes the plantar fascia to shorten as the winding of the plantar fascia shortens the distance between the calcaneus and metatarsals. This tightening of the

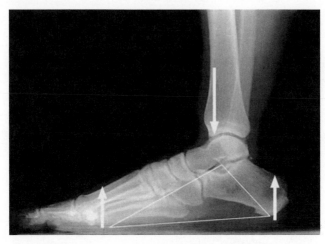

Figure 33-2. Radiograph of foot and ankle. The triangle outlines the truss formed by the calcaneus, midtarsal joint, and metatarsals. The hypotenuse (horizontal line) represents the plantar fascia. The upward arrows depict ground reaction forces. The downward arrow depicts the body's vertical force. The orientation of the vertical and ground reaction forces would cause a collapse of the truss; however, increased plantar fascia tension in response to these forces maintains the integrity of the truss. (Reproduced with permission from Bogla LA, Malone TR. Plantar fasciitis and the windlass mechanism: a biomechanical link to clinical practice. *J Athl Train.* 2004;39:77-82.)

plantar fascia helps to elevate the medial longitudinal arch. This windlass mechanism can also assist in supinating the foot during the late portion of the stance phase of the gait cycle (Fig. 33-2).

The specific causes of plantar fasciitis are poorly understood, but multiple factors likely contribute to the condition. Rome et al.[6] reported that plantar fasciitis accounts for 15% of all adult foot complaints requiring professional care and the condition is prevalent in both nonathletic and athletic populations. Riddle et al.[7] found that the risk of developing plantar fasciitis in a nonathletic population increased with a **decrease in ankle dorsiflexion range of motion.** Other independent risk factors include spending the majority of the work day standing and a body mass index (BMI) >30 kg/m^2.[7] A recent systematic review examining risk factors associated with chronic plantar heel pain affirmed the independent association between a BMI of 25 to 30 kg/m^2 and the development of plantar fasciitis.[8] This review also identified the presence of a calcaneal spur in a nonathletic population as a significant risk factor.[8]

Physical Therapy Patient/Client Management

Individuals suffering from plantar fasciitis may benefit from several physical therapy interventions including, but not limited to: modalities, manual therapy, taping, splinting, use of orthotic devices, and therapeutic exercise.[9] Most patients improve with such conservative treatment; however, up to 10% respond poorly, and require additional treatment.[10] Cortisone injections, nonsteroidal anti-inflammatory drugs, endoscopic plantar fasciotomy, and extracorporeal shockwave therapy are common interventions available for those who respond poorly to conservative treatment.[9,11–13] The goal of physical therapy for most patients with plantar fasciitis is to decrease pain and improve function.

Examination, Evaluation, and Diagnosis

Those at highest risk for developing plantar fasciitis, or those who already have the condition, often present with decreased passive ankle dorsiflexion[7], obesity, and tend to spend the majority of their work day on their feet.[9] Patients with plantar fasciitis often describe an insidious onset of sharp pain localized to the anteromedial aspect of the heel, or sometimes the center of the plantar aspect of the foot. Pain is most noticeable with initial steps after a period of inactivity (*e.g.*, first steps out of the bed upon wakening), but may worsen following prolonged weightbearing, especially toward the end of the day. During times of increased pain, an antalgic gait may be present.[9] Pain associated with plantar fasciitis often follows a recent increase in weightbearing activity (*e.g.*, increased walking or running distances). A common clinical presentation also includes immediate pain upon initial steps out of bed in the morning that may gradually decrease with increased activity.

The physical therapist should conduct a thorough investigation of the patient's past medical history and the current condition. Frequently, a patient reports a recent change in activity level, or employment change that requires more standing or walking. Clinically, the foot and ankle ability measure (FAAM) is a reliable and valid self-report questionnaire that assesses impairments, activity limitations, and participation restrictions associated with a patient's heel pain/plantar fasciitis.[9,14] The evaluation of a patient with plantar fasciitis should continue with a comprehensive musculoskeletal examination during which the therapist should be mindful of alternative diagnoses when activity limitations and clinical findings are inconsistent with plantar fasciitis. Key differential diagnoses include: calcaneal stress fracture, bone bruise, fat pad atrophy, heel spur, tarsal tunnel syndrome, Paget's disease of bone, Sever's disease, and referred pain due to an S1 radiculopathy.[9]

Table 33-1 describes common positive findings of patients with plantar fasciitis. These include: pain with palpation of the proximal plantar fascia insertion, decreased active and passive talocrural joint dorsiflexion, positive Tinel's sign with the tarsal tunnel syndrome test (dorsiflexion-eversion test), pain in the anteriomedial heel or midfoot with the windlass test, and decreased longitudinal arch angle.[9] Studies have demonstrated a significant correlation between individuals with plantar fasciitis and decreased passive ankle dorsiflexion with knee extended (gastrocnemius-soleus complex flexibility).[9,15] While stretching exercises for the gastrocnemius-soleus complex are nearly a universal intervention in a plan of care for plantar fasciitis, it has been recommended that hamstring length should also be assessed. If the hamstrings demonstrate limited length, stretching should be prescribed because increased hamstring

Table 33-1   FLEXIBILITY AND SPECIAL TESTS ASSOCIATED WITH PLANTAR FASCIITIS

Test	Patient Position	Positive Findings	Diagnostic Accuracy/ Reliability[9,19]
Active and passive talocrural joint (ankle) dorsiflexion	Patient lies supine on treatment table with feet over edge. Patient actively dorsiflexes ankle and then the therapist passively dorsiflexes the ankle. Therapist measures active and passive ROM with goniometer.	≤ 0° passive dorsiflexion	Intrarater reliability ICC: Passive—0.64-0.92 Active—0.74-0.98 Interrater reliability ICC: 0.29-0.81 Odds ratio: 23.3[7] (Those with ≤ 0° passive dorsiflexion compared to those with ≥ 10°)
Tarsal tunnel syndrome (dorsiflexion-eversion) test	Patient is seated with foot non-weightbearing, while therapist maximally dorsiflexes ankle, everts foot, and extends all toes for 5-10 s. Then, the therapist taps over the region of the tarsal tunnel.	Positive Tinel's sign or complaint of numbness suggests the diagnosis of tarsal tunnel syndrome.	*Based on numbness:* Sensitivity = 81% Specificity = 99% +LR = 82.73 −LR = 0.19 *Based on (+) Tinel's sign:* Sensitivity = 92% Specificity = 99% +LR = 84.07 −LR = 0.08
Windlass test	Test can be performed in two positions: (1) Patient sitting with ankle joint in neutral by therapist (non-weightbearing), or (2) Patient stands on step stool with metatarsal heads of foot over edge (weightbearing) Interphalangeal joints are allowed to flex and the first metatarsophalangeal joint is passively extended to end range or until the patient's pain is reproduced.	Pain in anteromedial heel or midfoot indicates plantar fasciitis	Non-weightbearing: Sensitivity = 18% Specificity = 99% +LR = 16.21 −LR = 0.83 Weightbearing: Sensitivity = 33% Specificity = 99% +LR = 28.70 −LR = 0.68
Longitudinal arch angle	Patient stands with equal weight on both feet. The therapist marks the midpoints of the medial malleolus, navicular tuberosity, and metatarsal head with a pen, and measures the resulting angle of the line with the navicular tuberosity as the fulcrum. (Fig. 33-3).	Decreased angle (< 130°) may correlate to development of plantar fasciitis.	Intrarater reliability ICC: 0.98 Interrater Reliability ICC: 0.67

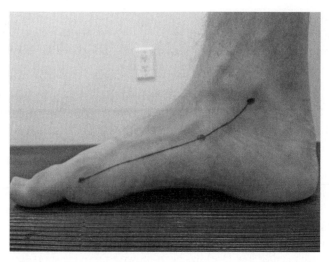

Figure 33-3. Measuring the longitudinal arch angle. Black dots on the midpoints of the medial malleolus, navicular tuberosity, and metatarsal head are connected by a line. Using the navicular tuberosity as the fulcrum, the angle of the line is the longitudinal arch angle.

tightness may cause prolonged forefoot loading with resultant increased tension on the plantar fascia.[16] Specific stretching of the plantar fascia is beneficial for decreasing pain in individuals with plantar fasciitis, regardless of the initial length of this tissue.[17] After determining that the cause of the patient's pain and dysfunction is secondary to plantar fasciitis, an evidence-based plan of care should be implemented, and the physical therapist should continually monitor the patient's progress through musculoskeletal reassessment and with a self-report questionnaire (*e.g.*, the FAAM).

Plan of Care and Interventions

Physical therapy interventions should address the subjective complaints and objective findings of the initial evaluation. A plan of care to address plantar fasciitis includes a combination of anti-inflammatory agents, modalities, and taping to provide short-term relief of symptoms (*i.e.*, less than 1 month), while manual therapy, orthotic devices, and night splints may be prescribed to deliver more long-term relief of symptoms (*i.e.*, greater than 1 month). Stretching of the gastrocnemius-soleus complex, and the plantar fascia itself, have been shown to provide both short-term and long-term relief, as well as functional improvements.[9]

Prescription and over-the-counter nonsteroidal anti-inflammatory drugs (NSAIDs), as well as glucocorticoid injections, are commonly used to address pain and inflammation related to plantar fasciitis. While these interventions are not within the scope of physical therapy practice, patients often ask the physical therapist for advice regarding these medications. Currently, no randomized control trials have been conducted to assess the efficacy of NSAIDs alone. Limited evidence supports the use of glucocorticoid injections as a source of short-term relief (2-4 weeks) of symptoms.[18] Ultimately, the physical therapist should refer the patient to his physician or a pharmacist for questions regarding the use, dosage, and efficacy of medications.

Modalities can be used on a short-term basis to treat plantar fasciitis symptoms. **Iontophoresis** of either 0.4% dexamethasone or 5% acetic acid, totaling 6 sessions over 2 to 3 weeks, has been shown to provide pain relief and subsequent improvement in function for 2 to 4 weeks.[9]

Manual therapy, including mobilization of soft tissue, nerves, and peripheral joints, has been supported by limited evidence to provide longer-term (1-3 months) pain relief and functional improvements. Peripheral joint mobilizations include posterior glide of the talocrural joint, lateral glide of the subtalar joint, anterior and posterior glides of the first tarsal-metatarsal joint, and distraction of the subtalar joint. The grade of mobilization was not specified for each of the joints.[9]

Taping (calcaneal or low-Dye) has been shown to provide short-term pain relief and improvements in function in multiple studies. However, specific parameters of taping duration for these benefits have not been specified.[19-21] The average duration of relief reported by patients was 7 to 10 days.

Orthotics are often prescribed to treat and help prevent recurrences of plantar fasciitis. The primary goal of orthotics is to reduce the amount of excessive pronation that increases stress on the plantar fascia. Prefabricated and custom orthotics have been shown to provide up to 3 months of pain relief and functional improvement for patients with plantar fasciitis.[9] There is currently no evidence to support the effectiveness of orthotics for treating plantar fasciitis for longer periods of time. It is unknown *why* orthotics are effective in treating plantar fasciitis because studies have been inconclusive.[8]

According to a recent review of literature, if patients are symptomatic for greater than 6 months, with or without concurrent treatment for plantar fasciitis, **night splints** may be effective in reducing pain.[9] Anterior, posterior, and sock-type night splints have all been shown to provide relief when worn by compliant patients every night for 1 to 3 months.[9]

There is sufficient evidence to support stretching as a short-term and long-term intervention for pain relief and functional improvement.[9] A number of studies have shown that **calf stretching** to increase ankle dorsiflexion correlates with decreased symptoms in patients. However, authors have not specified whether subjects in the studies had decreased dorsiflexion prior to stretching. Porter et al.[22] showed that dorsiflexion stretches in adults with plantar fasciitis improved pain and function. However, no difference was found between groups that performed intermittent stretching (5 sets of 20-second stretches twice per day) or sustained stretching (3-minute stretch performed 3 times per day).[24] Digiovanni et al.[17] showed that specific **stretching of the plantar fascia** was also effective at providing long-term (2 years) decreases in pain and improvement in function. The authors recommended a self-stretch in which the patient dorsiflexes the ankle and extends the toes with one hand while palpating for tension in the fascia with the other hand (Fig. 33-4). Patients were advised to hold the stretch for 10 seconds,

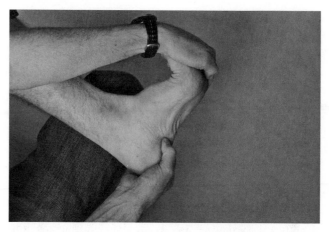

Figure 33-4. Plantar fascia stretching exercise. The patient crosses the affected leg over the contralateral leg. The patient is instructed to place the fingers across the base of the toes, pulling the toes back toward the shin until a stretch or tautness is felt along the plantar fascia.

repeating 10 times during a single set, and performing 1 set 3 times per day, with the first set performed before the patient takes his first step in the morning.

Evidence-Based Clinical Recommendations

SORT: Strength of Recommendation Taxonomy

A: Consistent, good-quality patient-oriented evidence
B: Inconsistent or limited-quality patient-oriented evidence
C: Consensus, disease-oriented evidence, usual practice, expert opinion, or case series

1. Limited ankle dorsiflexion ROM and high BMI (>30 kg/m^2) in nonathletic populations are intrinsic risk factors for the development of heel pain/plantar fasciitis. **Grade B**

2. Iontophoresis of 0.4% dexamethasone or 5% acetic acid provides short-term (2-4 weeks) pain relief and improvements in function for individuals with planter fasciitis. **Grade B**

3. Manual therapy and nerve mobilization procedures decrease pain and improve function in individuals with plantar fasciitis. **Grade C**

4. Low-Dye taping provides short-term (7-10 days) pain relief and improved function in individuals with plantar fasciitis. **Grade B**

5. Prefabricated or custom foot orthoses aimed at supporting the arch and reducing abnormal foot pronation provide short-term (3 months) improvements in function and reduction in pain in patients with plantar fasciitis. **Grade A**

6. Night splints should be considered as an intervention for patients with plantar fasciitis symptoms greater than 6 months. **Grade B**

7. Daily stretching, either sustained (1-3 minutes, 3 times per day) or intermittent (5 sets of 20 seconds, 2 times per day) targeting the gastrocnemius-soleus complex provides short-term (2-4 months) pain relief and improved calf muscle flexibility in individuals with plantar fasciitis. **Grade B**

8. Stretching of the plantar fascia can decrease pain and improve function in patients with plantar fasciitis. **Grade B**

COMPREHENSION QUESTIONS

33.1 A physical therapist examines a 40-year-old male with complaints of left heel pain for the last 6 months. His pain is worse in the morning when he first steps out of bed. Which intervention would be *least* effective in providing long-term relief (> 1 month) of his symptoms?

A. Low-Dye taping of the foot

B. Iontophoresis using 0.4% dexamethasone

C. Posterior night splint worn for 2 months

D. Prefabricated orthotics

33.2 A physical therapist examines a 55-year-old female with type 2 diabetes mellitus and recent development of heel pain. She has been diagnosed with plantar fasciitis. Which of the following is *most* likely to be a contributing factor to her pain?

A. Supinated resting foot posture

B. Pronated resting foot posture

C. BMI 24 kg/m^2

D. Decreased active dorsiflexion compared to normal values and her contralateral uninvolved lower extremity

ANSWERS

33.1 **A.** Low-Dye taping has been shown to provide only short-term pain relief, with patients reporting an average of 7-10 days of relief.[19-21] All of the other methods listed have been shown to provide months of pain relief to patients who suffer from symptoms of plantar fasciitis.[9]

33.2 **D.** According to Riddle et al.,[7] decreased dorsiflexion is the greatest risk factor for developing plantar fasciitis. While increased BMI has been identified as a risk factor for developing plantar fasciitis, a lack of dorsiflexion was shown to be a greater risk factor. A BMI < 30 kg/m^2 has not been consistently shown to contribute to plantar fasciitis (option C). While historically it was thought that decreased arch height leads to plantar fasciitis, this has not been consistently substantiated in the literature. Individuals with high and low arches may develop plantar fasciitis (options A and B).[1]

REFERENCES

1. Bogla LA, Malone TR. Plantar fasciitis and the windlass mechanism: a biomechanical link to clinical practice. *J Athl Train*. 2004;39:77-82.

2. Dutton M. *Orthopaedic Examination, Evaluation, & Intervention*. New York: McGraw-Hill; 2004.

3. Rose C, Gaddum-Rosse P, Hollinshead WH. *Hollinshead's Textbook of Anatomy*. Philadelphia, PA: Lippincott-Raven Publishers; 1997.

4. Kwong PK, Kay D, Voner RT, White MW. Plantar fasciitis. Mechanics and pathomechanics of treatment. *Clin Sports Med*. 1988;7:119-126.

5. Cornwall MW. Common pathomechanics of the foot. *Athl Ther Today*. 2000;5:10-16.

6. Rome K, Howe T, Haslock I. Risk factors associated with the development of plantar heel pain in athletes. *Foot*. 2001;11:119-125.

7. Riddle DL, Pulisic M, Pidcoe P, Johnson RE. Risk factors for plantar fasciitis: a matched case-control study. *J Bone Joint Surg Am*. 2003;85-A:872-877.

8. Irving DB, Cook JL, Menz HB. Factors associated with chronic plantar heel pain: a systematic review. *J Sci Med Sport*. 2006;9:11-24.

9. McPoil TG, Martin RL, Cornwall MW, Wukich DK, Irrgang JJ, Godges JJ. Heel pain-plantar fasciitis: clinical practice guidelines linked to the international classification of function, disability, and health from the orthopaedic section of the American Physical Therapy Association. *J Orthop Sports Phys Ther*. 2008;38:A1-A18.

10. Davis PF, Severud E, Baxter DE. Painful heel syndrome: results of nonoperative treatment. *Foot Ankle Int*. 1994;15:531-535.

11. Donley BG, Moore T, Sferra J, Gozdanovic J, Smith R. The efficacy of oral nonsteroidal anti-inflammatory medication (NSAID) in the treatment of plantar fasciitis: a randomized, prospective, placebo-controlled study. *Foot Ankle Int*. 2007;28:20-23.

12. Urovitz EP, Birk-Urovitz A, Birk-Urovitz E. Endoscopic plantar fasciotomy in the treatment of chronic heel pain. *Can J Surg*. 2008;51:281-283.

13. Malay D, Pressman MM, Assili A, et al. Extracorporeal shockwave therapy versus placebo for the treatment of chronic proximal plantar fasciitis: results of a randomized, placebo-controlled, double-blinded, multicenter intervention trial. *J Foot Ankle Surg*. 2006;45:196-210.

14. Martin RL, Irrgang JJ, Burdett RG, Conti SF, Van Swearingean JM. Evidence of validity for the foot and ankle ability measure (FAAM). *Foot Ankle Int*. 2005;26:968-983.

15. Drake M, Bittenbender C, Boyles RE. The short-term effects of treating plantar fasciitis with a temporary custom foot orthosis and stretching. *Journal Orthop Sports Phys Ther*. 2011;41:221-231.

16. Harty J, Soffe K, O'Toole G, Stephens M. The role of hamstring tightness in plantar fasciitis. *Foot Ankle Int*. 2005;26:1089-1092.

17. Digiovanni BF, Nawoczenski DA, Malay DP, et al. Plantar fascia-specific stretching exercise improves outcomes in patients with chronic plantar fasciitis. A prospective clinical trial with two-year follow-up. *J Bone Joint Surg Am*. 2006;88:1775-81.

18. Crawford F, Thomson C. Interventions for treating plantar heel pain. *Cochrane Database Syst Rev.* 2003:CD000416.

19. Osborne HR, Allison GT. Treatment of plantar fasciitis by Low-Dye taping and iontophoresis: short term results of a double blinded, randomised, placebo controlled clinical trial of dexamethasone and acetic acid. *Br J Sports Med.* 2006;40:545-549.

20. Hyland MR, Webber-Gaffney A, Cohen L, Lichtman PT. Randomized controlled trial of calcaneal taping, sham taping, and plantar fascia stretching for the short-term management of plantar heel pain. *J Orthop Sports Phys Ther.* 2006;36:364-371.

21. Radford JA, Landorf KB, Buchbinder R, Cook C. Effectiveness of low-Dye taping for the short-term treatment of plantar heel pain: a randomised trial. *BMC Musculoskelet Disord.* 2006;7:64.

22. Porter D, Barrill E, Oneacre K, May BD. The effects of duration and frequency of Achilles tendon stretching on dorsiflexion and outcome in painful heel syndrome: a randomized, blinded, control study. *Foot Ankle Int.* 2002;23:619-624.

Fibromyalgia

Jason Brumitt

CASE 34

A primary care provider referred a 45-year-old female to physical therapy with the diagnosis of back pain. The patient reports that she experiences pain in her back, but she also feels pain "all over her body." In addition to pain, she experiences fatigue, difficulty sleeping, poor memory, and frequent headaches. Her pain "never seems to get better" and "it gets worse with prolonged activity." Her symptoms started approximately 4 years ago after she fell down a flight of stairs. Repeated x-rays of the thoracic and lumbar spine were negative for fractures or bony abnormalities that could contribute to her symptoms. Previous physical therapy interventions (moist heat, massage, ultrasound, stretching) have not improved her symptoms. Her medical history is significant for irritable bowel syndrome and abdominal pain (both started 2 years ago). She works as a court reporter and describes her lifestyle as rather sedentary. Based on the patient's history, you suspect she may have fibromyalgia syndrome (FMS).

► Based on the patient's symptoms and medical history, what are the most appropriate examination tests to help confirm the diagnosis of FMS?
► What are the most appropriate physical therapy interventions?
► What are possible complications that may limit the effectiveness of physical therapy?

KEY DEFINITIONS

ALLODYNIA: Pain in response to a stimulus that would not normally cause pain

FIBROMYALGIA SYNDROME (FMS): Chronic widespread pain condition of unknown etiology marked by increased sensitivity to stimuli (*e.g.*, hyperalgesia, allodynia) and symptoms that may significantly impact functional capacity and quality of life

SICCA: Dryness of the mouth and eyes

TENDER POINT: Localized region on the body that is tender to digital pressure; FMS has been historically associated with 18 tender point locations (9 spots on each side of the body)

Objectives

1. Describe fibromyalgia syndrome and identify potential comorbidities associated with this diagnosis.

2. Describe American College of Rheumatology diagnostic criteria for FMS.

3. Prescribe a therapeutic exercise program designed to improve function and decrease pain in this population.

4. Understand common adverse drug reactions (ADRs) for medications used in the treatment of FMS that may affect physical therapy examination and/or interventions.

Physical Therapy Considerations

PT considerations during management of the individual with a diagnosis of fibromyalgia syndrome:

▶ **General physical therapy plan of care/goals:** Decrease pain; increase muscular flexibility; increase muscular endurance and strength; improve aerobic fitness capacity

▶ **Physical therapy interventions:** Patient education regarding potential pathogenesis of condition; massage/soft tissue mobilization techniques to decrease pain; muscular flexibility exercises; resistance exercises to increase muscular endurance capacity and functional strength; aerobic exercise program

▶ **Precautions during physical therapy:** Monitor vital signs; address precautions or contraindications for exercise based on patient's pre-existing condition(s)

▶ **Complications interfering with physical therapy:** Excessive fatigue, symptoms interfering with exercise tolerance, depression

Understanding the Health Condition

Fibromyalgia syndrome (FMS; also frequently referred to as fibromyalgia) is a chronic widespread pain condition of unknown etiology marked by increased sensitivity to stimuli and symptoms that may significantly impact one's lifestyle. Diagnosing FMS is challenged by a lack of clinical diagnostic tests. A patient may experience the symptoms of FMS for many months and/or years prior to receiving the diagnosis. In the United States, approximately five million people have been diagnosed with FMS; it is most common in adult women (3:1 ratio).[1,2] The prevalence of FMS increases with age and peaks during the fifth, sixth, and seventh decades of life.[2]

There is no cure for FMS. Providing effective treatment is challenging due to a limited understanding of the syndrome's pathophysiology. Several factors have been proposed in the pathogenesis: genetics, autonomic nervous system dysfunction, abnormal peripheral pain processing and central pain processing (central sensitization), neuroendocrine dysfunction, environmental factors, gray matter atrophy, psychological factors, and oxidative stress.[1,3–8]

Symptoms associated with FMS include chronic widespread pain, chronic fatigue, concentration and memory problems, headaches, muscular weakness, sleeping disorders (nonrestorative sleep), morning stiffness, sicca symptoms, and allodynia. Several comorbidities have been reported in patients with FMS: anxiety, depression, abdominal pain, chronic fatigue syndrome, migraine headaches, and bipolar disorder. The presence of comorbidities necessitates inclusion of therapies (e.g., cognitive behavioral therapy) in addition to those provided by the physical therapist.

Physical Therapy Patient/Client Management

The physical therapist may be one of many healthcare providers treating a patient with FMS. Exercise and cognitive behavioral therapy (CBT) are conservative treatments that have been shown to be effective in the treatment of patients with FMS.[9–15] Soft tissue mobilization and massage may help reduce symptoms in some individuals. Prescription medications may also be utilized.[16] The physical therapist should be aware of other treatments the patient has previously received or is currently receiving to help avoid redundancy and possibly reduce the risk of symptom aggravation. For example, if the patient is concurrently receiving services from a licensed massage therapist, soft tissue therapies should not be the focus of physical therapy interventions. The physical therapist must take a complete drug history from the patient, including prescription and nonprescription medications, as well as any supplements. Common prescription medications for the treatment of FMS include tricyclic antidepressants, selective serotonin reuptake inhibitors, serotonin norepinephrine reuptake inhibitors, gabapentin, cyclobenzaprine, tramadol, and pregabalin.[17] Table 34-1 presents the indications and ADRs associated with each drug (or class of drugs) that may affect physical therapy examination and/or interventions.

Examination, Evaluation, and Diagnosis

In 1990, the American College of Rheumatology (ACR) established the following diagnostic criteria for FMS: chronic widespread pain (pain involving all regions of the body) lasting longer than 3 months and pain with palpation at a minimum of

Table 34-1 INDICATIONS AND ADRS ASSOCIATED WITH COMMONLY PRESCRIBED MEDICATIONS FOR FMS

Drug (or Class of Drugs)	Indications	ADRs That May Affect Physical Therapy
Tricyclic antidepressants	Pain Depression Fatigue Sleep disturbance	Blurry vision Anxiety Dizziness Weakness Hypotension Tachycardia
Selective serotonin reuptake inhibitors (SSRIs)	Depression Anxiety	Fatigue Dizziness Increased risk of suicide Rash Insomnia Anxiety Mania/hypomania Nervousness Tremors Seizures
Serotonin norepinephrine reuptake inhibitors (e.g., duloxetine, milnacipran)	Depression Anxiety Pain	Tachycardia Hypertension Anxiety Nausea Insomnia
Gabapentin	Pain	Fatigue Ataxia Weight gain
Cyclobenzaprine	Depression	Drowsiness Myocardial infarction Stroke Sinus tachycardia Ataxia Hypotension Fatigue Headaches
Tramadol	Pain	Nausea Constipation Dizziness
Pregabalin	Pain	Dizziness Myalgia Ataxia Arthralgia Hypertension or hypotension

11 of 18 tender points.[18] Tender points are assessed by digital palpation (thumb pressure of 4 kg/cm^2 force, or force that would create nailbed blanching). Pain must be provoked during digital palpation to a tender point for it to meet the 1990 ACR diagnostic criteria.[18] The tender points are tested bilaterally in nine locations. They

are located at: the occiput at suboccipital muscle insertion sites, anterior low cervical region near the sternocleidomastoid muscles, the second rib (lateral to second costochondral junctions), the midpoint of the upper border of the trapezius, above the scapular spine in the supraspinatus muscle, the lateral epicondyle, the anterior edge of the gluteus maximus, the greater trochanter, and the medial joint line of the knee.[18]

It has been suggested that the 1990 ACR diagnostic criteria did not accurately account for the spectrum of signs and symptoms that may be present in patients with FMS.[19-21] The tender point criteria (requirement of pain with digital pressure to 11 of the 18 sites) were especially controversial.[19-21] For example, a patient can still have FMS in the presence of less than 11 tender points.[18] In addition, many primary care providers have diagnosed patients with FMS, but may have incorrectly performed the digital palpation or may have failed to test patients' tender points altogether.[18-20]

Twenty years after the initial FMS diagnostic criteria were published, the American College of Rheumatology has provisionally accepted new diagnostic criteria (Table 34-2).[21] A notable change from the 1990 criteria is that the use of tender point palpation has been removed. Now, FMS diagnosis is based on three criteria: history of widespread pain for at least 3 months, symptom behavior, and ruling out any other condition that could account for the patient's symptoms.[21]

Table 34-2 presents the scales used in the new 2010 ACR diagnostic criteria: the widespread pain index (WPI) and the symptom severity (SS) scale.[18] The WPI is used to identify the number of painful regions experienced by the patient during the past week. Each location that is identified as having been painful is scored with a 1 (absence of pain is scored a zero).[21] The maximum score possible on the WPI is 19. The SS scale assesses an individual's symptom experience during the previous week, including: fatigue, waking unrefreshed, cognitive symptoms, and the number of somatic symptoms.[18] The SS is scored on a 0 to 3 scale: 0 for "no problems" or "no symptoms," 1 for "a few problems (or symptoms)," 2 for "moderate, considerable problems (symptoms)," or 3 for "severe: pervasive, continuous, life-disturbing problems (or a great deal of symptoms)."[21] The combined WPI and SS scores, in combination with symptom history (no other condition can account for the patient's pain), are used to confirm a diagnosis of FMS. To be diagnosed with FMS, a patient must either have scores of: WPI ≥ 7 and SS ≥ 5 or a WPI = 3 to 6 and SS ≥ 9.[21]

A person with FMS is typically referred to physical therapy after having been diagnosed by a rheumatologist. However, a patient may access physical therapy via direct access (presenting to physical therapy without a physician's referral). Awareness of the ACR diagnostic criteria helps the physical therapist when evaluating a patient with chronic widespread pain who has accessed physical therapy directly. If a diagnosis of FMS is suspected, the physical therapist should refer the patient to a rheumatologist for comprehensive evaluation and treatment.

Whether the patient has a formal diagnosis of FMS or the therapist suspects the diagnosis, the physical therapist should obtain a traditional history from the patient. Identification of any activities that appear to cause a flare (symptom response) in the patient should be prioritized. The patient should complete additional measurement

Table 34-2   2010 AMERICAN COLLEGE OF RHEUMATOLOGY DIAGNOSTIC CRITERIA FOR FIBROMYALGIA SYNDROME

Criteria

A patient satisfies diagnostic criteria for fibromyalgia if the following three conditions are met:
1. Widespread pain index (WPI) ≥ 7 and symptom severity (SS) scale score ≥ 5 or WPI 3-6 and SS scale score ≥ 9.
2. Symptoms have been present at a similar level for at least 3 months.
3. The patient does not have a disorder that would otherwise explain the pain.

Ascertainment
1. WPI: note the number areas in which the patient has had pain over the last week. In how many areas has the patient had pain? Score will be between 0 and 19.

Shoulder girdle, left	Hip (buttock, trochanter), left	Jaw, left	Upper back
Shoulder girdle, right	Hip (buttock, trochanter), right	Jaw, right	Lower back
Upper arm, left	Upper leg, left	Chest	Neck
Upper arm, right	Upper leg, right	Abdomen	
Lower arm, left	Lower leg, left		
Lower arm, right	Lower leg, right		

2. SS scale score:
Fatigue
Waking unrefreshed
Cognitive symptoms
For the each of the three symptoms above, indicate the level of severity over the past week using the following scale:
0 = no problem
1 = slight or mild problems, generally mild or intermittent
2 = moderate, considerable problems, often present and/or at a moderate level
3 = severe: pervasive, continuous, life-disturbing problems
Considering somatic symptoms in general, indicate whether the patient has:*
0 = no symptoms
1 = few symptoms
2 = a moderate number of symptoms
3 = a great deal of symptoms

*The SS scale score is the sum of the severity of the three symptoms (fatigue, waking unrefreshed, cognitive symptoms) plus the extent (severity) of somatic symptoms in general. The final score is between 0 and 12.
Somatic symptoms that might be considered: muscle pain, irritable bowel syndrome, fatigue/tiredness, thinking or remembering problem, muscle weakness, headache, pain/cramps in the abdomen, numbness/tingling, dizziness, insomnia, depression, constipation, pain in the upper abdomen, nausea, nervousness, chest pain, blurred vision, fever, diarrhea, dry mouth, itching, wheezing, Raynaud phenomenon, hives/welts, ringing in ears, vomiting, heartburn, oral ulcers, loss of/change in taste, seizures, dry eyes, shortness of breath, loss of appetite, rash, sun sensitivity, hearing difficulties, easy bruising, hair loss, frequent urination, painful urination, and bladder spasms.

Reproduced with permission from Wolfe F, Clauw DJ, Fitzcharles MA, et al. The American College of Rheumatology preliminary diagnostic criteria for fibromyalgia and measurement of symptom severity. Arthritis Care Res. 2010;62: 600-610.

tools such as the fibromyalgia impact questionnaire (FIQ) and/or the continuous scale physical functional performance test. These outcomes measures should be administered again at a later date to assess changes in functional abilities that may reflect the effectiveness of the patient's therapeutic program.

A traditional physical examination should be performed; however, some measures (*e.g.*, goniometry, manual muscle testing) may not provide relevant clinical information to guide exercise prescription. Even though a patient may score a 5/5 on a traditional manual muscle test, this demonstration of isometric muscular capability does not provide clinically relevant information regarding muscular endurance. In addition, a single repetition of a manual muscle test does not reveal how a patient may respond to prolonged activity. In fact, many patients may have limited tolerance to repeated activity. For example, a patient may fatigue quickly during the training session and/or experience an exacerbation of FMS symptoms after completing the session (usually within 12-24 hours). Functional tests and measures may provide the therapist a quantitative and qualitative view of the patient's baseline fitness. Flexibility testing may be performed to identify regions that lack muscular flexibility. The Six-Minute Walk Test may be performed to appreciate changes in aerobic fitness over time. However, this test may be too demanding for some patients with FMS to perform during the initial patient evaluation. Functional tests, such as a lunge and a squat, allow the physical therapist to determine the individual's muscular strength in the lower extremities. One repetition maximum (1RM) testing may provide a quantitative assessment of an individual's strength. While researchers have measured strength using a 1RM test, patients with FMS should be initially tested with very low loads that can be used to closely approximate the 1RM using an online calculator.[22]

Plan of Care and Interventions

Physical therapy interventions frequently include patient education, **therapeutic exercise**, and soft tissue manual therapies. Numerous studies have demonstrated the effectiveness of improving strength and decreasing symptoms in this population.[22–29] There is some evidence to support the use of soft tissue mobilization.[30–32]

The Centers for Disease Control and Prevention (CDC) have established exercise recommendations to maintain or improve health for adults.[33] These guidelines should serve as goals for patients with FMS to achieve. However, the *initial* volume of prescribed exercise for a patient depends on several factors. For example, it would be premature to have a 50-year-old sedentary female with FMS initiate 30 minutes of moderate intensity aerobic exercise on the first day of a new exercise program. Exercise prescription for the patient with FMS should be based on the patient's subjective history, findings from the physical examination, and exercise programs prescribed to similar patient populations that have been reported to be successful.

The CDC recommends minimum training levels.[33] Adults (≥ 18 years of age) should, at a minimum, perform 2.5 hours of aerobic activity during the week and perform strength training exercises at least 2 days per week.[33] These exercise guidelines have been established for a general adult population and are not specific to a population with FMS. While individuals with FMS can attempt to meet these guidelines, progression toward these goals depends on each individual's tolerance. Table 34-3 presents the complete CDC recommendations including training recommendations based on intensity of exercise performed.[33]

Table 34-3 CDC'S EXERCISE RECOMMENDATIONS FOR ADULTS[33]			
Age Group	Aerobic Exercise	Exercise Intensity and Examples	Strength Training
Adults (18 years and older)	Moderate exercise: 2.5 h/wk or Vigorous exercise: 1.25 h/wk or A mix of vigorous and moderate intensity exercise	Moderate: bicycling, swimming Vigorous: running, sports competition, intense aerobic courses/activities	Two or more d/wk Train all muscle groups

Moderate intensity aerobic exercise is defined as that performed at an intensity of 50% to 70% of one's maximum heart rate (HRmax), which is typically estimated as 220 – one's age. Most studies investigating the effects of aerobic exercise on patients with FMS have prescribed programs within this training heart rate range. Vigorous-intensity aerobic exercises are those performed at 70% to 85% of one's maximum heart rate. Examples of vigorous-intensity exercise include swimming continuous laps, jogging/running, hiking, and bicycling greater than 10 miles per hour.[22] There is a paucity in the literature assessing vigorous-intensity exercise on subjects with FMS. This is likely due to a concern that vigorous-intensity exercises may cause an exacerbation of symptoms. Some researchers have been able to implement training programs for subjects with FMS with heart rates consistent with vigorous-intensity exercise (lower end of HRmax = 70%).[22] More research is warranted to determine the efficacy of this practice. For the patient in this case who was sedentary and experiencing significant pain, the short-term aerobic training goal would be a moderate-intensity program performed 3 days per week for 10-15 minutes each session. While the ultimate goal is for the patient to perform an exercise routine that meets CDC recommendations, gradual progression from a feasible baseline is practical.

Individuals with FMS may present to physical therapy with functional weakness resulting from decreased physical activity (secondary to fatigue and chronic pain). Individuals with FMS experience strength gains and improvements in symptom behavior after participating in a resistance training program or a comprehensive program featuring strength training exercises.[22–29] Strengthening exercises, aerobic exercises, Tai Chi, whole body vibration, and stretching exercises have been prescribed to patients with FMS.[22–29] Table 34-4 presents randomized controlled trials that have assessed the **effect of exercise programs on strength, pain, and other functional measures in subjects with FMS.** Despite the heterogeneity among the exercise programs (length of programs, types of exercises prescribed, training volume), improvements in some domains were realized by a large percentage of subjects with FMS. Additional research is warranted to determine the most effective therapeutic exercise program. A physical therapist treating a patient with FMS should gradually progress the training program, utilizing exercise modes that the patient will be most likely to perform and adhere to. For the patient in this case, a training program initially consisting of 4 to 6 resistance exercises for the

Table 34-4   PRESCRIBED EXERCISE ROUTINES FOR PATIENTS WITH FMS

Author (Year)	Training Period	Aerobic Exercise	Resisted Training Exercise	Flexibility Exercise
Hakkinen et al. (2001)	21 wk (2 times per wk)		Exercises for upper and lower extremities performed initially with high reps (15-20) at low loads (40%-60% of 1RM) progressing up to low reps (5-10) at high load (70%-80% 1RM)	
Kingsley et al. (2005)	12 wk (2 times per wk)		1 set of 8-12 reps 11 exercises for muscles of trunk, upper extremities, and lower extremities	
Wennemer et al. (2006)	8 wk (3 times per wk)	Low-impact exercise performed (no details or dosing parameters provided)	Core stabilization, upper body strengthening, Tai Chi or Feldenkrais	Stretching exercises
Alentorn-Geli et al. (2008)	6 wk (2 times per wk)	30 min		25 min
Alentorn-Geli et al. (2009)	6 wk (2 times per wk)	30 min of walking or dancing (65%-85% HRmax)	Exercises on a whole body vibration machine	25 min (5 reps of each stretch, 30-s holds, 30-s rest between stretches)
Kingsley et al. (2010)	12 wk (2 times per wk)		3 sets of 8-12 reps 5 exercises	
Sanudo et al. (2010)	24 wk (2 times per wk)	45-60 min	8 strengthening exercises	
Garcia-Martinez et al. (2011)	12 wk (3 times per wk)	20 min (initially dosed at 60%-70% of maximal heart rate (MHR) and progressed to 75%-85% MHR, as able	20 min of strengthening and stretching (individualized exercise program)	Individualized stretching program (unspecified)

upper and lower extremities could be prescribed (1 to 2 sets of 15 repetitions per exercise).

A variety of **soft tissue mobilization techniques** have been evaluated for their effectiveness in reducing pain and improving function in patients with FMS. In a study with adults with FMS, 30 subjects (mean age 49 ± 11 years) received weekly 90-minute sessions of a massage-myofascial release program directed toward the 18 tender points for 5 months.[30] The control group (29 subjects with mean age 46 ±12 years) received one 30-minute treatment per week, consisting of magnotherapy (turned off). At the end of the 5-month intervention, subjects in the experimental group experienced significant improvements in pain, quality of life, sleep (latency and duration), and anxiety. Pain (measured by a visual analog score) also improved significantly in the experimental group compared to the control group. The experimental group also experienced a significant decrease in pain at four tender point sites (algometer was used to assess pain). Compared to the control group, the experimental group reported a significant decrease in anxiety at the 6-month postintervention follow-up. The experimental group demonstrated significant within-group improvements in sleep duration and a decrease in pain at only one tender point.[30]

Ekici et al.[31] compared manual lymph drainage therapy (MLDT) to connective tissue massage (CTM; a technique that is performed by applying a shearing force to the skin) in a population of women with FMS (MLDT group = 25 subjects, mean age 39 ± 6 years); CTM group = 25 subjects, mean age 37 ± 9 years). Both groups demonstrated significant improvements in quality of life and pain; but, the MLDT group showed significant between-group improvements for some FIQ functional measures.

Field et al.[32] compared massage therapy versus relaxation therapy in a sample of 20 women with FMS (mean age = 51 years). Subjects in the experimental group received 10 sessions (2 sessions per week for 5 weeks) of a 30-minute massage therapy program (Swedish and Shiatsu techniques). The relaxation group received 30-minute relaxation therapy sessions (2 sessions per week for 5 weeks). Both groups experienced significant reductions in anxiety and depression at the end of the treatment period. However, the massage therapy group had greater improvements in reducing depression scores, improving sleep, decreasing pain, decreasing fatigue, and total number of tender points. Further studies are warranted to identify the optimal techniques and treatment intensities.

Evidence-Based Clinical Recommendations

SORT: Strength of Recommendation Taxonomy

A: Consistent, good-quality patient-oriented evidence
B: Inconsistent or limited-quality patient-oriented evidence
C: Consensus, disease-oriented evidence, usual practice, expert opinion, or case series

1. Therapeutic exercise programs (strengthening and stretching exercises) decrease pain and/or improve function in patients with FMS. **Grade B**

2. Aerobic exercise programs may decrease fatigue and improve function in patients with FMS. **Grade B**

3. Soft tissue mobilization techniques may decrease pain and improve quality of life in patients with FMS. **Grade B**

COMPREHENSION QUESTIONS

34.1 The original 1990 American College of Rheumatology (ACR) diagnostic criteria for FMS included the assessment of 18 tender points. Why has the ACR eliminated the assessment of tender points from the latest (2010) diagnostic criteria?

A. Non-pharmacological treatments do not reduce pain at the tender points.

B. The 18 tender points are asymmetrically located throughout the body.

C. Physicians' assessments of the tender points were believed to be incorrectly performed.

D. Location of the tender points was not agreed upon by therapists.

34.2 Which of the following exercise types should be included in an exercise program for an individual with FMS?

A. Moderate intensity aerobic exercise, plyometric exercises, stretching exercises

B. Vigorous intensity aerobic exercise, strengthening exercises, stretching exercises

C. Vigorous intensity aerobic exercise, plyometric exercises, whole body vibration exercises

D. Moderate intensity aerobic exercise, strengthening exercises, stretching exercises

34.3 The Centers for Disease Control and Prevention recommend that adults (general population) should perform either 150 minutes of moderate intensity or 75 minutes of vigorous intensity aerobic exercise each week. Which of the following *best* describes a moderate intensity aerobic exercise?

A. Running at 75% of one's estimated HRmax

B. Walking at 75% of one's estimated HRmax

C. Swimming laps at 80% of one's estimated HRmax

D. Walking at 65% of one's estimated HRmax

ANSWERS

34.1 **C.** One of the reasons that the tender point criteria was not included in the current 2010 ACR diagnostic guidelines is because it was believed that some physicians were either inaccurately assessing patients' tender points or failing to assess them altogether.

34.2 **D.** Several modes of exercise (*e.g.*, moderate intensity aerobic exercise, strengthening exercises, stretching exercises, whole body vibration, and Tai Chi) have been shown to improve pain and function in subjects with FMS. Vigorous intensity aerobic exercise and plyometrics have yet to be adequately assessed for their ability to improve FMS symptoms and increase function *without* exacerbating symptoms.

34.3 **D.** A moderate intensity aerobic exercise is performed at 50% to 70% of one's estimated maximum heart rate. Examples of moderate intensity aerobic exercise include walking quickly, bicycle riding, and playing doubles tennis.

REFERENCES

1. Finan PH, Zautra AJ. Fibromyalgia and fatigue: central processing, widespread dysfunction. *PM R.* 2010;2:431-437.

2. Lawrence RC, Felson DT, Helmick CG, et al. Estimates of the prevalence of arthritis and other rheumatic conditions in the United States. Part II. *Arthritis Rheum.* 2008;58:26-35.

3. Bradley LA. Pathophysiology of fibromyalgia. *Am J Med.* 2009;122:S22-S30.

4. Iqbal R, Mughal MS, Arshad N, Arshad M. Pathophysiology and antioxidant status of patients with fibromyalgia. *Rheumatol Int.* 2011;31:149-152.

5. Cordero MD, Moreno-Fernandez AM, Carmona-Lopez MI, et al. Mitochondrial dysfunction in skin biopsies and blood mononuclear cells from two cases of fibromyalgia patients. *Clin Biomech.* 2010;43:1174-1176.

6. Cordero MD, De Miguel M, Moreno Fernandez AM, et al. Mitochondrial dysfunction and mitophagy activation in blood mononuclear cells of fibromyalgia patients: implications in the pathogenesis of the disease. *Arthritis Res Ther.* 2010;12:R17.

7. Iannuccelli C, Di Franco M, Alessandri C, et al. Pathophysiology of fibromyalgia: a comparison with the tension-type headache, a localized pain syndrome. *Ann N Y Acad Sci.* 2010;1193:78-83.

8. Ozgocmen S, Ozyurt H, Sogut S, Akyol O. Current concepts in the pathophysiology of fibromyalgia: the potential role of oxidative stress and nitric oxide. *Rheumatol Int.* 2006;26:585-597.

9. Busch AJ, Schachter CL, Overend TJ, Peloso PM, Barber KA. Exercise for fibromyalgia: a systematic review. *J Rheumatol.* 2008;35:1130-1144.

10. Cazzola M, Atzeni F, Salaffi F, Stisi S, Cassisi G, Sarzi-Puttini P. What kind of exercise is best in fibromyalgia therapeutic programmes? A practical review. *Clin Exp Rheumatol.* 2010;28:S117-S124.

11. Gowans SE, deHueck A, Voss S, Richardson M. A randomized, controlled trial of exercise and education for individuals with fibromyalgia. *Arthritis Care Res.* 1999;12:120-128.

12. Gowans SE, deHueck A, Voss S, Silaj A, Abbey SE, Reynolds WJ. Effect of a randomized, controlled trial of exercise on mood and physical function in individuals with fibromyalgia. *Arthritis Care Res.* 2001;45:519-529.

13. Gowans SE, deHueck A, Voss S, Silaj A, Abbey SE. Six-month and one-year follow-up of 23 weeks of aerobic exercise for individuals with fibromyalgia. *Arthritis Care Res.* 2004;51:890-898.

14. Hassett AL, Gevirtz RN. Nonpharmacologic treatment for fibromyalgia: patient education, cognitive-behavioral therapy, relaxation techniques, and complementary and alternative medicine. *Rheum Dis Clin N Am.* 2009;35:393-407.

15. van Koulil S, van Lankveld W, Kraaimaat FW, et al. Tailored cognitive-behavioral therapy and exercise training for high-risk patients with fibromyalgia. *Arthritis Care Res.* 2010;62:1377-1385.

16. Jones KD, Burckhardt CS, Deodhar A, Perrin NA, Hanson GC, Bennett RM. A six-month randomized controlled trial of exercise and pyridostigmine in the treatment of fibromyalgia. *Arthritis Rheum.* 2008;58:612-622.

17. Smith HS, Barkin RL. Fibromyalgia syndrome: a discussion of the syndrome and pharmacotherapy. *Dis Mon.* 2011;57:248-285.

18. Wolfe F, Smythe HA, Yunus MB, et al. The American College of Rheumatology 1990 Criteria for the Classification of Fibromyalgia. Report of the Multicenter Criteria Committee. *Arthritis Rheum.* 1990;33:160-172.

19. Fitzcharles MA, Boulos P. Inaccuracy in the diagnosis of fibromyalgia syndrome: analysis of referrals. *Rheumatology* 2003;42:263-267.

20. Buskila D, Neumann L, Sibirski D, Shvartzman P. Awareness of diagnostic and clinical features of fibromyalgia among family physicians. *Fam Pract.* 1997;14:238-241.

21. Wolfe F, Clauw DJ, Fitzcharles MA, et al. The American College of Rheumatology preliminary diagnostic criteria for fibromyalgia and measurement of symptom severity. *Arthritis Care Res.* 2010;62:600-610.

22. Hakkinen A, Hakkinen K, Hannonen P, Alen M. Strength training induced adaptations in neuromuscular function of premenopausal women with fibromyalgia: comparison with healthy women. *Ann Rheum Dis.* 2001;60:21-26.

23. Kingsley JD, Panton LB, Toole T, Sirithienthad P, Mathis R, McMillan V. The effects of a 12-week strength-training program on strength and functionality in women with fibromyalgia. *Arch Phys Med Rehabil.* 2005;86:1713-1721.

24. Wennemer HK, Borg-Stein J, Gomba L, et al. Functionally oriented rehabilitation program for patients with fibromyalgia: preliminary results. *Am J Phys Med Rehabil.* 2006; 85:659-666.

25. Alentorn-Geli E, Padilla J, Moras G, Haro CL, Fernandez-Sola J. Six weeks of whole-body vibration exercise improves pain and fatigue in women with fibromyalgia. *J Altern Complement Med.* 2008;14:975-981.

26. Alentorn-Geli E, Moras G, Padilla J, et al. Effect of acute and chronic whole-body vibration exercise on serum insulin-like growth factor-1 levels in women with fibromyalgia. *J Altern Complement Med.* 2009;15:573-578.

27. Kingsley JD, McMillan V, Figueroa A. The effects of 12 weeks of resistance exercise training on disease severity and autonomic modulation at rest and after acute leg resistance exercise in women with fibromyalgia. *Arch Phys Med Rehabil.* 2010;91:1551-1557.

28. Sanudo B, de Hoyo M, Carrasco L, et al. The effect of 6-week exercise programme and whole body vibration on strength and quality of life in women with fibromyalgia: a randomised study. *Clin Exp Rheumatol.* 2010;28(Suppl 63):S40-S45.

29. Garcia-Martinez AM, De Paz JA, Marquez S. Effects of an exercise programme on self-esteem, self-concept and quality of life in women with fibromyalgia: a randomized controlled trial. *Rheumatol Int.* 2011;32:1869-1876.

30. Castro-Sanchez AM, Mataran-Penarrocha GA, Granero-Molina J, Aguilera-Manrique G, Quesada-Rubio JM, Moreno-Lorenzo C. Benefits of massage-myofascial release therapy on pain, anxiety, quality of sleep, depression, and quality of life in patients with fibromyalgia. *Evid Based Complement Alternat Med.* 2011;561753.

31. Ekici G, Bakar Y, Akbayrak T, Yuksel I. Comparison of manual lymph drainage therapy and connective tissue massage in women with fibromyalgia: a randomized controlled trial. *J Manipulative Physiol Ther.* 2009;32:127-133.

32. Field T, Diego M, Cullen C, Hernandez-Reif M, Sunshine W, Douglas S. Fibromyalgia pain and substance P decrease and sleep improves after massage therapy. *J Clin Rheumatol.* 2002;8:72-76.

33. Centers for Disease Control and Prevention. Physical activity for everyone. Available at: http://www.cdc.gov/physicalactivity/everyone/guidelines/index.html. Accessed August 15, 2011.

Listing of Cases

Listing by Case Number

Listing by Health Condition (Alphabetical)

Listing by Case Number

Listing by Health Condition (Alphabetical)

NOTE: Page numbers followed by *f* or *t* indicate figures or tables, respectively.